Medicine Is War

SUNY series, Studies in the Long Nineteenth Century
———————
Pamela K. Gilbert, editor

Medicine Is War

The Martial Metaphor in Victorian Literature and Culture

Lorenzo Servitje

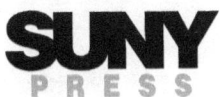

Published by State University of New York Press, Albany

© 2021 State University of New York

All rights reserved

Printed in the United States of America

No part of this book may be used or reproduced in any manner whatsoever without written permission. No part of this book may be stored in a retrieval system or transmitted in any form or by any means including electronic, electrostatic, magnetic tape, mechanical, photocopying, recording, or otherwise without the prior permission in writing of the publisher.

For information, contact State University of New York Press, Albany, NY
www.sunypress.edu

Library of Congress Cataloging-in-Publication Data

Names: Servitje, Lorenzo, [date]- author.
Title: Medicine is war : the martial metaphor in Victorian literature and culture / Lorenzo Servitje.
Description: Albany : State University of New York Press, 2021. | Series: SUNY series, studies in the long nineteenth century | Includes bibliographical references and index.
Identifiers: LCCN 2020017342 | ISBN 9781438481678 (hardcover : alk. paper) | ISBN 9781438481685 (pbk. : alk. paper) | ISBN 9781438481692 (ebook)
Subjects: LCSH: English fiction—19th century—History and criticism. | Medicine in literature. | Diseases in literature. | War in literature. | Medicine, Military—Great Britain—History—19th century. | War—Medical aspects.
Classification: LCC PR878.M42 S47 2020 | DDC 823/.8093561—dc23
LC record available at https://lccn.loc.gov/2020017342

10 9 8 7 6 5 4 3 2 1

Medicine Is War is dedicated to my wife, Mary Servitje, and my daughter, Loriana Servitje.

Contents

Acknowledgments ix

Introduction 1

PART 1

1. Denaturing the Emergent Martial Metaphor in Mary Shelley's *The Last Man* 29

2. Charles Kingsley Meets Cholera Face-to-Face 69

PART 2

3. Military Pasts and Medical Futures in Bram Stoker's *Dracula* 109

4. Arthur Conan Doyle's Imperial Armamentarium 145

5. Modernist Refractions of Tropical Medicine in Joseph Conrad's *Heart of Darkness* 193

Collateral Damage: An Afterword 227

Addendum: A Surge of Epilogics in the Midst of the War against COVID-19 239

Notes	249
Bibliography	293
Index	321

Acknowledgments

I wish there were an adequate way to recognize the scores of people who made this work possible in the manner that they deserve. If I have learned anything, it is that knowledge production does not happen in a vacuum. It is with great pleasure (and some anxiety that I will miss someone) that I take time to recall and express thanks to the friends and colleagues who have helped make the three words that comprise the title into the monograph that follows.

I would like to express my sincere appreciation for my dissertation chair, Susan Zieger, who challenged me and encouraged my work from my first day in graduate school. Her work on addiction and nineteenth-century literature was my first introduction to the intersections of literature and medicine as an undergraduate, and it spurred my interest in graduate study. The idea for this project emerged from a single paper for her "Victorian Media" seminar. Sometime in 2013, in an office meeting to discuss the paper after she had already given extensive feedback, Susan asked me to think about how military history might play into the metaphorical construction of "medicine is war" and its literary history—blood transfusions, field hospitals, and the like. This led me down a most productive line of inquiry for the years to follow. I wince a little, now, trying to recall how many versions of the Stoker, Kingsley, and Conrad chapters she read in their various forms (be they for a seminar, for my PhD exam, my dissertation, or before I submitted one to a journal). Her guidance, feedback, and attention to countless drafts and anxious emails were instrumental in the development of this project and me as scholar.

I would like to thank Sherryl Vint for her help on much of the theoretical grounding of this project in biopolitical theory. Her consistent and extended feedback on all chapters in each of their stages has helped me expand my thinking about this project beyond the Victorian era. I am also truly grateful for all her additional help and encouragement on the various related side-projects on medical discourse more broadly that informed my methodological approaches and interests, and, in turn, helped shape this project's revisions. For many of the ideas in the afterword, in particular, I am truly indebted to her.

Joe Childers devoted countless hours to my exam planning and dissertation, and has given me enough professional advice to comprise a substantive how-to manual on academic work. His insistence on a comprehensive understanding of Victorian literature and history has truly strengthened this project and my scholarship in countless ways. He should know where my recently identified penchant for asking students about metonymy, the Poor Law, the Corn Laws, Chadwick, and Althusser's definition of ideology can be traced back to.

I would also like to extend special thanks to Devin Griffiths for serving as my extralocutor for this project's defense as a dissertation. He has been incredibly supportive in many ways, but most recently, I must express my appreciation for Devin making himself available for long phone calls relating to functional antibiotic resistance genes, and citational demands in interdisciplinary work.

My colleagues at Lehigh University in the English and the Health, Medicine and Society Program have supported me in so many ways: in short conversations about ideas, reading groups, answering my varied queries from their areas of expertise, or providing helpful advice on the project itself. Perhaps even more so, just by being the most welcoming department/program that anyone could ask for. To Michael Kramp, your feedback and encouragement has made all the difference in the world.

I'd like to express an extra special thanks to my friends and colleagues who have provided invaluably specific feedback and insight into the history of medicine. Encountering Michael Brown's work for the first time at the 2015 Military Masculinities Conference introduced me to the vast scholarship that provided some of the historical evidence for many of my hunches, inducted from fiction or from literary or cultural studies scholars. His work, if my citations do not adequately intimate, directed me to many primary sources and taught more about the specific field of medical history, and how it is researched, than I can express. Along with Michael, Stephen Casper has been so very generous with his time and expertise, providing helpful sources, frameworks, and writing advice. I owe both of them a debt of gratitude for their support at key moments in this project's development.

There are so many other scholars at other institutions who were generous enough to take time and interest in this work. I would especially like to thank Pamela K. Gilbert, whose research inspired and helped me narrow my interest in infectious disease and whose advice and guidance over the past few years has been invaluable. I'm also grateful for the feedback and encouragement from those who have been generous in their engagement and collaboration on this work and related projects, in particular, Catherine Belling, Emilie Taylor-Pirie (née Taylor-Brown), Tabitha Sparks, Meegan Kennedy, Louise Penner, Colin Milburn, Priscilla Wald, Juliet McMullin, Nathan Hensley, Martin Willis, Hannah Landecker, and Sarita Mizin.

My friends and colleagues at UCR have heard and helped me improve countless iterations of these chapters and ideas in various forms. I must single out Anne Sullivan, Ann Garascia, Jessica Roberson, and Sarah Lozier for their insight, encouragement, and support. Among other fond memories, we will always have Chicago style, and its allowance (or demand, if you were in the Archive seminar) for discursive footnotes. I'm also grateful to Addison Palacios, Stina Attebery, and Josh Pearson, among others, who came to so many presentations and provided such thoughtful insights.

I am indebted to Gillian Andrews for her resolve in the face of esoteric research inquiries and innumerable footnotes with (my) questionable formatting. Her incisive copyediting (over and over again) was instrumental in making the manuscript presentable. If the reader judges a particular sentence in this book to be especially effective in its concision and clarity, it is very likely a product of Gill's suggestions. Her acuity in chasing down obscure leads with periodical sources was nothing short of indefatigable. Ashlee Simon, likewise, improved this manuscript with her close attention to detail when I was doing final revisions. Her research on pre-nineteenth century humoralism, and nineteenth-century antibiotic discourse was extremely helpful. Thank you, Gill and Ashlee.

I am grateful for the anonymous reviewers of this manuscript in its early form, the time they devoted, their generous comments, and their attention to detail. Additionally, the feedback from editors and reviewers at *Literature and Medicine*, *Victorian Studies*, and the *Journal of Victorian Culture* has truly helped shape earlier versions of a number of chapters for the better. I would also like to thank my colleagues at the North American Victorian Association, Modern Language Association, and Society for Science Literature and the Arts, who have provided probing questions and thoughts on conference presentations. If they haven't been named above, my thanks also goes out to the other scholars working in literary studies, medical history, Victorian studies, and medical humanities who have given me invaluable advice or provided support for this project.

To those whom I do not know or am unable to express my gratitude personally, I thank you for your important and influential work. At the risk of being characterized as excessively citational in my referencing, I have done my best to responsibly credit every piece of evidence or idea that I learned from your work. I hope my notes and bibliography lead others to consult the scholarship that I have learned so much from.

Mary Servitje, PharmD provided unwavering help and interest over the past several years made this work possible. Her inspiration, encouragement, and medical expertise helped shape this project through its various stages. I had never even thought of the history of medicine as a specific field of inquiry until that one day so many years ago, when she asked me if I knew anything about frontier medicine. On a handful of occasions, the discussions of pharmacology referenced in my work have been characterized in some favorable way. I will continue to stress that if there is an appreciable amount of accuracy in my work in this capacity, it is because of the wealth of knowledge Mary holds and gratuitously shared at all hours of the night.

Loriana Servitje, with her tenacity, spirit, curiosity, and love of learning continues to inspire my scholarship and teaching every day. At six years old, she asked me what research is and if mine is like science and its experiments. I have never thought about my research methods and forms of evidence I provide the same way since. My stepson, David Marquez, like his mother, has been an invaluable copy editor and audience for this work, and I am very grateful for his time and attention.

I would also like to thank my parents, Lorenzo and Mariana Servitje for their support throughout my education. While every time they asked me how my work was going since I began graduate school, I usually responded "not great," I will say that, at least at the moment I write these acknowledgments, things are, "pretty good." Thank you both for pushing me to go back to college.

Toiling through medical school while I did the same in graduate school, my friend Paul Kanaby has probably answered basic and obscure questions about microbiology and pathology in the order of hundreds. He might, however, have received a more expansive acknowledgment if he would have chosen a specialty more conducive to my research interests such as tropical medicine, toxicology, or epidemiology.

I would not be writing these acknowledgments without an editor who took a chance to listen to a pitch from a soon-to-be finished graduate student. I hope other authors are fortunate to work with Amanda Lanne-Camilli, who made a very stressful period as stress-free as possible.

If readers are at all familiar with the academic twitter scene, they will no doubt be familiar with the Rebecca Colesworthy, who I had the great fortune to work with after the manuscript was accepted. Rebecca is well known for demystifying the world of academic publishing (as a process and profession). The stories are, in fact, true: her fans on social media should know she is every bit as committed, attentive, and generous to her authors as she seems. Rebecca, you truly made sure the hard part was over.

This project has benefited from significant institutional support. The Office of the Vice President and Associate Provost for Research and Graduate Studies at Lehigh University has provided multiple grants that have afforded me the time and means to revise this manuscript. I would like to thank Graduate Division, University of California, Riverside, and the UC system more broadly for the Graduate Research Mentor and Dissertation Year Fellowships that supported much of the archival work required for this project, in addition to the time needed to revise chapters. I would also like to thank the Centers for Ideas and Society Research Grants for also supporting these efforts.

A version of chapter 5 is published *Literature and Medicine*: Lorenzo Servitje, "'Triumphant Health': Joseph Conrad and Tropical Medicine," *Literature and Medicine* 34, no. 1 (2016): 132–57, doi:10.1353/lm.2016.0007.

Introduction

When Sabeti learned that Ebola had reached Sierra Leone, she called a meeting in what she and her colleagues had begun to refer to as the Ebola War Room.

—Richard Preston, "The Ebola Wars" (2014)

First, we must be in a position to discover the infective material easily and with certainty; and, secondly, we must be able to destroy it.

—Robert Koch, "The Crusade against Typhoid Fever" (1903)

One could meet cholera face to face, as one does with those Russians.

—Charles Kingsley, *Two Years Ago* (1857)

A clear thread ties these quotations together: the common understanding of medicine through the conceptual domain of war. The connection might seem to go without saying: isn't it only natural to talk about medicine as war because medical technology kills pathogens and fights disease and because the immune system works in defense of our corporeal health? Each of the authors quoted above follows that familiar pattern in framing infectious disease at a specific historical moment. In the first quotation, Richard Preston, author of *The Hot Zone* (1994), refers to a computational biologist who led the sequencing of the Ebola virus in the 2014 pandemic. In the second quotation, from "Crusade against Typhoid Fever," the famed bacteriologist Robert Koch discusses his attempt to develop a treatment for the tuberculosis bacillus that he discovered a decade earlier. The third, from *Two Years Ago*, a popular Victorian social-problem novel by Charles Kingsley, addresses a military officer taking measures against a deadly cholera outbreak in a small Cornish town by comparing the disease to Britain's enemy during the Crimean War, a conflict in which the British military was ravaged by cholera.

The martial metaphor is not natural; it emerged from of a set of historical relations between actors, ideologies, and cultural productions. The connections between wars of public health, personal battles against disease, and disease as a threat to national security are related not simply by using the shorthand of the martial metaphor, but by being scaled iterations of how medicine operates as politics by other means. We can trace the metaphor's contemporary pervasiveness back to the nineteenth century, and specifically look to Victorian fiction. In doing so, we can understand how literary form negotiated—reflected, reinforced, and critiqued—the entanglements of the military and medical science in British culture.

Instead of focusing on the accuracy of the metaphor, or arguing for more precise representation of the relationships between humans, microbes, and medical technologies, I consider how this metaphor was naturalized and how the process was related to larger social, political, and cultural contexts that were mediated through literature. *Medicine Is War* explores military encounters with disease, their political and rhetorical constructions, and how military encounters made their way into the dominant language through which civilian medicine and the general public understood infectious disease.[1] I suggest that literature played a constitutive role in the martial metaphor's emergence from the institutions, bureaucracies, and material conditions of military medicine.[2] While military medicine encompasses hygiene, therapeutics, and the surgical treatment of wounds, even in the nineteenth and twentieth centuries most monographs on the subject, such as Edmund Park's *Practical Hygiene* (1864), foregrounded the importance of preventing and treating disease. In their introductions, authors like Park write of the primacy of prevention and treatment of disease, rather than wound care, even though military medical practitioners were mainly surgeons.[3] The military surgeons writing about infectious disease during wartime imbued the context of their practice with the discourse of their profession by discussing medicine and war in a metonymic capacity: soldiers were dying of disease and combat operations were affected, so disease was framed as an enemy. Those writings, however, had a limited audience and fairly fixed rhetorical purpose: instruction for other medical professionals, and both military and civilian governmental officials. Literature allowed for a broader reach and for orders of complexity through which to permute the martial metaphor to various venues and audiences.

Medicine Is War examines how nineteenth-century authors considered the British military's encounter with disease as they reflected on the developing politics of public health, hygiene, and medicine more broadly. Specifically, it explores the role of fiction in the constitution of the martial metaphor as it gained traction as a tool of governance through linking medical systems of thought with national defense. Military medical practice preceded the subversion of martial vocabulary into the metaphor, which was then popularized in the fiction written by Mary Shelley, Charles Kingsley, Bram Stoker, Arthur Conan Doyle, and Joseph Conrad. These authors reflected on significant events and concerns of military medicine, reimagining them in the figurative construction of medicine as war. As it helped forge the metaphor, literature occluded the material connections between the military, medical science, and public health by means of a metaphorical substitute. At the same time, however, in a few instances, it provided opportunities to critique this processual metaphorical militarization.

Metaphors are useful for understanding disease processes, along with the institutional efforts to mitigate them. This is especially true of infectious disease. The complexity of physiological processes and bureaucratic structures of public health are often more easily conveyed and understood in metaphorical terms, using another conceptual frame in which life is at stake. In terms of rhetorical power, it can unite diverse interests and audiences through a common cause, and for the individual, it can provide a sense of agency, optimism, and attribute meaning to illness.[4] At the same time, metaphorizing disease can be problematic, as other scholars across disciplines have suggested.[5] The martial metaphor is no exception. Unlike Susan Sontag's *Illness as Metaphor*, and other studies in the medical humanities, *Medicine Is War* focuses less on individual pathography, abstract experience of illness, or solely on epidemics and more on the broader cultural work performed by the specific metaphor of war as it developed historically. The ubiquity of the metaphor in all registers has led to its naturalization and, furthermore, its invisibility. The martial metaphor's continued noncritical use has materially problematic effects beyond the oft-cited critiques related to doctor-patient communication, such as exacerbating antibiotic resistance resulting from the "total war" against bacteria and the fostering of health for some at the expense of others—most often, nonnormative, racialized, and foreign bodies. The metaphor uses war's states of emergency to justify potentially questionable medical practices, like heroic measures and high-risk procedures or treatments, often deployed in emergency situations as well as end of life care. By attending to the history of the martial metaphor, we can denaturalize the inimical relationship between humans and infectious disease and disclose the conditions that have shaped the politics of medicine in the present moment. While the medical humanities often use literature as a mode to prompt bioethical questions, this investigation, rooted in nineteenth-century cultural study, urges us to think about the broader implications of historical medical representations in literature.

The Metaphor We Cure and Kill By

It is important to clarify how the martial metaphor structures our thinking about medicine. One example of the metaphor's ubiquity lies not just in medical practice but also in scholarship about medicine and, specifically, histories of infectious disease. This is not to condemn the use of metaphor by historians and interdisciplinary scholars. As the narrator of George Eliot's *The Mill on the Floss* (1860) reminds us, it is lamentable "that intelligence so rarely shows itself in speech without metaphor—that we can so seldom declare what a thing is, except by saying it is something else."[6] Rather than simply challenging other scholars' use of the martial metaphor, we must understand the implications, history, and politics that underlie it so scholars can reflect critically not only on its nineteenth-century literary and cultural history but also on its role in medical historiography, ethics, and practice.

I follow the medical humanists who have suggested that "medicine is war" is a conceptual metaphor, what George Lakoff and Mark Johnson define as the fundamental understanding of one idea in the conceptual domain of another.[7] That is, it is difficult to think about medicine and disease in non-militarized terms. The metaphor is conceptual because we don't even think of it as a metaphor: the construction's logic registers immediately, without our having to process how medicine *is* or even *is like* war. This is different from metaphors that are less aligned with the hostile connotations of war such as thinking of medicine as a balance, dance, or a symbiosis or ecology between various actors, environments, and processes.[8] This language matters, in a very material sense. The conceptual metaphor of medicine as war has shaped how we have overused antibiotics since their inception during the mid-twentieth century. Consequently, there is now an urgent need, especially in the case of pharmacological selective pressures on bacteria, to rethink the martial metaphor. The National Academies of Science, Engineering, and Medicine's 2005 Forum on Microbial Threats summarizes the need to change paradigms. In *Ending the War Metaphor: The Changing Agenda for Unraveling the Host-Microbe Relationship*, the editors of the postforum publication urge that "the metaphor of 'war' on infectious disease—characterized by the systematic search for microbial 'cause' of each disease, followed by the development of antimicrobial therapies—can no longer guide biomedical science or clinical medicine."[9] The threat has become so pressing that humanists as well as biomedical researchers have urged a reconceptualization of the language we use in infectious disease discourse. To think differently, however, we must acknowledge the martial metaphor's subtleties and ramified enmeshments in Western culture more broadly.

The martial metaphor shapes material conditions and social determinants of health. The power of the metaphor over conceptual understandings and material practices lies in the fact that the vehicle (*war*) amplifies some aspects of the tenor (*medicine*) while deemphasizing others.[10] The figure makes it easier to know and experience some aspects of illness and health while making it harder to see others. As Charles Rosenberg suggests: "Disease is at once a biological event, a generation-specific repertoire of verbal constructs reflecting medicine's intellectual and institutional history, an aspect of and potential legitimation for public policy, a potentially defining element of social role, a sanction for cultural norms, and a structuring element in doctor/patient interactions."[11] It is with Rosenberg's definition of disease in mind that I understand medicine in somewhat broader terms as not only the pharmacological or surgical intervention in the body, but as the shaping of the material conditions of existence that forestall death, including modifications to hygiene, architecture, infrastructure, and public health. It is precisely in these varied registers that Rosenberg suggests disease operates, that the martial metaphor shapes life and its conditions. In that vein, I follow a genealogical approach to medical history to unravel the medical certainties that are bound to the present. This "medical complex," as Nikolas Rose defines it, is composed of "the valorization of health and the sanitization of suffering, the powers ascribed to medical personages in relation to the disquiets of the body, soul, and social order, the sense of ourselves as perfectible through the application of medical techniques."[12]

These imperatives scale the politics of medicine from the individual to the nation, often in problematic ways. Given war's ability to incite populist and nationalist sentiment and foster related cultural anxieties, it makes sense that an appeal to metaphorical war is an effective means of persuasion in political campaigns such as the late-twentieth-century US. "War on Drugs." In this war, however, the health of the white, middle-class body was protected at the expense of Black people, immigrants, and the poor. Similar biases and structural processes operate in wars against infectious disease and have done so since the nineteenth century. Like the outbreak narrative, the martial metaphor brings some people together and pushes others apart.[13] *Medicine Is War* illustrates how this violent process and rhetorical appeal to medicine's social ordering has its roots in Victorian literature and culture.

There are many lineaments to this story, which historians of medicine, cultural studies and literary studies scholars have made visible. Scholars in bioethics and medical humanities have spoken to the existence of the effects of the metaphor in terms of doctor-patient relationships, health-care decisions, and, since the early 2000s, the ecological dynamics of the host-microbe relationship.[14] While Sontag's oft-cited *Illness as Metaphor* suggests that the martial metaphor is a controlling metaphor for talking about disease and that it originated in the 1880s with the rise of bacteriology,[15] the metaphor has a history before germ theory. I borrow Graham Mooney's characterization of ascribing such kinds of changes solely to germ theory as a form of "technoscientific determinism."[16] Focusing on epidemics specifically, Roger Cooter has previously denaturalized what he calls "the war-and-epidemics couplet," showing how it was used to make retrospective statistical comparisons between casualties from combat versus those from disease between the 1830s and to the 1940s. This coupling, he suggests, can veil how the conflation of the two represented and expressed "different sets of social mediated interests: including pacific laissez-faire political economy, public health, military medicine, and the disciplining of demography and epidemiology."[17] Medical practitioners were certainly in a unique position to act on these socially mediated interests. Exploring the cultural dimensions of the linguistic enjoinment of medicine and war, as it related to medical professionals themselves, Michael Brown shows how practitioners deployed the metaphor in a masculine ethos of heroism and self-sacrifice, citing some specific contemporaneous literary expressions by authors like Kingsley. These specific social and professional histories should also be considered in the context of another key discourse that is often taken for granted and commonly premised on bellicosity: the immune system. Ed Cohen has examined how immunity moved from a juridical to a biomedical register, highlighting the precursors of bodily self-defense vis-à-vis biological immunity in law and Enlightenment political philosophy which can be traced through biopolitical governance.[18] Studies in nineteenth-century literature and medicine have provided unique perspectives on these and adjoining histories. They have traced epidemiological, social, and political fissures and convergences, as expressed through literary forms and other cultural productions. Pamela Gilbert details the mobilization of the country in response to cholera as a significant process in nation-building and citizenship.[19] Laura Otis tracks how the development of cell theory and the subsequent metaphors of invasion participated in the imperial projects of England and Germany.[20] Erin O'Conner exposes the material and metaphoric crossovers between pathology and Victorian culture.[21] More recently, Tina Young Choi has explored the coproduction of medico-scientific prose, literature, and corporeal social relations of belonging and participation, speaking to the site of conflict wrought by germ theory.[22]

Much of the extant scholarship, however, has not considered the conditions of the metaphor's emergent cultural work with respect to the literary expression of military history throughout the nineteenth century and across multiple genres in a sustained way. *Medicine Is War* traces the metaphor throughout the Victorian era, showing how it only became dominant through literature's engagement with military medicine beginning in the first quarter of the century, and developed through the fin de siècle. It is crucial to address the influence of the military logics on the metaphor that continues to structure medical systems of thought or "regimes of truth": the language, theories, technologies, institutions, and material practices that make disease thinkable and describable and allow its treatment to be actionable, justifiable, and authoritative.[23] A brief outline of the specific medical histories over the long nineteenth century will help ground recurrent themes in the chapters that follow as to how disease itself was conceptualized under changing professional and epidemiological conditions.

Disease Agents and the History of Medicine

While the martial metaphor does predate the early nineteenth century, it does not fully emerge in medical discourse and the popular imaginary until then. Its use, mostly in terms of how disease is figured as an enemy, can be traced back at least as early as the seventeenth century.[24] John Donne described his illness as a "siege" in *Devotions upon Emergent Expressions* (1623).[25] The seventeenth-century English physician Thomas Sydenham proclaimed that "[A] murderous array of disease has to be fought against, and the battle is not a battle for the sluggard," while his contemporary Robert Fludd represented the body as a castle in his cosmological medical engravings, "The Invasion of the Fortress of Health" from *Medicina Catholica*.[26] Though the martial metaphor appears in these earlier works, their figuration of disease as an inimical agent does not quite fit with the reigning system of medical thought of the time as congruently as it would after the nineteenth century. Moreover, these iterations do not do the same cultural work. Earlier forms of militaristic metaphors like those in Donne, Fludd, and Sydenham's works appear before 1800 as a heuristic device to convey an idea, but there are a number of reasons beyond the metaphor's representation in literary fiction in the nineteenth century, that those earlier figurations did not gain the same kind of traction later uses would.[27] These conditions include the increased circulation of published material on medicine, in professional and lay venues; the changes in the medical professions and its relation to the state; the debates surrounding what constitutes the normal and the pathological; and what ontological form diseases that affected populations took.

The social, cultural, and political changes in the medical profession and medical journalism, especially from the early to the mid-nineteenth century, were conducive to escalating the use of war as a figuration for medicine.[28] The Medical Act of 1858, which legislated the requirements of qualified medical practitioners, helped create a vision of a national body of practitioners who could delimit its ranks from the corrupting influence of "quacks." Populated by clinically trained physician-surgeons, general practitioners, Poor Law medical officers, and—notably—demobilized military surgeons, this body of middle-class practitioners positioned itself against the book-trained physician-gentleman. We can also look to medical periodicals, especially the *Lancet* (founded in 1823), to see how a growing contingent of these men would increasingly unify themselves in epistemological, ideological, and political terms against the "Old Corruption" of medical elites that had dominated the higher ranks up until the late eighteenth century.[29] Michael Brown has demonstrated how this group formed an "imagined community," in the *Lancet*'s "textual space," were they could synchronically debate, reform, and apply their expertise to public service. This group imagined itself as a professional medical body that defended the social body against disease.[30] As the decades progressed, the discourse these practitioners used to represent themselves in medical publications would very explicitly invoke an ethos of militarized masculinity in the middle-class vision of professional identity.[31] Like the different political vision of the newer generation of practitioners that developed from the first quarter to the middle of the century, the epistemologies, ontologies, and etiologies that structured their practice were congruent with militaristic thinking when viewed in contrast to what kind of language and logic came before them.

Earlier forms of humoral medicine focused on the fluid equilibrium between the microcosm of the body and the macrocosm of the environment (often further detailed in terms of temperature and moisture—hot/cold and wet/dry). As fibers and solids, and the study of their movements, became an area of more interest over fluids themselves in iatromechanical medicine, the body was often metaphorically described in terms of machines, textiles, woven/webbed fibers, and string.[32] In health, these structures were understood as the harmonious vibration and undulation—one might say frequency—of elastic fibers that moved fluids like blood.[33] In diseased states, they became spasmodic or lax, but were still, like humors, conceptualized in contiguity with the environment surrounding the body. Even beyond the discourse of a single body's impairment, the language of epidemics was largely environmental rather than militaristic. While the language of attacks and invasions was present in pre-nineteenth-century writings, it more often presented the occurrence of larger-scale disease in frameworks of theology through figurations of gardening, even in the case of military medicine: "'visitations,' 'rages,' 'infestations,' together with 'seeds' (germs) sown and brought under maturity under the appropriate 'soil.'"[34]

The shift in medical epistemes that occurred during the transition from the late-eighteenth to the early-nineteenth century facilitated conceptualizing disease as an entity while at the same time recognizing it as a process. During the late eighteenth century disease was an idiosyncratic, psychosomatic, environmental, and spiritual condition of individuals and their relation to their milieu, both in humoralism and iatromechanism. Toward and during the nineteenth century, the primary objects of medical inquiry became lesions, cells, and eventually, proteins and molecular compounds. The transition was one of "medical cosmologies" that N. D. Jewson characterizes as forming different periods in the production of medical knowledge from roughly the 1770s to the 1870s. The conceptualization of disease moved from the whole person ("Beside Medicine") to the tissue ("Hospital Medicine"), to the cell ("Laboratory Medicine").[35] These last two transmutations of conceptual form gave disease a concrete existence separate from the body, a contingency that allowed for the figuring and emplotment of disease as an inimical agent.[36] Prior to emergence of the medical gaze, disease was not localized in the manner of lesions in tissue to the same degree. Before Xavier Bichat's pathological anatomy, disease was most often thought of as a constellation of signs rather than a thing in and of itself.[37] The reification of disease specifically allowed for the possibility of fighting against it to become a more logical proposition than the previously dominant humoral and iatromechanist medical systems of thought.

While the martial metaphor can be broadly conceived as a resistance to death, following Bichat's definition of life as "the totality of those functions which resist death,"[38] the movement from pre-nineteenth-century Bedside Medicine to the Hospital medicine's clinical gaze and, consequently, to "disease objects" narrowed the scope of what it meant to resist death in the period of Laboratory Medicine.[39] Fighting disease does fall into the spectrum of Bichat's resistance, but as medical cosmologies shifted from Bedside to Hospital medicine, and Hospital to Laboratory, the antagonist to resist was conceptualized as a knowable entity that was not of the body. That resistance became thinkable as an active *fight*, in defensive (preventative) and offensive (allopathic) capacities against an invader. That invader took different physical forms in the nineteenth century with respect to disease that affected individuals and populations: contagion, pestilent miasma, and microbe. Those three forms and their conflation played a central role in literature's mediation of the martial metaphor.

During the nineteenth century, the three physical forms of disease became three different etiologies: contagionism, anticontagionism or miasma theory, and germ theory. Though the cause of disease had been debated for centuries, and all three theories existed previously in various forms, these scholarly and medical discussions had never grown as contentious as they did after the matter garnered a politically polarizing meaning in the nineteenth century.[40] While the three theories invoke different causal factors, a nuanced understanding of their interrelationships shows that it is difficult to parse them as entirely discrete from each other, either in concept or periodization. Many medical practitioners and social commentators believed in various conceptual blends of those theories, such as contingent contagionism, as I show in the first chapter on Mary Shelley.[41] When sides were taken, it was often more a matter of politics than of medical science and hinged on what could be done to ameliorate or prevent the spread of disease, particularly in terms of governmental intervention. In the history of the martial metaphor, medical professionals and authors continually conflate the three theories, a trope perhaps most memorably remembered in *Bleak House*'s (1853) Jo, who embodies and spreads Tom-All-Alone's pestilential ecology.[42] For the sake of clarity, however, some points of reference for each etiology allow for a rough but helpful context for the debates that frame the traction of the martial metaphor. Contagion theory provides a particularly helpful initial inroad to this history.

Contagionists posited that disease was transmitted by bodies. They debated the ultimate causes of disease but their shared position was that human bodies were the proximate source of it. Numerous historical examples, most prominently venereal disease, gave credence to contagionism. In the late eighteenth century, one of the most notable affirmations of contagion theory was smallpox, in large part due to the prophylactic variolation—the application of smallpox-infected human material to a patient—introduced by Lady Mary Wortley Montagu from her travels in the Ottoman Empire. Variolation was followed by the development of vaccination—the application of cowpox-infected material to a patient— by Edward Jenner, at the end of the eighteenth century.[43] Poets such as Wordsworth and Coleridge advocated on Jenner's behalf, describing him in military terms in the early nineteenth century, to promote vaccination as the healing power of nature.[44] Quarantine, the medical intervention that defined contagionism, was military in origin and implementation. As a technology of public health, a quarantine delimits a *cordon sanitaire*, a guarded border defining the boundary between the healthy and the (potentially) contagious. The physical boundary restricts the movement of exposed populations by mandate, creating a cordon held by soldiers, police, or other guards. The practice of quarantine dates at least as far back as the Middle Ages. For most of the nineteenth century, quarantine was considered outdated because it was contrary to liberal principles, as it restricted both personal freedom and free trade through the closure of trade routes and the quarantining of ships carrying imported goods. However, as I show, quarantine remains a structuring tenet of the violence and coercive force associated with the martial metaphor.

Anticontagionists, also sometimes known as sanitarians, suggested that quarantine was not only wrong, outdated, and "illiberal," but dangerous insofar as it exacerbated disease by crowding people together in unsanitary, confined conditions as suggested by well-known proponents of miasma theory such as Thomas Southwood Smith, Edwin Chadwick, and Florence Nightingale.[45] Anticontagionism, which was generally equated with miasma theory, pointed instead to environmental conditions as the source of disease, and thus held that the filth, lack of ventilation, and concentration of bodies produced by quarantine and, likewise, the overcrowding of urbanization, would foster disease. Pestilent vapors were generated in foul environments, such as filth, decay, contaminated water, and excrement—often lumped under the broad rubric of "nuisance"—and spread through the air. Miasmic infectivity varied depending on air quality and wind, among other factors, often including an individual's constitution, harkening back to humoral medicine. Miasma conceptually aligned with disease as an inimical external agent and, consequently, with the martial metaphor during the first half of the nineteenth century as it invaded the body from without. Furthermore, in its relationship to biopolitics, it worked to conduce populations and mobilize governmental apparatuses through military rhetoric.

Given that anticontagionists focused on environmental conditions, their medical interventions were reformative in nature. Sanitarians pushed for drainage and ventilation and focused on impoverished populations, linking their disease theory to social reform and making it more a movement than a theory, although the mid-century sanitary movement was far from straightforwardly progressive.[46] As Edwin Ackernecht notes in his influential history of that etiology, anticontagionism was focused on "fighting for the freedom of the individual and commerce against despotism and reaction."[47] The use of bellicose metaphor to describe that historical movement aside, I suggest that given those liberal aspirations, sanitarians nonetheless reinscribed the martial metaphor through discourses on hygiene that encouraged individuals to internalize the larger mechanisms of the state and military through the inculcation of disciplinary techniques. Moreover, although in some capacities it was considered progressive and conducive to improving living conditions by cleaning up slums, miasma theory tended to reinforce classist and racist essentializing discourses that metonymically identified the poor by their insalubrious environments,[48] racializing them in the same way as peoples of tropical and colonial environments were seen as primitive, unhygienic and filthy.[49] Anticontagionism was solidified in the political sphere during the mid-century, populated by sanitarians like Chadwick and Smith. Chadwick's influential *Sanitary Report* (1842) and the Public Health Act of 1848 that followed contributed to the ascendancy of anticontagionism as the dominant disease theory for the majority of the nineteenth century, roughly from the 1830s to the 1880s.

Although there had been earlier theories of living germs, the work of Rudolph Virchow, Louis Pasteur, and Robert Koch from the mid-century approached its apotheosis with Koch's discovery of *Mycobacterium tuberculosis* in 1882, and his publication two years later of the criteria for determining whether a microorganism causes a disease.[50] From the 1880s on, conversations about infectious disease tended toward the microorganismal idiom, which drew the attention of writers such as Conan Doyle, Stoker, and Conrad. Often cited with respect to germ theory and microscopy, Conan Doyle's Sherlock Holmes claims a threat "cease[s] to be dangerous if we [can] define it."[51] Microbiology served this function, but it often did so through the grammar of war. In one sense, the martial metaphor ameliorates the existential threat posed by infectious disease propagated by invisible and innumerable microbes by giving a narrative frame, agency, and meaning to an entity or process that has no motive, only a drive to reproduce. That legacy did not arise simply from the visibility of bacteria through microscopy but reformed the military legacies and politics of contagion and miasma theory in a new way that magnified the rhetoric of war in medical discourse. Yet, germ theory was, indeed, a notable point of inflection in the development of the martial metaphor, as it personified diseases as living and self-reproducing agents. It brought together some of contagion and miasma theory's conflicting premises, as disease could be communicated between bodies and arise from environmental conditions in an identifiable way. While it is understandable that scholars such as Sontag and Alfred Tauber date the martial metaphor to the 1880s and the rise of germ theory, discounting the earlier nineteenth-century history of the martial metaphor further occludes its attachment to the military and earlier cultural work with respect to British identity, empire, race, and gender.[52] Earlier medical discourse created the conditions for the construction of germs (disease) as enemy and bacteriology (the new scientific field informing medicine) as war. Germ theory animated the form and narrative of disease, as microbes breached the boundaries of the body and attacked its cellular life. That visibility further naturalized the militarization of medicine. The contest between humans and disease was condensed down to the cellular level, linking attributes like walls, membranes, mass reproduction, and invisibility to the level of social and international relations. The "gospel of germs" was comforting, showing scientific progress and promising new treatments; it also gave new force to the martial metaphor. Although the microbe came under the microscopic medical gaze, it remained invisible to the naked eye, in contrast to the seemingly perceivable filth of miasma.[53] If disease was ubiquitous, colonizing both the body and the quotidian environment regardless of one's social position, then the martial metaphor was a way to understand and respond to the new order of the world. Germ theory gave disease a conceivable "face" and new possibilities for being anthropomorphized, providing new specificity to Bichat's definition of life as resistance.[54] The medical gaze moved from tissue to cell; its focus, from object to target.

Bichat's notion of life as resistance against death certainly took on another inflection with the rise of evolutionary theory and Darwin's "struggle for life." Darwin used war as a metaphor to discuss the relationships between species and resources, and sexual selection in *On the Origin of Species* (1859) and *The Descent of Man* (1871).[55] While remaining relevant to the broader cultural context of science and medicine, Darwin's use of the metaphor did not reference the military as an institution in the same way as the literary authors discussed in the chapters that follow did. Struggle, like resistance, very broadly characterizes violent efforts in contest, whether in sports or combat. Moreover, as a whole, this book addresses medicine and war, rather than the semantic hyponyms life and struggle, although those broader concepts do inform certain iterations of the metaphor of war such as the definition of life in Kingsley's writings, discussed in chapter 2, and the discourse of eugenics, discussed in chapter 3. The texts I examine are not just instances of struggle in general, but they also track how literary authors more specifically reflect on the relationship between medicine—the technology to foster life in the face of disease—and the military—the institutions, bureaucracies, logics, and imperatives of state-sponsored armed forces. Undoubtedly, natural selection and competition, reformulated from zoology and botany to the social forms of humans through the work of Herbert Spencer, were significant determining concepts to the prominence of filtering medicine through the metaphorics of war. With the increasing cultural emphasis on rivalry, "war came to be seen by some as the ultimate expression of collective human endeavor."[56] Like immunity and germ theory, evolution is one important, but not the sole, dimension to the history of the martial metaphor. As the shifting notions of race and heredity became increasingly biologized in the nineteenth century and inherited conditions were conflated with infectious disease, both mistakenly and for argumentative purposes, biopolitical thinking was inflected through the discourse of degeneration. Degeneration is evident in fiction and medical prose even as early as Kingsley, but through the influence of Herbert Spencer, Max Nordau, Francis Galton, and Karl Pearson in the last quarter of the nineteenth century, among others, it played a larger role in the writings of authors such as Conan Doyle, Stoker, and Conrad. Under the paradigm of degeneration, foreign and internally racialized Others, such as the working class and the poor, became threats to national identity while the middle-class body indexed the nation's health.[57] The effort to maintain racial purity in these terms was often expressed through the martial metaphor. That mind-set has a long history in terms of the broader, governmental interest in intervening in and mitigating biology.

The Martial Metaphor "in Theory"

The martial metaphor worked as a tool of biopolitical governance: a mechanism to regulate populations and foster the self-fashioning of individuals, which together mitigated the biological obstacles to expanded urbanization, industrialization, colonization, and the consequential increased risk of disease. Biopolitics refers to a shift in political thinking and operation where life itself became the object of governance. Life became abstracted from individuals and directed, calibrated, and shaped at the level of populations through the operation of disciplinary apparatuses for determining how individuals fashioned themselves as healthy and productive subjects. The governmental targeting of life—in terms of mortality, morbidity, and birth rates, for instance—was co-constitutive with the rise of biological science, statistics, and biomedicine.[58] Those kinds of calibrations secured the labor force and state itself against disease and scarcity, as preemptions and calculated allowances for Malthusian checks. This was especially the case with endemic and epidemic disease. Foucault provides a way to understand the biopolitical implications of endemic versus epidemic thinking.

> At the end of the eighteenth century, it was not epidemics that were the issue, but something else—what might broadly be called endemics, or in other words, the form, nature, exten-

> sion, duration, and intensity of the illnesses prevalent in a population. These were illnesses that were difficult to eradicate and that were not regarded as epidemics that caused more frequent deaths, but as permanent factors which . . . sapped the population's strength, shortened the working week, wasted energy, and cost money . . . In a word, illness as phenomena affecting a population. Death was no longer something that suddenly swooped down on life—as in an epidemic. Death was now something permanent, something that slips into life, perpetually gnaws at it, diminishes it and weakens it.[59]

Foucault's characterization of endemicity might seem contrary to the logic of the martial metaphor, as in this paradigm disease is no longer an angel of death that "swoops down on life" and the concern is no longer epidemics. Of course, epidemics were still a major problem. The point to take from Foucault is that the permanent presence of epidemic disease, among other biological determinants, became part of the governance and definition of life itself.[60]

Infectious disease waged a war of attrition that must be perpetually held at bay. The reason illness became a central concern of the state was the shift in focus to fostering population. Governmental power became productive rather than deductive, aiming to "make live" and "let die."[61] This imperative shaped the political tensions between the one and the many, between individual freedom and social control.

Liberalism and individualism framed the modern social body made up of individuals, leading to biopolitical formations as individual health became necessary to its maintenance.[62] The way the middle-class body became the index for the nation during the mid-century was in line with the rise of sanitary reform, for which middle-class domesticity and morality became the model, and in prose related to public health such as in Chadwick's and Nightingale's work. Middle-class reformers imposed their orders of morality, domesticity, and hygiene on the working classes to make them proper, healthy subjects.[63] That project was often carried out in the language of the martial metaphor, which became a mode of empowerment, a technique for producing an individual's healthy subjectivity, most evident in Kingsley's writings. The representation of medicine as war incorporated individual health with aggregate public health, linking the different orders of cell, body, and society.[64] If life is the set of functions that fight against death, then each individual life is always already at war with death and must actively produce its own health, often through techniques derived from the needs and practices of the military. That construction, however productive, shaped liberal subjectivity as inherently pathological and always sick, if not actually, then potentially.

The liberal war against disease was not always as affirmative in producing life or so passive in allowing it to die. The inherent pathology of the liberal subject fosters the conditions for what Julian Reid calls "logistical life": that is, "life that is lived under duress to be efficient." Logistical life comes not from the actual shifting of regimes of war to those of peace, but from the logistical orders in which life is shaped by the organizational needs of the modern state to prepare for war. In this vein, making life live under liberalism requires waging war on its behalf.[65] The history of disciplinary techniques shows that the production of individualizing subjectivities as a mode of control can be traced to military practices such as hygiene, self-surveillance, regularized schedules, and proper divisions of bodies in space. Nathan Hensley, who makes a more developed and historically precise claim, contends that Victorian political modernity is based on an equation between peace and war, despite the espousal of law and contract in contrast to physical coercion. Violence was not an exception to liberal modernity but rather the premise, a contradiction negotiated through the expanded possibilities of literary form.[66] Insofar as the martial metaphor is semantically and genealogically tied to violence despite being deployed to foster life, its history is likewise tied to liberal modernity.

Biopower certainly entails violence insofar as in its productive capacities it creates conditions for the material demise of those who are allowed to die; in its deductive, thano- or necropolitical iterations, the violence is overtly more explicit and active, often deploying military weaponry and tactics. That said, Hensley astutely cautions against abstracting the relation between biopolitics and violence, erasing historical and categorical specificity. It is tempting, first, "to fold different degrees of and genres of violence, such that peacetime's violence *in potentia* is construed as somehow equivalent to the physical injuries actuated in what we would be forgiven for calling real warfare." Second, it is easy to "conflate diverse historical moments—diachronic processes of unfolding and contestation—into a single, eternal antagonism: modernity as an endless combat."[67] Attending to this critical and historiographic acuity, *Medicine Is War* differentiates the violence of "real war" with the metaphorical and nonmilitary violence of regulatory biopolitics operating under medical aegis. However, I trace connections between both kinds of violence, the violence in representation and the material force exerted on human bodies.[68] In effect, that violence highlights the relations between the different degrees of violence occasioned by metaphorical war.

The idea of the state defending its own way of life through a disciplinary apparatus as well as regulatory biopolitics, has roots in immunity's role in social ordering. Cohen contends that "immunity emerges at the end of the nineteenth century to naturalize the military model as the basis for organismic life."[69] I follow Cohen's genealogy and agree that the fin de siècle marks a particularly aggressive traction of the metaphor of immunity, but this specific formulation is just one of the martial metaphor's points of inflection, where the previous logics of miasma and pregerm contagion were internalized in the body and provided an oppositional ontology to counter microbial life. Victorian literature was constitutive to this rendering. It helped render the martial metaphor in a way that occluded its military origins, making the connections between the use of medicine to defend the body's life qua immunity and the use of war to defend the state's way of life mutually inclusive, self-evident propositions. Consequently, the metaphorical abstraction helped make the violence embedded in biopolitics invisible. The paradox here, then, is that the erasure makes the metaphor real and fictional at once, suggesting that war is the true logic of medicine and immunity while disavowing any material connection to the military as an institution or its violence. The use of figuration as mode of concealment follows the very work of the state of exception, as Jasbir Puar suggests, "to hide or even deny itself in order to further its expanse, its presence and efficacy, surfacing only momentarily and with enough gumption to further legitimize the occupation of more terrain."[70] When we trace the martial metaphor's history through the relationships between literature, medicine, and the military, it becomes clear that military language and thought is a tool for inciting populist and nationalist sentiment, for killing to make life live, often against foreign and internal Others. "Biopolitical strategies," suggests Priscilla Wald, are "neither self-evident nor are they static; they must be meaningfully made and continually reproduced."[71] This is precisely one of the central underpinnings of the martial metaphor: replicating the production of "us" versus "them" under medical auspices.

Literature participated in this occlusion by naturalizing the connection between medicine and war. It catalyzed the metaphor's inculcation in the individual, and emplotted them within the larger national biopolitical defense of the state. Material manifestations of the metaphor, most notably the martial quarantine, function overtly as legal states of exception while covertly countenancing the affirmative, productive imperatives of biopower. This development was not a clear break but a gradient, with both the material and figurative medical wars remaining mutually constitutive while the martial metaphor circulated in the popular imagination in literary forms. The military fight became entangled with public health, which informed the personal, disciplinary battle for health; in the age of immunity, the proposed natural operation of the body's relationship to disease became its defense system. In the shift from metonymy to metaphor in degrees, we see how the martial metaphor condensed the national and the military to the cellular and was materialized as the natural order of the body. The authors and works discussed in the following chapters mark those degrees in various intellectual, political, and medico-scientific shifts, and through significant moments in the military and cultural history of the Victorian era. *Medicine Is War* illustrates how literature mediated the way in which medicine, from individual hygienic practices to public health, from the Victorian era to the present, wages a perpetual war against disease.

Overview

Considering the cultural work of literature allows for a fuller understanding of the consequences of science and technology than a narrower focus on dimensions that medical prose, with its generic conventions and specific audiences, tends to prioritize. By using literature to understand the cultural work of medical science, we can reveal the complex, ambiguous, and overdetermined implications medicine has in other, ostensibly nonmedical, aspects of life; we can unravel the complexities in the medicalization of society.

The multidimensional and expansive qualities that literature affords is especially present in the case of medicine and the Victorian novel, given the rise in the social status of the medical profession, the emergence of the doctor as a frequent hero of Victorian fiction, and the mechanism by which the novel served as a vehicle for the production of subjectivity.[72] Through the diversity of perspectives, narrative engagements, and dialogical operations, reading fiction alongside medical prose reveals the tensions that emerge from the martial metaphor: what it meant to be a healthy British citizen and nation at various points in the nineteenth century; the implications of medical interventions for social justice, personal liberty, and political economy; and the problematic use of medical knowledge as a tool for colonization and a weapon to diffuse the strength of enemy armies and their supporting populations. I focus on novels, and in the case of Conan Doyle, short stories as well, that develop extended meditations on the relationship between military medicine and civilian health. Each chapter details how specific authors incorporate the martial metaphor and draw from contemporaneous developments of military medicine, be they full-scale conflicts such as the Napoleonic, Crimean, and Boer Wars, or supportive deployments for colonial endeavors in India and Africa.

Medicine Is War is divided into two parts that sketch a genealogical shape of the martial metaphor through the debates over disease theories, the shifting question of national identity in racialized terms, and the expansion of empire. Texts are grouped according to their most influential etiology and diseases. The first part pertains to authors responding to miasma and contagion theory in the face of the first three cholera epidemics. The authors in part 2 respond to bacteriology, parasitology, immunity, and eugenics. While *Medicine Is War* follows a chronological order, even authors writing in the age of germ theory continually look back to older etiologies, most often to racialize foreigners' bodies by conflating them with foreign lands. In part 1, I discuss how Shelley and Kingsley conflated the cholera epidemics of the first half of the nineteenth century with war in the context of the debates between contagionism and anticontagionism. Cholera catalyzed the martial metaphor's co-constitution with the discourses of public health and hygiene. After the 1817 pandemic, Britain suffered four major cholera outbreaks. Until the mid-1860s, cholera was at the center of the development of public health, the modernization of government, and the defining of the nation in the public imagination, leading into the racial and gendered paradigms in the middle of the nineteenth century and hypernationalism at the beginning of the twentieth.[73]

When epidemic cholera "invaded" England in 1831 and was suddenly no longer relegated to colonial territories, it challenged the naturalized salubrious identity of Britain. In chapter 1, I show how the recurrence of military language in discussions of disease and the narrative function of war in Shelley's *The Last Man* (1826) respond to the emergence of the metaphor in the medical prose of the early nineteenth century on the 1817 cholera pandemic. Shelley's novel also marks a significant moment in the rise of the metaphor by emblematizing a movement from humoral to the ontological valences of contagionist and anticontagionist etiologies. Her novel articulates the movement away from "Romantic medical discourse," influenced by pre-nineteenth-century disease theories, and toward Victorian imperatives of purity and defense.[74] Yet, *The Last Man* challenges the martial metaphor, while also contributing to its use. It circulates the metaphor as a central and recurring theme and fosters a bellicose response to the proposition that Britain is not constitutionally more resilient to disease than colonial lands. The militant definition of British health in the novel is concordant with a national identity that was in part forged by British military campaigns over the long eighteenth century, especially the Napoleonic Wars (1803–1815).[75] At the same time, the novel undercuts this position and critiques warfare as an amplifier of disease, specifically commenting on how Britain enabled the spread of the first cholera epidemic through military movement. Published in 1826, the novel's temporal proximity to the first major epidemic to hit England in 1831 illuminates how the discourse of military medicine primed England's adoption of the language of war to respond to cholera as a foreign invasion.

In chapter 2, I show how Kingsley develops the relationship between cholera and the martial metaphor by linking the disease's effects on military efforts during the Crimean War to England's third cholera outbreak. Kingsley writes the martial metaphor across various sermons, pamphlets to soldiers in Crimea, and sanitary lectures. I read these texts in concert with his post-Crimean, Condition-of-England novel *Two Years Ago* (1857), which uses the martial metaphor as a central plot device. In the novel, military surgeon Tom Thurnall defends a small Cornish town against a cholera outbreak at the advent of the Crimean War. *Two Years Ago* not only narrativizes the metaphor in an extended form, it also indexes the way Kingsley uses the metaphor to weave English history, the Church, the domestic space, the battlefield, and the public sphere together, treating it as a biopolitical tool. His texts empower individuals as self-fashioning agents and guides their conduct through the reification of gendered scripts. He develops the unified battle of men and women against disease by situating the biological science of anticontagionism within the familiar Christian framework of original sin. Kingsley cuts across class and gender lines by giving citizens an agent against which to develop their subjectivities in the form of cholera. Those middle-class sanitary practices empowered subjects to self-govern their own health, and made that self-governance a duty, both to God and the nation.

Part 2 addresses the links between empire, race, and germ theory in the second half of the nineteenth century as articulated in the writings of Stoker, Conan Doyle, and Conrad. I investigate epistemological changes to the understanding of disease as caused by living, replicating organisms, and to the understanding of the body's response in terms of the counteracting logic of immunity toward the end of the century. The development of germ theory, immunity, and organic chemistry gave medicine a weapon in the form of modern pharmacology. Regarding the trend toward pharmacology in 1881, Thomas Huxley wrote in the then relatively new journal *Science*: "It will, in short, become possible to introduce into the economy a molecular mechanism which, like a very cunningly-contrived torpedo, shall find its way to some particular group of living elements, and cause an explosion among them, leaving the rest untouched."[76] Huxley's "torpedo"—later characterized as a "magic bullet"—emblematizes the movement toward the use of drugs as the primary medical interventional technology; these compounds fit into the schema of the martial metaphor as the main weapon of the doctor's armamentarium.

Chapter 3 explores how Bram Stoker delves into military history to reflect on and respond to anxieties over the fin-de-siècle and the future of the British as a people. In its recurring use of the martial metaphor, explicitly and as a narrative logic, *Dracula* (1897) sublimates racial threats to the purity of the nation into both an ancient military threat and a modern form of disease. While the former draws on the mythic narrative of the Crusades, the latter constructs the vampire as an anachronistic, overdetermined disease: at once contagion, miasma, and microbe. In this history, I consider the contemporaneous writings of physicians such as William Budd and James Young Simpson on the extirpation of rinderpest and smallpox as they inform how the Crew of Light narratively contests Dracula's biological invasion. Reading these texts in conversation exposes the rhetorical process of the broader metaphorical militarization of medicine in Victorian Britain that appropriated the exigencies of war while eliding negative connotations associated with its violence from the mid-to-late nineteenth century.

In looking back to a specific moment in the history of British military medicine—the Crimean War—the novel speaks to the conflict's civilian implications through its representation of women's sexuality as a response to the Contagious Diseases Acts (1864, 1866, 1869), legislation that policed female sex workers in an effort to curb the high rate of syphilis among enlisted men. Stoker narrates the aggressive response to the CD Acts' repeal, reflecting on the words of feminist and social reformer Josephine Butler, who called the Acts a "war waged against impure women."[77] Developing the institutional influence of the military on Victorian life, *Dracula* also alludes to the contemporaneous reflection of the British military's involvement in the developing field of tropical medicine through the figuration of blood and the vampire as parasite. In these capacities, Stoker's novel imbues military logics into the anxieties of reverse colonization and degeneration attached to the foreign vampire, making the fight for the nation one fought by doctors.

Looking more specifically at Koch's bacteriological research into tuberculosis and the developing field of immunology, Chapter 4 considers how Conan Doyle writes the martial metaphor in his fiction and prose in markedly different ways before and after the turn of the twentieth century. Before the Second Boer War (1899), the metaphor operates as a subtle guiding logic in his detective fiction through Sherlock Holmes's forensic and toxicological work and the military medical background of John Watson, especially when read in conversation with Conan Doyle's popular prose on medical science. Bacteria, as well as diseased military personnel, begin to appear in Doyle's fiction after the Second Boer War, with Doyle himself embodying Watson's medical military background by serving as a surgeon in South Africa. Doyle experienced the failed vitality and martial prowess of the British military and the governmental institutions that were supposed to support them. In response, he narrativized them into bacterial weapons, as in "The Adventure of the Dying Detective" (1913), and into soldiers who become diseased, as in "The Adventure of the Blanched Soldier" (1926). By tracing Doyle's shifting representations of the intersections of the military and medicine, we can see the anxieties of degeneration imposed on national defense, and an uncertainty about the power of bacteriology to secure the nation against imperial threats. Doyle drew attention to the facile allayment of anxieties over the weakening of the British race, which bolstered the need to think of medicine as war. In his changing manner of representation, Doyle's writings show the metaphor's progressive legitimization.

In the final chapter, I suggest that Joseph Conrad responds to the discourse of degeneration by showing how the medical evolution wrought by the development of British tropical medicine facilitated the atrocities in the Belgian Congo and the fostering of disease in native populations. Making use of modernist indeterminacy, Conrad's *Heart of Darkness* (1899) challenges the martial metaphor promoted in both medical and public circles by tropical medicine specialists like Ronald Ross. In Conrad's treatment, European health functions as a weapon of empire, turning the "white man's grave" into a grave for the native Congolese. I conclude the chapter with a discussion of the Congo's sleeping sickness epidemic (1899–1905), which served as a laboratory for testing atoxyl, a precursor to pharmacologist Paul Ehrlich's famous "magic bullet." This pharmacological ideal facilitated the development of the first antibiotic drug, Salvarsan. The link is highlighted in *Heart of Darkness*'s representations of tropical disease in the Congo and health in the form of the preternatural vitality of the notorious General Manager. Understanding Conrad's novel and the history of pre-penicillin antimicrobial chemotherapy in this way reveals how the military history of tropical medicine was central to the emergence of antibiotic pharmacology. This technology ultimately solidified the metaphor's attachment to the development of penicillin in the mid-twentieth century, arguably one of the most significant technological developments in medical history.

The afterword, "Collateral Damage," reflects on the martial metaphor's impact on contemporary medical concerns, specifically antibiotic resistance, the continued conflation of immigration with infectious disease, and the war on cancer in pharmacological, individual, and structural terms. This contextualization brings this project's intervention in Victorian studies to bear on the health humanities. I suggest that historicizing the metaphor enables a more critical understanding of how military language and rhetoric in medicine operates, retaining the martial discourse of its origins.

I close this study with a brief addendum that documents how this monograph (written and edited from approximately 2015 to the beginning of 2020) and its conclusions held up in the face of COVID-19. Written from March to August 2020, during the first wave of the pandemic, it details the flood of events—political, epidemiological, personal—and discourse that resonated with *Medicine Is War*, in the form of epistolary fragments. In those final pages, I had the opportunity to engage with the sudden visibility and mass criticism of the martial metaphor. At once mimicking the form of *Dracula* and reflecting the role of twitter in science communication, I hope to preserve some of the complicated sentiments, thoughts, and sense of surreality that arose from seeing the object I have studied from the safety of historical (and fictional) distance materialize in 2020.

Medicine Is War's sketch of the martial metaphor's arc from Shelley to Conrad reflects a movement from Romanticism to Modernism not simply following conventional literary periodization, but rather articulating how authors reacted to and propagated the martial metaphor even as they critiqued its effects. In the opening and concluding chapters, I show that in using the language of the martial metaphor both Shelley and Conrad mark the way militarism breeds disease, and also circulated and reinscribed its cultural hegemony. In this genealogy, the relationship between different literary representations of the changes in medical science and in military-inflected medical politics is evident from humoral theory to contagionism and anticontagionism; from miasma to the germ and from anecdotal and idiosyncratic treatments to evidence-based pharmacological torpedoes.

❧

Tracing the martial metaphor through Victorian literature and culture lets us answer the question of what war has made thinkable and actionable in medical systems of thought, in both affirmative and adverse capacities: making health a moral responsibility, cosigning reform, using medicine as a tool of governance, linking individual health to aggregate public health, justifying dividing practices, and internal state racism. These operations develop a medical spectrum of the normal and the pathological that makes the impossible yet desirable dream of the hermetic subject and nation a necessary fantasy. This study also provides us a way to consider the possibilities and dangers in terms of medicine's fictional and nonfictional representation.

Max Weber famously articulated the progress of Enlightenment rationalism in modernity: the movement toward a secularized worldview that values scientific knowledge over religious and superstitious belief systems. In a similar vein, Foucault concludes that with the rise of the medical gaze, "Disease breaks away from the metaphysic of evil; and it finds in the visibility of death its full form in which its content appears in positive terms."[78] While the discourses of evil do not go away completely in the nineteenth century, the movements from humoral medicine through the debates between contagionism and anticontagionism, all the way to germ theory, would certainly disenchant theocentric understandings in which disease is a form of divine punishment. Twentieth-century refinements of microbiology would surely dispel the racial and classist biases of nineteenth-century disease theories. Positivist science and clinical and evidence-based medicine would seem to have objectified disease theory and freed it of cultural mythologies. *Medicine Is War* illustrates that while the understanding of disease was modernized through the development of scientific medicine, it was simultaneously reenchanted in and through literary form.

PART 1

1

Denaturing the Emergent Martial Metaphor in Mary Shelley's *The Last Man*

In reference to the arrival of a foreign pandemic that had been sweeping across tropical and colonial regions, Lionel, the narrator-protagonist of Mary Shelley's 1826 *The Last Man*, contends that England will "fight the enemy to the last. Plague will not find [it] ready prey, as [the English] will dispute every inch of ground."[1] In an emblematic deployment of the martial metaphor, Lionel equates the incursion of a disease into a new population and region with an invasion by a foreign military coming, as the English had come so many times before the novel was written, to conquer and colonize. Opposing the weaponized threat that the disease presents, Lionel expresses confidence that the English will "blunt the arrows of pestilence" (*LM*, 214). By the end of the novel, however, it becomes clear that this kind of thinking is more than just optimistic; it is a fantasy: "Death had never wanted weapons wherewith to destroy life, and we, few and weak as we had become, were still exposed to every other shaft with which his full quiver teemed" (*LM*, 340). Despite being the first nineteenth century novel to deploy the martial metaphor in an extended narrative, *The Last Man* also pushes the metaphor to its limit. The novel not only draws attention to the fictiveness of the construction; it also challenges metaphor's efficacy and questions its ethical and epidemiological implications. In the early nineteenth century, the metaphorization of medicine as war was not quite as idiomatic as it would be by the mid-century. Its presence in Shelley's corpus signals a point of inflection at which medical discourse, informed by colonialism, militarism, biopolitics, and the tension between what we now, however questionably, call the Victorian and the Romantic, began to change the popular understanding of the relationship between disease, the individual, and the social body.

The Last Man's publication in the early nineteenth century situates it among several significant moments in military, cultural, medical, and literary history, making it particularly well-attuned to conditions that shaped the relationship among medicine, statecraft, and war. With respect to war, although at this moment in time Great Britain had never experienced a foreign invasion, militarism played a prominent role in the forging of British identity over the eighteenth century. The Napoleonic Wars encouraged Britons to define themselves collectively against a hostile Other, as they would also do against the colonial peoples their increasing military superiority would allow them to conquer. The pressures of war resulted in the need rethink the logistics of laboring manpower to support its armed forces, along with the impetus to reinvigorate the image of the ruling class as a responsible and patriotic body of leadership. These, among a number of other variables led to a larger national investment in militarism in the first decades of the nineteenth century. This cultural identity of "nationhood and belonging" in terms of "remarkable strength and resilience" developed a binary "us" versus "them" mentality.[2] Culturally primed for militance, the early 1800s would also be concomitant with the rise of the imaginative construction of the social body, defined by mortality, morbidity, and reproduction.

In this increasingly militarized culture, the question of how disease was thought to operate in the body and the population was also mutating. The movement away from the conceit of balance from humoralism during the first quarter of the nineteenth century, toward disharmonious irritation and inflammation and eventually disease agents, retained an environmental determinant. This condition influenced how foreign people and places were discursively constructed. The period also saw anxieties over inoculation and its general acceptance, in both variolation and vaccination; at the time, inoculation was the most significant intervention medicine had made to curtail infectious disease. Edward Jenner himself was touted as a military hero for his development of the smallpox vaccine in 1796,[3] using the martial metaphor in at least one instance, when he refers to smallpox as "that formidable foe to health."[4] Because inoculation was such an effective protection against smallpox, it was certainly a significant factor in the framing of medicine in bellicose terms; indeed, the discourse of vaccination plays a notable role in Shelley's novel. These events and epistemological shifts shaped the metaphor's development, but when Shelley was writing *The Last Man* cholera was especially influential to the metaphor's traction.

Writing and publishing the novel between the first (1817–1824) and second (1829–1851) cholera pandemics gave Shelley a very specific medical context for fashioning her fictional plague in the language and narrative of war. In *The Last Man*, she drew from the British military's response in India to the 1817 pandemic, and its role in propagating it. The novel attests to the use of military discourse as a cognitive resource for medicine in the first quarter of the nineteenth century, which primed the English response to the epidemics that would recur in England throughout the rest of the century. While England did escape the first global pandemic, another arrived in 1831, becoming the first English pandemic.[5] The liminal period between these outbreaks prompted contrary positions: on the one hand, the idea that something constitutional about England protected it from disease; on the other hand, that it was only a matter of time before the "Asiatic" cholera appeared there, too. Yet, both positions cultivated the martial metaphor—either England had natural defenses, or it needed to mount artificial ones. In both cases, the novel's metaphorization of disease as a foreign enemy reflected the way colonial logics and the military were mutually constitutive factors in the kind of thinking that framed cholera as a hostile invader. This framing helps us understand how therapeutic and biopolitical interventions developed out of martial thinking. Furthermore, it reveals the problematic implications of the relationship between medicine and war, such as dividing practices, xenophobia, racial alterity, and the way military action itself is a catalyst of disease, creating and expanding epidemics. With respect to racial identity, the deployment of colonial choleric discourse to characterize certain places and populations shaped the racialization of the lower classes in Britain. Places were similarly stigmatized: slums and factories were often "tropicalized." India, for instance, time and again served as an analog of the urban space.[6] Imperialism was essential to shaping Englishness by defining it not only against other countries and peoples, but against threatening elements within itself. While race becomes especially medicalized during the age of the germ, eugenics, and the New Imperialism as part 2 of this book details, the pathologization of lower classes and racialized Others was clearly operative during the early-nineteenth century. In Anne McClintock's words, "Imperialism is not something that happened elsewhere. . . . Rather, imperialism and the invention of race were fundamental aspects of Western, industrial modernity." She suggests that "the invention of race in the urban metropoles" was "central not only to the self-definition of the middle class but also the policing of the 'dangerous classes.'"[7] Unraveling the complexities surrounding early-nineteenth century cholera, Shelley defamiliarizes these processes—invention, self-definition, policing, and fighting—bringing to light their enactment through medical discourse.

The period between the pandemics was also significant for the debates over the etiology of diseases like cholera, typhus, and yellow fever—whether they were contagious or infectious via polluted air. Each position carried distinct political implications related to the governmental management of diseases affecting the population, and to the imaginative construction of Englishness. Shelley's novel indexes the way the language of war draws from the politics of both theories, and it condenses the graduated transition from pre-nineteenth-century humoral and climatological dyscrasia into miasmic and contagious antagonists.

The Last Man reflects the martial metaphor's emergence in degrees during a time of flux and contradiction. It does so in three specific ways: first, in Shelley's engagement with changes in disease theories, their biopolitical implications, and their relationships to military medicine; second, in her aesthetic and ethical critique of the martial metaphor with respect to the Romantic politics of Percy Shelley and William Godwin; and finally, in the dialectical position she takes to both challenge the martial metaphor while effectively fostering it as a shorthand for extended use in her novel. On the one hand, considering *The Last Man*'s distinct martial and medical threads raises questions about how literary form transduced the martial metaphor into the popular imagination; on the other, it reveals how reading literature in the context of that medical history unravels the naturalized, ideological function and history of the martial metaphor, illustrating the way in which it wrought the violent and nationalistic qualities of the military into medical modernity.

Shelley's text provides insight into the epidemiological effects of colonialism and its supporting military apparatus,[8] and more pressingly, how these medico-military intersections occurred through the imposition of the language of militarism into medical discourse. I demonstrate this navigation of the nebulous conceptual boundaries between contagionism and anticontagionism as they proceeded from pre-nineteenth-century medical theories. Furthermore, though Shelley's novel espouses what Fuson Wang terms "Romantic medical discourse"—an affirmative biopolitics, embracing the Other and the abnormal as well as vaccinated contamination—I show that *The Last Man* also presents an extended expression of a confrontational ethos that helped forge Victorian sanitary imperatives. Though the novel challenges the idea of medicine as war, it also reflects the metaphor's early traction and demonstrates the graduated movement from Romantic immunity and affirmative contamination to Victorian purity and defense.

This chapter begins by exploring Shelley's representation of her plague in relation to the 1817 cholera epidemic and Britain's military presence in India during its initial outbreak, priming the imaginative construction of the 1832 cholera epidemic in England. *The Last Man*'s representation of the contagion theory of disease shows how medical practitioners in the British military who were writing about cholera began thinking of disease as an enemy army. Shelley follows some contemporary commentators' accounts of the initial cholera outbreak attributing it, in contagionist terms, to the movement of British troops. This follows an account of how she links military actions, to the propagation of both the metaphor and disease itself. Shelley, moreover, shows us how the notion of imbalance in earlier medical theories morph into miasma as an inimical agent. In doing so, she indicates miasma's ties to colonialism, and calls into question the reformative imperatives of the anticontagionist movement.[9] In the final section, I examine how the aesthetics of the sublime, the feeling of awe and terror evoked by that which is incomprehensible, encourages contradictory ways of responding to disease as a hostile natural force. Shelley's deployment of the sublime denatures the confluence of medicine and war; moreover, it explodes the biopolitical calculus of human suffering, thus revealing her resistance to the belief in inherent human progress held by both her husband and father. Shelley is not completely pessimistic, however; in attributing Lionel's immunity to his encounter with the "[N]egro half clad," she presents an affirmative politics to form empathetic bonds with the Other in an effort to live *with* rather than *against* disease. While the scene itself is problematic in its instrumentalization of the Black body, within the context of the novel's representation of disease, it draws attention to the martial metaphor's costs, specifically the idea of making some live at the expense of letting Others die. Reading *The Last Man* through this critical trajectory complicates the relationship between literature, medicine, and the martial metaphor. In voicing her critique of medicine as war, Shelley provides an accessible language to expose how it can be used as narrative anodyne to the existential crises of infectious disease. At the same time, however, by consistently foregrounding the medical politics and military history of the time, her novel reveals the metaphor's entangled ideological, cultural, and material structure and components.

Cholera, Contagionism, and Military Medicine

The cholera epidemics of 1817 and 1832 were crucial to the adoption of the martial metaphor, not only because of their material links to the military but also because theorizations of the disease's causality formed an epistemological framework for understanding disease agents as enemies. *The Last Man*, published between the epidemics, reflects the debates as they relate to framing medicine as war. Although some political and literary writers expressed concern over disease "attacking" British troops,[10] it was mainly military surgeons who deployed the metaphor before the nineteenth century. What is significant about these early iterations is that they point to the grounding of the figurative martial metaphor in the material intersection of medicine and the military, one of the central claims of this book. While other tropical diseases were certainly a concern, it was cholera that mobilized colonial military medicine and prompted its sublimation into a widely adopted metaphor. Reading *The Last Man*'s military language and plot elements within the history of the 1817 cholera outbreak, military medicine, and contagionism illuminates how the novel accounts for the epidemiological consequences of military and colonial activities.

The 1817 epidemic challenged older medical concepts and provoked tensions in the imaginative construction of cholera. The disease was at once new and old. *Cholera* did not denote the *vibrio cholera* bacterium until 1882.[11] The term comes from humoral medicine and could have also referred to *choler*, or yellow bile, one of the four humors, or the Greek word *cholerda*, meaning gutter, signaling the disease's primary symptom: the forceful evacuation of fluids from the bowels. Before the nineteenth century, when Europeans spoke of cholera they were generally referring to gastroenteritis—basically, any irritation of the GI tract—with vomiting or diarrhea.[12] But as news of it spread early in the century, the "Asiatic cholera" or "blue cholera" of 1817 seemed a completely different beast from the cholera endemic to England, known as *cholera morbus*. Some medical commentators suggested that the new disease was a different one, but others thought it was simply a more potent strain of cholera due to its birth in the tropics. Even before the 1832 pandemic hit England, historians of cholera commented on the public's perception of the disease, noting that the 1817 epidemic had not initially caused much concern. The authors of a widely circulated 1831 *Lancet* article suggested that "Misled thus by the identity of a name of hurried and almost popular imposition, the cholera of India was confusedly deemed identical with the disease of that title familiar to the English practitioner; and, arguing from the rare mortality, and the evidently non-contagious nature of the latter, the public erroneously flattered themselves with the notion, that the Indian pestilence had received exaggerated attributes."[13] Moreover, they noted that much of the public felt secure "that it would doubtless remain within the cradle of its birth, and never manifest the power of extending its virulence to other climates."[14] The nature of cholera itself was fitting to the emergence of the martial metaphor. Its violent symptoms—uncontrollable fecal expulsions to the point of death by dehydration or hyponatremia—and its rapid progress—usually twenty-four to forty-eight hours from the onset of symptoms to death, but sometimes as few as eighteen—likely contributed to its characterization as an "attack." Of the most influential texts on the subject is James Jameson's *Report on the Epidemick Cholera Morbus: As It Visited the Territories Subject to the Presidency of Bengal, in the Years 1817, 1818 and 1819*, published in 1820, where he almost exclusively uses the term *attack* to refer to the onset of symptoms.[15] To consider this pathology as the central cause of cholera's influence on the martial metaphor, however, would be to oversimplify the metaphor's history and contribute to its naturalization. A number of factors beyond symptomology were involved in making the disease an antagonist under the institutional discourse of the military, such as theories regarding the nature of the ultimate and proximate cause of disease.

The three major etiological proposals in circulation in the nineteenth century theorizing the cause of diseases like cholera were contagionism, anticontagionism, and germ theory, with the dispute between contagionism and anticontagionism being the most relevant to Shelley. Contagionism posited that disease was transmitted by bodies, and metonymically made a person a disease agent. It was associated with conservative ideologies that proposed quarantines as public health measures on the model of the *cordon sanitaire*, a quarantine secured by force. Anticontagionists considered the practice outdated and illiberal, as it involved the closure of trade routes and the restriction of personal freedom. Anticontagionism's miasma theory, pointed instead to air quality and filth.

Before the 1831 epidemic, medical practitioners in England tended toward contagionism.[16] The epidemiological maps that Anglo-Indian medics developed in the 1820s and 1830s were inclined to support the contagionist model, even as the tide began turning in favor of anticontagionism in the late 1820s. Many practitioners in England were able to link the 1817 cholera epidemic to contagion, and military medical practitioners in India were much more inclined to contagionism.[17] One contagionist publication that stands out is the 1831 *Lancet* article previously mentioned, "History of the Rise, Progress, Ravages, &c. of the Blue Cholera of India," which maps the disease's progress and articulates how British military movements, alongside other displacements of populations, spread the disease. This article is a historical correlative to Shelley's reflections on how the Empire, through the military, biologically affected the parts of the world it inhabited. Although anticontagionism and contagionism are now categorized as two rival historical disease theories, it is important to realize that in many cases, the distinction between the two theories was not so clearly defined at the time.[18] Likewise, medics' beliefs in etiology during the period cannot be easily placed into that binary, which was in large part devised in response to political pressure to take a clear stand on social and economic consequences, especially regarding trade and quarantines.[19] With respect to Shelley's novel, while most critics follow Ann McWhir's contention that Shelley's draws on anticontagionism to write the miasmic character of the plague in *The Last Man*,[20] it is important to consider her use of contagionism on its own terms, because it reflects the different politics each theory imbued into the martial metaphor.

Contagionism had come to be intimately linked to military medicine through military-enforced quarantine, in which armed force was used to contain infectious bodies in defense of national boundaries or military troops. But the 1817 epidemic was an influential event in the transmutation of military medicine into the martial metaphor. Cholera became a prominent concern both of physicians in the East India Company Army and of British regulars who supported the company's rule. While the job of military physicians and surgeons was certainly to provide aid during military operations, the health of soldiers living in the barracks was their primary concern: disease casualties were the main cause of military inefficiency.[21] By killing soldiers and inhibiting troop movement, it made sense that cholera was imagined as an enemy for those working within and writing about the military.

In contagionist logics, cholera's relationship with the British military in India was not unidirectional: the military itself affected the course of the epidemic. A number of scholars and medical commentators at the time suggested that British soldiers were a primary vector in the spread of cholera across India. Alan Bewell makes this case in his extended study of the relationship between Romanticism and the global exchange of disease. He shows how literary and medical authors of this period "attempted to understand their own biomedical identities in relation to these new, more dangerous environments that colonial contact brought into being."[22] Bewell contends that the most influential context of *The Last Man* was the British military facilitating the spread of cholera in India, and how armies helped the local cholera epidemic become a global pandemic.[23] With respect to the martial metaphor, then, medicine is war not only because disease is an enemy, but also because war always includes and frequently amplifies disease. *The Last Man* draws specific attention to the way military operational support in India reconfigured the ecology—the relationships between pathogens, hosts, and their environment—of cholera.

The intersection between defense and propagation is evident in the way medical practitioners described cholera. In both military and civilian medical writings, the 1817 cholera was often referred to as if it were an army, in nominal and predicate capacities. When tracing the disease's path across India, especially through British military camps, surgeons and physicians often described it as "marching." The authors of the *Lancet* article from 1831, for instance, make numerous references to cholera's martial traverses: "We have now followed this disease in its marchings and countermarchings in every direction of the compass."[24] It leads them to conclude that the movement of contagion, rather than air, was the cause: "We associate this explanation with the indisputable fact that the rapidity of the march of cholera from place to place, is exactly augmented in the ratio of the increase in celerity of intercommunication, of places."[25] The authors follow *contingent* contagionism, a qualified contagion theory, which posited that noxious exhalations or emanations arising from the body could be transferred from person to person under the right circumstances. Specifically, they emphasize the close relationship between the movement of soldiers and the disease.[26] One effect of the martial metaphor in the rhetoric of cholera *attacking* and *marching* as a military force is that it obscures the role the military actually plays in the propagation of the disease by naturalizing the connection between medicine and war. The metaphorical march of the disease displaces the actual march of the army and its role in circulating cholera.

In most instances, the fictional plague's etiology in *The Last Man* follows miasmic understandings of disease, but many also hint at a contagionist contingency. Much like the British military's spreading of cholera, an attack on Constantinople by the novel's Byron-inspired military adventurer,[27] Lord Raymond, opens the door to the besieged and plague-ridden city, allowing disease to spread. Even before describing Raymond's campaign, however, Shelley critiques the ideology behind his desire to go to war. Through Raymond's actions and motivations, Shelley indicts Britain's exceptionalism and imperial drive for their role in amplifying the plague.

Raymond's governance of England and his colonial militarism, impulsive nature, and association with the Turkish princess Evadne are closely tied to the plague's outbreak. Raymond begins governing in place of the rightful heir, Adrian, who has abdicated. But before the major turning point in the novel, when the plague makes its appearance in Constantinople, Raymond has lost interest in governing England and decides to fight in the war of Greek independence. He boasts his Napoleonic imperial drives early in the novel: "My first act when I become King of England, will be to unite with the Greeks, take Constantinople, and subdue all Asia. I intend to be a warrior, a conqueror; Napoleon's name shall vail to mine . . . magnify[ing] my illustrious achievements" (*LM*, 44). His words allude to the significance of disease in military efforts during the Napoleonic Wars, such as the role typhus played in halting Napoleon's advance into Russia. Like Napoleon in Antoine-Jean Gros's *Napoleon Visiting the Pesthouse at Jaffa* (1804), Raymond sees the threat of plague as a "base superstition."[28] It is normal, he says, for the "plague [to] rage each year in Stamboul" (*LM*, 154), essentializing the East as an immanently pathological geography.

Raymond's Napoleonic tendencies lead to the failure of his rule in England, a comment on the side effects of colonial imperatives in the homeland. When he abdicates his role as Lord Protector to fight in Greece, he asks Lionel to join him and "witness the mighty struggle there going forward between civilization and barbarism; behold and perhaps direct the efforts of a young and various population for liberty and order" (*LM*, 121–22). Raymond's call to arms expresses not only the colonial imperative of advancing civilization against barbarism, but also the interest in deploying governance on foreign populations and acquiring land and resources. The othering of foreign bodies, characterizing them as inhabiting inferior racial positions—in this case barbarism—eventually leads to turning the same biopolitical logic inward.

Shelley associates Raymond's imperial purpose with disordered self-interest, as he shows himself to be "gallant and imperial" (*LM*, 143) when he takes command of the Greek army. But Raymond has already started losing interest in governing and improving the populace of England, taking recourse instead to parties and drink. In an incisively ironic statement that highlights Britain's own history in the slave trade, he complains that his service to society inhibits his personal desires: "Because I am Protector of England, am I to be the only slave in its empire?" (*LM*, 120). Raymond's inability to control himself, and his impulsive egoism that projects that inability outward, are analogous to the imperial conquest's origin in the failure of England's domestic politics.[29] His rhetorical question is certainly a broad critique of Britain's imperialism, and highlights the way those practices displace resources from a nation's population and can ultimately lead to internal public health consequences.

Raymond's egoism and Byronic militarism leave him the sole bearer of the Greek flag, seeking to conquer the city himself. But he is killed when the buildings collapse and a city-wide fire erupts along with a "turbid cloud" (*LM*, 159), fulfilling Evadne's prophecy of fire, war, and plague.[30] The miasmic connections between the dark cloud and pestilence are obvious; however, it is important to consider what happens after the event to understand the spread of the disease. Back in England, Adrian, Lionel, and Ryland, Raymond's successor as protector of London, hear that the plague that facilitated the Greek victory has spread.

> It seems that the total destruction of Constantinople, and the supposition that winter had purified the air of the fallen city, gave the Greeks courage to visit its site, and begin to rebuild it. But they tell us that the curse of God is on the place, for every one [sic] who has ventured within the walls has been tainted by the plague; that this disease has spread in Thrace and Macedonia; and now, fearing the virulence of infection during the coming heats, a cordon has been drawn on the frontiers of Thessaly, and a strict quarantine exacted. (*LM*, 176)

The scene follows contingent contagionism. The Greeks enter the ruined city to rebuild it as Greek territory. They had earlier discussed "in lofty terms the prosperity of Greece, when Constantinople should become its capital" (*LM*, 148). Even after they think the city is safe, everyone who enters becomes sick. It is no coincidence that the disease spreads across the Greek territories: it is carried by people who entered the city and carried the effluvia out with them. Furthermore, the Greeks do think it is contagious, which is why they enact a cordon: they don't have the knowledge at that point, as Lionel later recounts that "the plague was not what is commonly called contagious, like the scarlet fever, or extinct small-pox" (*LM*, 185). This position, however, is based on a stricter contagionism that didn't allow for the contingency of transmission by effluvia. The westward advance of the epidemic can thus be read as an invasion from the East. The narration of Raymond's siege, a military attack, an attempted colonization, and the passage of bodies in and out of the city highlight how Shelley's novel condemns the military and colonial practices that enabled the movement of the 1817 cholera.

The effluvious contingency reappears in the martial language of invasion when Lionel recounts his histrionic meeting with the "[N]egro half clad." Lionel writes how the man was ". . . writhing under the agony of disease, while he held me with a convulsive grasp. With mixed horror and impatience I strove to disengage myself, and fell on the sufferer; he wound his naked festering arms round me, his face was close to mine, and his breath, death-laden, entered my vitals" (*LM*, 268). This scene is often read both as Lionel's infection and inoculation: he takes ill soon after but does not die, and subsequently appears to be immune. The "festering" limbs and "death-laden" breath evoke the different iterations of contingent contagionism, of effluvia as arising from breath or body. But even as the disease takes the form of a miasma, as an air that "enters [his] vitals," its invasive quality bespeaks its status as a penetrative disease agent: an invasive, abject force that arises from one racialized body and enters another. While the ultimate cause is the diseased body, the proximate cause is pathogenic air. With the blurriness between contagionism and anticontagionism, and the presentation of contingent contagionism, Shelley not only reflects the transition and bridging between two disease theories but also demonstrates the way they both can draw on and reinscribe xenophobic ideologies. By the end of the novel, however, Lionel's complete embrace of racial otherness, together with his developed immunity,[31] affirms the positive possibility of embracing the Other, of engaging difference with sympathy rather than through the narrative of defense. In this scene, Shelley challenges both the contagionist politics that quarantined foreign bodies and the anticontagionist sanitary imperatives that associated poor and racialized individuals with colonial filth. Lionel's brief illness, recovery, and immunity counter the assumption that defense and purity are the best medicines. We must not, however, discount the cost of Lionel's survival. The "[N]egro half clad" is in effect a sacrificial vessel that enables both Lionel's recovery and the possible upending of readers' stereotypical, naturalized associations of racialized others with disease. Thus, even in its affirmative capacity, this scene's narrative arc follows a biopolitical logic: the immunological resolution and impetus for ideological reflection it affords the reader, which presumably can spur larger cultural change, is only made possible at the expense of a specific kind of body that has a long history of exploitation and expendability.

Along with effluvia and contingent contagionism, Shelley links miasma, in the general sense of oppressive air and unhygienic circumstances, to the material consequences of war. The primal scene in Constantinople shows how miasma, the related influence of the weather, and the conditions of battle can have a combined pathological effect. While Raymond and the Greek army hold the siege, the fire of weaponry is conflated with the noxious air and heat that produce the conditions for miasma to fester.

> Each day the soldiers of the garrison assaulted our advanced posts, and impeded the accomplishment of our works. Fireboats were launched from the various ports, while our troops sometimes recoiled from the devoted courage of men who did not seek to live, but to sell their lives dearly. These contests were aggravated by the season: they took place during summer, when the southern Asiatic wind came laden with intolerable heat, when the streams were dried up in their shallow beds. . . . In vain did the eye strive to find the wreck of some northern cloud in the stainless empyrean, which might bring hope of change and moisture to the oppressive and windless atmosphere. All was serene, burning, annihilating. We the besiegers were in the comparison little affected by these evils. . . . The sun's rays were refracted from the pavement and buildings—the stoppage of the public fountains—the bad

> quality of the food, and scarcity even of that, produced a state of suffering, which was aggravated by the scourge of disease; while the garrison arrogated every superfluity to themselves, adding by waste and riot to the necessary evils of the time. (*LM*, 151)

Hoping for an element of Britain's weather to counter the threat, the soldiers "strive to find the wreck of some northern cloud." Although the miasmic plague was already present in Constantinople, the siege concentrated and exacerbated it. The drainage problems, low quality and quantity of food, poor ventilation, and heavy work combined with the miasma from the East was aggravated by the hot weather, which in many anticontagionists' theories increased disease's virulence. While the scene frames the material relationship between battle and disease, it also signals the social construction of associating disease with the foreign. The original disease agent is traced to the "Asiatic wind" in contrast to the "northern cloud," following climatological disease theories as they figured in colonialism.

Lionel's dream of a miasmic phantom figure helps us understand how in war, even a war on disease, everybody loses. After the city collapses on Raymond's entry, Lionel has a dream that portends the coming plague through an imagining of Raymond's military campaign: "Methought I had been invited to Timon's last feast; I came with keen appetite, the covers were removed, the hot water sent up its unsatisfying steams, while I fled before the anger of the host, who assumed the form of Raymond; while to my diseased fancy, the vessels hurled by him after me, were surcharged with fetid vapour, and my friend's shape, altered by a thousand distortions, expanded into a gigantic phantom, bearing on its brow the sign of pestilence (*LM*, 161)." The threat of mutually assured infection that emerges from war's miasmic pollution resonates with iconic illustrations of cholera in 1829, at the beginning of the second pandemic before it made its way to England. Raymond's association with the figure of Pestilence alludes to an image of the grim reaper that recurs in written and visual depictions of miasma such as "King Cholera," who is often pictured hovering in an ether of pestilential air in Victorian periodical prose. The image of Raymond as a phantom is eerily similar to Robert Seymour's *Cholera Tramples the Victor & the Vanquish'd Both* (fig. 1.1), published just five years after the novel in *McLean's Monthly Sheet of Caricatures*, which depicts the disease attacking both sides of the Polish insurrection at Warsaw early in the 1831 cholera pandemic.

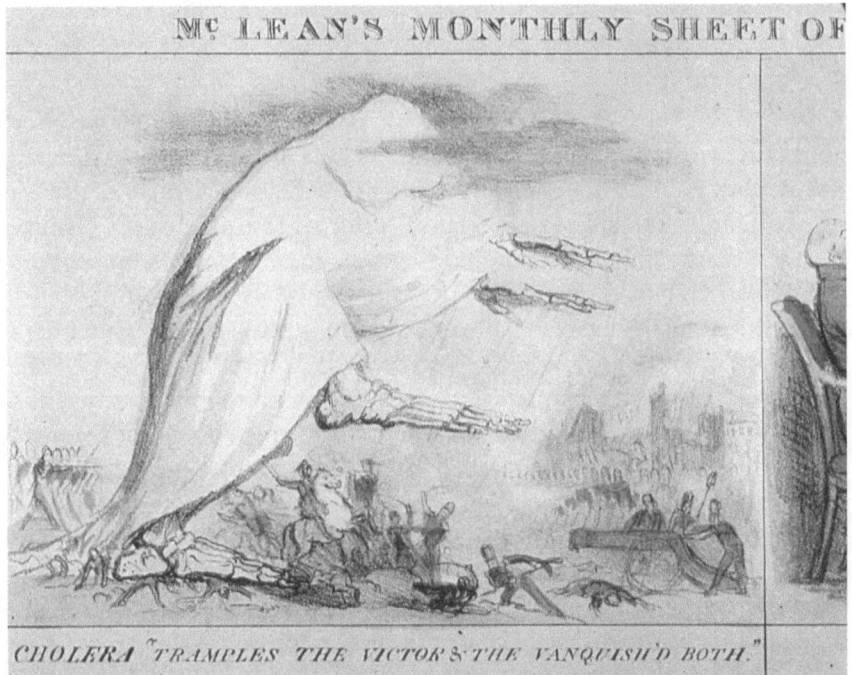

Figure 1.1. Robert Seymour, *Cholera Tramples the Victor & the Vanquish'd Both*, 1831, print. Public domain. Originally published in *McLean's Monthly Sheet of Caricatures*, London, October 1, 1831. Courtesy of the US National Library of Medicine.

The smoke from the cannons and rifles merges with the cholera as much as Raymond's siege fostered the pestilence in Constantinople. Shelley deploys almost the exact wording of Seymour's title later, when Lionel recalls the meeting between the makeshift English army and the foreign invaders, reminding the reader that "plague still hovered to equalize the conqueror and the conquered" (*LM*, 238). The resonance of the Warsaw image with the language of universal destruction falls in line with Shelley's critique of war's epidemiological effects. Shelley presents that apocalyptic connotation through the sublime. But in order to fully grasp Shelley's pestilential sublime, it is important to first clarify the associations between military discourse and miasma in terms of pre-nineteenth-century medical theories that identified environment as a determining factor for health and disease.

The Humoral and Climatological Genealogy of Miasma as Invasion

Although the physical containment of bodies by the military cordon contributed to the logic of medicine as war by giving it a material manifestation, the anticontagionist theory of miasma also came to bear on the martial metaphor's emergence. Prior to the nineteenth century, humoral theory was framed around the coextensive relationship between the human body and its milieu. After the first quarter of the nineteenth century, miasma theory tended toward positing the environmental conditions of noxious air and filth as something external that invaded the interior of the body, making it fit conceptually with the ideas of invasion and defense. Shelley's novel draws attention to this etiological gradient. Reading *The Last Man* in terms of that gradient, marks the shift from metaphors of balance to metaphors of contest, of war; it unveils the humoral and climatological residues of the racial alterity imbricated in anticontagionism. This reading also highlights the political and economic effects of war and its figuration in medicine, revealing contradictions in England's identity with respect to the rest of the world.

The novel's representation of disease as foreign reveals the internal regulatory biopolitics imbricated in anticontagionism. In most iterations of the theory, the pathogenicity of air was a result of filth and thus linked to poverty. This belief led the sanitary movement to make the specifically urban environments and the lives and routines of the people who lived there its primary target, in an effort to sanitize the poor through hygienic measures and government intervention. For anticontagionists, the idea of filth and airborne infection compelled not just an inquiry into how disease might spread or be contained, it also posed the question as to the extent of the obligation disease imposed on society to care for its more precarious members.[32] In reference to the obligation of care, Melville addresses the way hospitality operates in *The Last Man*, especially for foreigners seeking refuge from the plague in England, which becomes a hospital in both the medical and relational domestic senses of the word.[33] Ryland, who ultimately renounces his own responsibilities as Lord Protector out of fear of the plague, explicitly refuses to "hospitaliz[e]" England, asserting, "I neither pretend to protect nor govern an hospital—such will England quickly become" (*LM*, 194–95). Adrian stands in contrast to this isolationist policy when he challenges Ryland's renunciation of his duties, invoking the martial metaphor when he becomes Lord Protector: "It is not by flying, but by facing the enemy, that we can conquer. If my last combat is now about to be fought, and I am to be worsted—so let it be!" (*LM*, 195). Whether to welcome the diseased citizens of that "other nation" within England is a question of how the concepts of *hospital* and *hospitality* operate within the politics of anticontagionism. While this reformative impulse of hospitality seems distant from militarism, over the course of the novel the image of England as hospital becomes tainted with war and violence.

Part of what made miasma comprehensible as an enemy was the difficulty of containing it. Lionel himself suggests that the disease's "chief force" was "derived from the pernicious qualities of the air" (*LM*, 196). However, one conceptual difference between miasma and contagious bodies is the possibility of containment. Lionel puts it this way: "If infection depended upon the air, the air was subject to infection. As for instance, a typhus fever has been brought by ships to one sea-port town; yet the very people who brought it there, were incapable of communicating it in a town more fortunately situated. But how are we to judge of airs, and pronounce—in such a city plague will die unproductive; in such another, nature has provided for it a plentiful harvest" (*LM*, 185). A state can cordon contagious bodies, but how can force and structure contend with a noxious atmosphere? Anticontagionism allowed for two solutions. The first addressed living conditions such as overcrowding, hygiene, drainage, and ventilation. In the novel, once the plague begins spreading across the world, and expatriates and foreigners flood into England, Lionel hints at epidemiological concerns about population density. He refers to London as an "overgrown metropolis" (*LM*, 196). Lionel's concerns can only be alleviated if "the cleanliness, habits of order, and manner in which our cities are built, [are] all in our favor" (*LM*, 196). This follows Percy Shelley's belief that disease was a result of social disorder, one that could be remedied by political reform.[34] The same thinking appears in Kingsley's work, as discussed in the following chapter, where he expresses his sanitarian agenda for social ordering through the language of war against both cholera and Russians in Crimea. In *The Last Man*, England attempts to fight the disease with biopolitical governance, evident when Lionel asserts that "Perhaps in no part of the world has [disease] met with so systematic and determined opposition" (*LM*, 196). He then rallies anxious Londoners by appealing to both masculinity and militarism, calling for the deployment of those metaphorical barriers against miasma: "If manly courage and resistance can save us, we will be saved" (*LM*, 196). In doing so, he charges the anxious crowd to have faith in, and actualize, those particular qualities of English identity. Raymond's actions contradict that plan, as it is precisely his militaristic drive that fosters the spread of the plague. While we might be quick to condemn Raymond's militaristic drive as exacerbating matters, the scene's call to arms also gestures toward Lionel's more affirmative political, anticontagionist reforms. In an echo of the quotation that opened this chapter, Lionel draws on the martial metaphor still more explicitly: "We will fight the enemy to the last. Plague shall not find us a ready prey; we will dispute every inch of ground; and by methodical and inflexible laws, pile invincible barriers to the progress of our foe" (*LM*, 196). The methodological and inflexible laws to which he refers are sanitary principles based on the science of nature, principles, and barriers that public policy and individuals can materialize into defensive action. Yet, insofar as the martial metaphor in Lionel's speech associates his rhetoric with Raymond's material exacerbation of disease, Shelley calls into question this martial framing.

More informs Lionel's speech than confidence in intercession by the state and cooperation amongst individuals, which marks the second, and equally problematic, solution that anticontagionism offers for the plague: the assumption that England is an essentially healthy territory. He contends that "perhaps no country is naturally so well protected against our invader," suggesting that England can rely on the geography provided by nature: the best defense is to live in the most "naturally" salubrious territory, England itself. Lionel adds that nature has not "anywhere been so well assisted by the hand of man" (*LM*, 196). England is naturally hygienic, but it still needs the civilizing work of the English social order to make it livable. As Adrian puts it, "The labour of hundreds of thousands alone could make this inclement nook fit habitation for one man" (*LM*, 258). As the novel progresses, Shelley dismantles the ideology that naturalized the struggle with epidemic disease in colonial societies yet credited European societies with resistance to it.[35] This framing, posited by Adrian but debunked by the plague over the course of the narrative, emerges from the vestiges of humoralism in anticontagionism as they are folded into the logic of war.

Persisting until the mid-nineteenth century, humoral medicine had an essential environmental component. The humoral medical discourse on "the tropics" was thus climatological insofar as weather and temperature affected European bodies depending on their constitution.[36] The climatological and geospatial conceptualization of humoralism, which Mary Floyd-Wilson terms "geohumoralism," was popular for much of the early modern period.[37] Bodies were prone to different disease states depending on race, diet, and other factors, a point Shelley alludes to when Lionel asserts that "bodies are sometimes in a state to reject the infection of malady, and at others, thirsty to enbibe it" (*LM*, 185). A person's humoral balance could be thrown off by a region's temperature, and certain people were prone to particular imbalances that made them incompatible with certain locales. As previously discussed, there was some epistemic movement toward the idea of the external invading the internal in geohumoral discourse, but that belief did not quite reach the threshold of the inimical framing that appears in nineteenth-century contagionist and anticontagionist theories. By the late eighteenth and early nineteenth century, medical topography began to supplant geohumoral theories per se, as it developed concordantly with British consolidation of colonial rule in India.[38] In contrast to the analog quality of imbalance, the whole-person in situ of humoral theory, nineteenth century miasma and contagion theories were tending more toward binary logic of invasion or repellence. During the nineteenth century, the human organism begins to imagine itself as distinct, separate, and even oppositional from the environment. The climatological-environmental dimensions of medical topography and miasmatic disease theories became more conducive to the martial metaphor for two reasons. First, in terms of conceptual constructions, miasma was becoming framed more as disease object external to the body and consequently often described as a kind of invading force, with either the weather of a foreign land invading the colonizer or the pestilent wind of the East traveling to invade England. Second, in material terms, these changing environmental understandings of disease were shaped by British military and colonial efforts, beginning in the early nineteenth century.

Shelley's novel pivots around this graduated enjoinment of medicine and militarism, in her various descriptions of setting, characters, and of the plague as an antagonistic, climatic force of nature. In doing so, she draws attention to the significance of environment as it framed the biomedical identities and boundaries of the modern world. In Bewell's words, the "'Tropics' shifted from being a climatic term to a being a social, biological, and medical construction."[39] In *The Last Man*, Lionel's description of miasma follows this logic in an Orientalist idiom. Alluding to Percy Shelley's "Ode to the West Wind" (1820), Lionel apostrophizes,

"Then mighty art thou, O wind, to be throned above all other vicegerents of nature's power; whether thou comest destroying from the east, or pregnant with elementary life from the west" (*LM*, 183). In the vein of colonialist-informed debates about disease, the pathogenic wind comes from the East, much like the Asiatic cholera in Shelley's time. This is in contrast to the West wind, which is characterized in both fecund and virile terms, a figuration Stoker later mutates to describe Dracula's microbial infection of the air as a pathogenic embryo. In Shelley's novel, miasmic wind is a function of the weather, notably adopting environmental figures of the sublime, such as the snow and the ocean. This disparity between East and West figures prominently in the isolationism Lionel projects in the early part of the novel.

The Last Man presents and then undercuts an ideological construction of England as a naturally healthy country and people; however, even the latter belief could further catalyze the martial metaphor by requiring synthetic defenses. The isolationism at work in the British response to the 1817 epidemic is present through the first half of *The Last Man*. For instance, in the earliest reactions to rumors of the plague's invasion of Athens, isolation, order, and salubrity are used to frame the "natural" condition of England. Operating under what Emily Lyon's calls a "pastoral illusion," Lionel says, "We, in our cloudy isle, were far removed from danger" (*LM*, 179).[40] Though England requires social order to make its state of nature habitable, its location and weather make it pathostatic, not conducive to the production of disease. Lionel's reference to "cloudiness" thus does not connote miasma; instead, the romantic fantasy of England's natural superiority to the forces of nature is justified by height in a metaphor of relative positionality. The arrogance underlying that position speaks to the role of climate, environment, and constitution in the essentializing of place, people, and culture. Recall the speech Lionel gives to quell the anxious citizens, in which England's "cleanliness, habits of order, and the manner in which [its] cities were built" will provide protection (*LM*, 196). The figure of England as a cloudy isle immune to colonial and Asiatic disease is based on a number of traits of superiority the English possess, in their understanding: not only the country's status as an island and its cold climate, but an assumed naturally civilized, hygienic social order. To this effect, England's salubrity is differential, its immanent vitality contingent on the naturally pathogenic construction of the East.

England's separation from the East by other countries and its adamantine wall of water gives it additional protection, contributing to the naturalization of defense from foreign disease: "England was still secure. France, Germany, Italy, Spain, were interposed, walls without a breach" (LM, 185). Showing some humility before the sublimity of nature, Lionel redoubles on the sentiment of security, suggesting that others' vessels, both nautical and bodily, "truly were the sport of the wind and waves, even as Gulliver was the toy of the Brobdignagians, but we on our stable abode could not be hurt in life or limb by these eruptions of nature. We could not fear—we did not. Yet a feeling of awe, a breathless sentiment of wonder, a painful sense of the degradation of humanity was introduced into every heart" (LM, 185). Upon reflection of the plague after it wipes out humankind, Lionel revisits the sublimity of disease with more deference when he addresses Shelley's notion that, contrary to Godwin's espousal of progress and the ultimate perfection of humankind,[41] the fight against disease is ultimately futile. Deploying the martial metaphor through the language of boundaries and quarantine, he rallies the English spirit which he assumes will immanently overcome any barrier to liberal prosperity: "The English spirit awoke to its full activity, and, as it had ever done, set itself to resist the evil, and to stand in the breach which diseased nature had suffered chaos and death to make in the bounds and banks which had hitherto kept them out" (LM, 187–88). The ethos of Englishness stands to fill the breach in the hermetic, insular identity of the isles. In doing so this identity draws conceptual boundaries and defenses against biopolitical disorder, figured here as the foreign Other.

The military language used to describe England's climatological resiliency to the plague often figures disease as weaponry, suggesting that disease may be stopped by human intervention; however, it is later revealed that only nature itself can provide a sufficient shield. As the narrative progresses, England's environment turns out not to be strong enough. After the plague breaches the cloudy isle, England's climatological advantage stymies the progress of the miasmic apocalypse. Winter is thought to be a "never-failing physician" (LM, 190) on both climatological and miasmic grounds: "Winter was coming, and with winter, hope. In August, the plague had appeared in the country of England, and during September it made its ravages. Towards the end of October, it dwindled away, and was in some degree replaced by a typhus, of hardly less virulence" (LM, 214).[42] Lionel expresses hope that the English frost "would blunt the arrows of pestilence, and enchain the furious elements; and the land would in spring throw off her garment of snow, released from her menace of destruction" (*LM*, 214). But though the disease recedes during the winter, it returns with the warmer months: "Summer advanced, and, crowned with the sun's potent rays, plague shot her unnerving shafts toward the earth" (*LM*, 220).

The isolationism that holds England to be naturally pathostatic as it appears in *The Last Man* is analogous to a popular belief about the 1817 cholera epidemic. When Asiatic cholera was discovered to be different from the English *cholera morbus*, many people concluded that it could not survive in the English climate.[43] Lionel represents that attitude when he recalls trying to convince himself that the plague was only endemic to colonial spaces.

> The vast cities of America, the fertile plains of Hindostan, the crowded abodes of the Chinese, are menaced with utter ruin. . . . Countrymen, fear not! In the still uncultivated wilds of America, what wonder that among its other giant destroyers, Plague should be numbered! It is of old a native of the East, sister of the tornado, the earthquake, and the simoon. Child of the sun, and nursling of the tropics, it would expire in these climes. It drinks the dark blood of the inhabitant of the south, but it never feasts on the pale-faced Celt. If perchance some stricken Asiatic come among us, plague dies with him, uncommunicated and innoxious. Let us weep for our brethren, though we can never experience their reverse. (*LM*, 186–87)

Lionel's description of the plague as an "old native of the east" and a "nursling of the tropics," like his linking of it to the uncultivated America, not only follows the belief that Indian cholera was different from English cholera, but also deploys the rhetoric of time and history to contrast it with advanced European civilization. Moreover, Lionel draws on both climatological and contagionist logic to ameliorate concerns of the disease spreading to England. In a notable pre-germ theory agentification and vitalization of disease, he contends that the disease will "expire" in England's climate and addresses the possibility of contagion by predicting its death within the "stricken Asiatic." Using anthimeria, the rhetorical conversion of one part of speech to another, he metonymically associates the hypothetical invading foreigner with the parts of the world where the disease was thought to naturally occur. In addition to etiology, Lionel's speech stresses the entanglements among empire, economics, and disease.

The Last Man contests England's natural isolation with the economic consequences of plague, a concern that reflects anticontagionist anxieties relating to quarantine, the main weapon in the contagionist armamentarium. Shelley reflects those concerns in the novel while linking them to broader notions of national identity related to the martial metaphor and the pre-nineteenth-century roots of anticontagionism. Following the models of Boccaccio's *Decameron* (1353), Defoe's *Journal of a Plague Year* (1722), and other plague narratives in which epidemics unravel the social fabric, Lionel describes the economic harm that England suffers even before the disease biologically touches the English. The plague has halted international trade "by the failure of the interchange of cargoes as usual between us, and America, India, Egypt and Greece" (*LM*, 186). Compounding the wide-ranging effects of the plague is the wave of immigrants fleeing it. Foreigners arrive penniless and cannot be supported by state relief, in line with concerns similar to Chadwick's argument about the relief of the poor before the 1834 Poor Law, the legislation that created the workhouse system to replace outdoor relief for poverty. Lionel comments that many of the new arrivals "were utterly destitute; and their increasing numbers forbade a recourse to the usual modes of relief" (*LM*, 186). The economic distresses "were occasioned by the fictitious reciprocity of commerce, increased in due proportion. Bankers, merchants, and manufacturers, whose trade depended on exports and interchange of wealth, became bankrupt" (*LM*, 187). The ultimate effect is that

> the prosperity of the nation was now shaken by frequent and extensive losses. Families, bred in opulence and luxury, were reduced to beggary. The very state of peace in which we gloried was injurious; there were no means of employing the idle, or of sending any overplus of population out of the country. Even the source of colonies was dried up, for in New Holland, Van Diemen's Land, and the Cape of Good Hope, plague raged. O, for some medicinal vial to purge unwholesome nature, and bring back the earth to its accustomed health! (*LM*, 187)

In Shelley's representation of the plague's portents before its actual arrival, she articulates the political and economic investments in the debate over cholera's contagious nature. *Health,* in this passage, signals proper, colonial economics, controlled immigration into the homeland, and consistent income from the colonies. The framing of England's dependence on Eastern and colonial lands does not present those lands in a strictly positive light. Although Lionel challenges Ryland's isolationist position, which equates the plague with foreign fruit,[44] and wants to "lament over and assist the children of the garden of the earth" (*LM,* 187), in his own description of the economic losses, Lionel highlights the danger of colonial contact by alluding to the popular association of disease with the colonies. Just before he reports of the colonies "being dried up," he writes that "[of] late we envied their abodes, their spicy groves, fertile plains, and abundant loveliness. But in this mortal life extremes are always matched; the thorn grows with the rose, the poison tree and the cinnamon mingle their boughs" (*LM,* 187). The chimeric entanglement of the poison and cinnamon trees figuratively frames colonial contact as a doubled-edge sword: profitable and luxurious, yet dangerous and pathogenic. This contradiction between openness to trade and fear of poisonous contact suggests that despite Lionel's progressive politics, he retains conservative anxieties over tropical disease.

In keeping with the challenge to England's social, rather than economic, isolationism, Shelley invokes the martial metaphor when affixing the disease's arrival with the arrival of foreigners. While the construction of the foreigner as an enemy threat resembles the previous linkage between medicine and the military, insofar as *The Last Man*'s plague alludes to the British military's encounters with cholera, it goes a step further in the abstraction of the martial metaphor. Shelley's following of the anticontagionist paradigm does not so much suggest that foreigners brought the disease with them, a sentiment held both in the Victorian period as much as our own moment. Instead, the passage reveals the fallacy of assumed English superiority as constructed through medical discourse.[45] Critics often understand the movement of foreign bodies into English territory through images of invasion and anxieties about reverse colonization,[46] a discourse that appears later in the century in Stoker and Conan Doyle's writings. Yet in Shelley's novel, the disease is already present in England prior to when foreigners incite social unrest. In this ordering of emplotment, Shelley stresses that England's socioeconomic health is contingent on hierarchical colonial relations. Without them, the English have no constitutional defense against disease. Their presumed superiority is based on the social determinants of colonialism. Once the families that had been "bred in opulence and luxury" were "reduced to beggary," Lionel laments, the previous peace and "accustomed health" of England was naught.

The manifest conflict between classes creates an opportunistic climate for the burden and social disorder brought by foreigners, especially when the immigrants prove to be militant. Lionel recounts Americans pillaging and quartering themselves in Irish homes after sailing east to avoid the plague. This disruption leads some of the Irish to join the Americans and embark for England: "[The American] incursion would hardly have been felt had they come alone, but the Irish collected in unnatural numbers, began to feel the inroads of famine, and they followed in the wake of the Americans for England." The Irish and American incursions "struck the English with affright . . . [the invaders'] lawless spirit instigated them to violence" (LM, 219). In blending the English lower classes with the foreigners, Lionel writes that they "swept the country like a conquering army, burning—laying waste—murdering. The lower and vagabond English joined with them" (LM, 237). The relation of national and class difference in this characterization is indicative of how the martial metaphor becomes deployed internally as a way to regulate potentially threatening members of the population. In response to alliance between the foreigners and the lower classes, "some few of the Lords Lieutenant who remained, endeavored to collect the militia—but the ranks were vacant, panic seized on all, and the opposition that was made only served to increase the audacity and cruelty of the enemy. They talked of taking London, conquering England—calling to mind the long detail of injuries which had for many years been forgotten" (LM, 237). This reconciliation of the foreign with the domestic Other certainly reflects not only the fears of Foreign incursion by the French during the Napoleonic Wars; it also follows the anxiety of the very possibility of that the lower classes could catch the revolutionary fever that swept France and the United States decades earlier. By raising this narrative confluence in the context of disease, *The Last Man* undercuts the martial logics of external and internal defense deployed under medical auspices, capitalizing on British anxieties of revolution and colonial vengeance.

The plague not only reverses the social order in England, it reconfigures the imperial order that had been secured by the material, economic, and ideological support of England's superiority. Read in the context of the plague and its colonial origins, that revolution challenges the military discourse underwriting England's imperial power, which could seemingly establish connections for profit while remaining impervious to colonial exposure. The reversal of the imperial order also leads to military encounters, which have two potential consequences: the amplification of military defense and the inimical construction of foreigners, who do not carry disease per se but take advantage of its destabilizing effects; or, a change to exceptionalism by embracing the Other in the face of shared vulnerability to disease.

Shelley creates a scenario with both options, where Lionel and Adrian attempt to foster an embracement of the Other—notably, however, with the threat of military force—only to have national difference and colonial desires of conquest reemerge. The foreign invasion of England is ultimately quelled by Adrian's oratorical prowess, supported by his aggressive display of force. In a reversal of earlier events, Shelley's catalog of the invasion of England also follows a pattern similar to the chapter in which Raymond seizes Constantinople. Artillery and arms are collected, troops led, banners carried, and as in the Warsaw cholera illustration and the siege of Constantinople, smoke from the cannons "filled up the horror of the scene" (*LM*, 240). Adrian aggressively raises his sword and orders the invaders to surrender: "We shall conquer, for the right is on our side; already your cheeks are pale—the weapons fall from your nerveless grasp. Lay down your arms, fellow men! brethren! Pardon, succor, and brotherly love await your repentance. You are dear to us, because you wear the frail shape of humanity; each one among you will find a friend and host among these forces. Shall man be the enemy of man, while plague, the foe to all, even now is above us, triumphing in our butchery, more cruel than her own?" (*LM*, 240). The ultimate sign of alliance is a single, fallen soldier whom Adrian approaches as he laments: "It was if the fate of the whole world seemed bound up in the death of this single man" (*LM*, 241). This is a crucial point, for it signals Shelley's rejection of the statistical calculus of life that is inherent in both Malthusian prediction and biopolitical governance. The armies proceed to join "hand-in-hand" and "assist each other." In the scene, the English are reminded of their "community in death" with the foreign, which can "inspire both fear and sympathy,"[47] and that the plague as "the enemy of man" can unite all people under the auspices of a vital precarity, "the frail shape of humanity." England is eventually deserted by the remaining human population, a mix of Americans and Western Europeans. The peace secured by Adrian, however—like the realization that the Greeks were fighting the plague and not the Turks—does not put an end to the military conflicts that arise from the shattered social order in the wake of the plague. Later in the novel, the English emigrate and colonize Paris in two waves (*LM*, 299). The waves become two rival factions led by a fanatical religious zealot, who "enlists under his banner" men from "the lower ranks of society" and "panic struck . . . high-borne females" (*LM*, 308). After attempts to form peace and integrate with the rival factions, the group of English and French who aligned themselves with Adrian and Lionel, their "muster[ed] company" (*LM*, 316), flee France for Switzerland. This reemergence of political, religious, and social divisiveness, even in the face of the shared frail shape of humanity, challenges the utopian hope that the fight against disease has a necessarily unifying effect and that under its aegis the martial metaphor will "make [all] live." This presumed pessimism notwithstanding, Shelley's figuration of disease as a sublime force provides the possibility of affirmative inclusion, but at the same time can also lead to the divisive and exclusionary logics of the martial metaphor, revealing its dialectical work in *The Last Man*.

On the Nature of the Pestilential Sublime and Shipwrecked Humanity

Shelley's association of disease with the sublime forces of nature makes it tempting to read *The Last Man* as a pessimistic outlook in contrast to other Romantics' utopian optimisms. If disease is a figure of awe and terror—like a deity or pantheistic nature that is incalculable and inconceivable in magnitude—can the subject or the state respond martially with any efficacy at all? In the novel, the miasmic cloud, shapeless, unquantifiable, and threatening, a product of nature exacerbated all the same by human social conditions, is a figure of the sublime.[48] On first reading, the presentation of the disease as a sublime force of nature seems to oppose the martial metaphor. When disease is equated with natural forces and oceanic storms, there is little purpose in fighting it; one can endure a storm, but not fight it, much as one cannot do anything but endure a disease that one sees as a punishment from God. As Edmund Burke suggests, however, the sublime can also trigger a bellicose response by inciting the instinct of self-preservation. In a Kantian understanding, the sublime makes subjects feel limitless in their ability to grasp and overcome nature.[49] Yet, the relationship between the sublime and the martial metaphor, much like that between the novel and disease, is far from straightforward. Perhaps the best for which the afflicted can hope for is to navigate the turbulence of the plague with an ethical action that does not conflate the one with the many or the foreign with the diseased. In Shelley's *Last Man*, the sublime force of the sea functions as a topos to explain her blending of disease theories, her rejection of her husband's and her father's faith in Romantic, utopian progress, and her understanding of the martial metaphor's danger and futility. Ultimately, the novel's repeated use of the sublime and the martial metaphor inflects the apocalyptic in a way that prevents the plague from being used to make concordant patterns out of the natural history of disease, which by means of provisioning an ending, produce "satisfying consonance between the origin and the middle."[50] The sublime spotlights how the narrative of war functions to make sense of the precarity of human life and its proleptic demise in problematic ways. At the same time, it dissolves the boundary between the real and the fictional, attesting to how despite being a fiction, the martial metaphor has material consequences in the biopolitical ordering of the social.

Disease is sublime insofar as it invokes terror and awe at its immeasurability as a force of nature; it is difficult to conceptualize in scale, particularly in, as the idiom goes, "epidemic proportions." For Burke, the sublime is "whatever is fitted in any sort to excite the ideas of pain and danger. . . . Whatever is in any sort terrible, or is conversant about terrible objects, or operates in a manner analogous to terror is a source of the sublime."[51] The sublime is experienced when one encounters something dangerous that triggers a fear of pain, particularly natural objects that seem vast and infinite; a kind of terror is evoked by the inability to fully comprehend the object. This feeling precipitates bodily reactions in turn, as Vanessa Ryan has suggested in terms of Burke's "physiological sublime."[52] This phenomenological grounding in the body provides a basis to see how the sublime mediates medicine and disease. Burke discusses material changes in the nervous system, and describes the sublime as evoking delight, "the sensation which accompanies the removal of pain or danger."[53] He also gives the example of health: "When we recover our health, when we escape imminent danger, [it is] with a sense of joy we are affected." This, we are told, is why looking over a precipice is a sublime experience. It also means that the object cannot be too near or presenting too immediate a threat, because "When danger or pain press too nearly, they are incapable of giving delight."[54] The body experiences terror of certain circumstances "without being in such circumstances."

In *The Last Man*, the sublimity of the plague is overdetermined: how it is able to travel across continents; the way it inspires pain and danger; the way it threatens life; the difficulty of delimiting it conceptually; and the impossibility of controlling it. This incompressible scale of disease with respect to cholera was not lost on British commentators when the disease hit industrialized England in the decades following the novel.[55] Erin O'Conner characterizes one author's 1848 description of the massive landscape of night soil, manure, and topsoil as a "sublime wasteland."[56] Similarly, as Canadian health commissioner Richard Nelson so poetically renders in his 1866 history of the early nineteenth century cholera pandemics, the disease is simply "stupendous": "stupendous in its widespread malignancy over ever content; stupendous from the missions of victims it has swallowed; stupendous from the rapidity of its spread; stupendous from the few brief moments of life it allows to those it attacks." Authors like Nelson, among so many others throughout the nineteenth century, figuratively, explicitly, or implicitly inosculate cholera, colonialization, and industrialization, as a kind of master trope for modernity.[57]

The aesthetic use of the sublime in the above example to articulate disease helps us understand the martial metaphor as an expression of the social reconfiguration of the environment. The plague's connection with war, as described during Raymond's siege on Constantinople, is another. A number of phenomena other than natural forces fall under the rubric of the sublime, such as technology or, relatedly, war.[58] Referring to Benjamin West's painting *Death on the Pale Horse* (1803),[59] Lionel recounts the sublimity of the encounter with death through the narrative frame of war.

> I have heard a picture described, wherein all the inhabitants of earth were drawn out in fear to stand the encounter of Death. The feeble and decrepit fled; the warriors retreated, though they threatened even in flight. Wolves and lions, and various monsters of the desert roared against him; while the grim Unreality hovered shaking his spectral dart, a solitary but invincible assailant. Even so was it with the army of Greece. I am convinced, that had the myriad troops of Asia come from over the Propontis, and stood defenders of the Golden City, each and every Greek would have marched against the overwhelming numbers, and have devoted himself with patriotic fury for his country. But here no hedge of bayonets opposed itself, no death-dealing artillery, no formidable array of brave

soldiers—the unguarded walls afforded easy entrance—the vacant palaces luxurious dwellings; but above the dome of St. Sophia the superstitious Greek saw Pestilence, and shrunk in trepidation from her influence. (LM, 152–53)

Lionel describes the aftermath of war like that portrayed in Benjamin West's, *Death on the Pale Horse*, with the conditions prime for disease. The painting (fig. 1.2) depicts the Four Horsemen of the Apocalypse—Death, War, Famine, and Pestilence—in a scene where humans stand against Death who assaults them in the midst of fighting warriors, tangled and pestilence-ridden bodies, smoke, and dark clouds.

The painting's composition resonates with the image of miasmic cholera qua Death in the Seymour illustration discussed earlier in this chapter. It is also consistent with Evadne's dying curse on Raymond: "Fire, and war, and plague, unite for thy destruction" (LM, 145). In all of these examples, the technologies of war and the forces of nature unite materially to the detriment of both the victors and the vanquished. The specific allusion to West's painting invokes what Morton Paley has called "the apocalyptic sublime": the apocalyptic renderings and scenes composed with a distinctly sublime aesthetic in late-Romantic art of painters like West, John Martin, and J. M. W. Turner.[60] War, sublime in its vastness, can scale to a degree that is incomprehensible and evokes terror as a human-made analog of the destructive forces of nature. West's

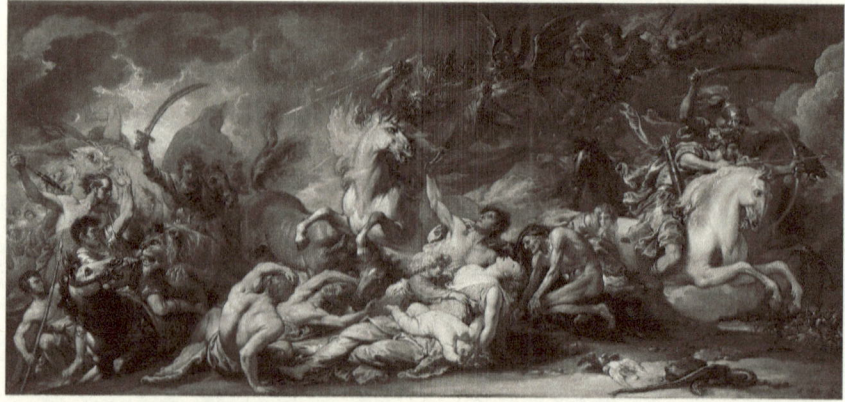

Figure 1.2. Benjamin West, *Death on the Pale Horse*, 1796, oil on canvas. Courtesy of the Detroit Institute of Arts, Founders Society Purchase, Robert H. Tannahill Foundation Fund, 79.33.

iteration of the sublime links Biblical figurations of divine revelation and judgment (along with the plague it rings in) with war to produce a thrill and a terror, a sense that effervesced out of the period of the French Revolution, the Napoleonic Wars, and the agitation for reform.[61] Reversing the direction of the martial metaphor, Mary Shelley also famously characterizes war as a disease with respect to those two wars in her travel narrative through Europe in 1817 with Percy: "The distress of the inhabitants, whose houses had been burned, their cattle killed, and all their wealth destroyed, has given a sting to my detestation of war, which none can feel who have not travelled through a country pillaged and wasted by this plague, which, in his pride, man inflicts upon his fellow."[62] Thus, even if disease is a sublime natural force, it is one exacerbated by human social and political failures. Her invocation of the sublime, especially in its connection to militarism, informs the way Shelley manifests war as an amplifier of disease; it evokes the historical context of the British military encounter with cholera, where war produced ecological changes to humankind's relationship to nature.

The most prominent way Shelley formulates the plague as sublime is through her figuration of the sea. The ocean, and, in particular, the oceanic storm, may be the most emblematic instance of the sublime, as Burke and other contemporary critics suggest.[63] The connections between the plague and the sublimity of storms at sea are congruent with climatological and miasmic disease theories by virtue of forces like the wind and barometric pressure, which affects temperature and other factors of nineteenth century understanding of epidemiology. Following Shelley's association of the plague as a force of nature with the sublime manifestations of the sea, humankind and its social structures are figured as a ship. With Lionel's repeated references to England as the center of humankind and its progress before the plague, the novel opens with a naval figuration which follows that imaginative construction: "England, seated far north in the turbid sea, now visits my dreams as a well-manned ship, which mastered the winds and rode proudly over the waves . . . the earth's very centre was fixed for me on that spot, and the rest of her orb was a fable" (*LM*, 5). Lionel is writing after the plague has left him as the last man, and he now dreams only of what was. Toward the end of the novel, there is a point at which the idea of English mastery has changed. Lionel gazes on a sea storm, an analog of the plague that works coextensively with it, and, as he recalls, "A sublime sense of awe calmed the swift pulsations of my heart—I awaited the approach of the destruction menaced, with that solemn resignation which an unavoidable necessity instils" (LM, 270). The image of naval mastery signals the presumed superiority of the Royal Navy and, more broadly, England's ability to subdue nature. Shelley goes on to suggest this itself is the fable.

This depiction of nature is paradoxical, undercutting the picture of English superiority that Lionel and Adrian first present, because nature is Janus-faced. In the time before the plague, nature is at once a force to be reckoned with—"the turbid sea"—and one that is ultimately divertible for societal ends—"master[ing] the winds." At the same time, nature in its threatening aspect provides England with a socially valuable "natural" defense against military and biological threats. Hinting at the fable even before the plague makes its way to England, Lionel writes,

> We wept over the ruin of the boundless continents of the east, and the desolation of the western world; while we fancied that the little channel between our island and the rest of the earth was to preserve us alive among the dead. It were no mighty leap methinks from Calais to Dover . . . Yet this small interval was to save us: the sea was to rise a wall of adamant—without, disease and misery—within, a shelter from evil, a nook of the garden of paradise—a particle of celestial soil, which no evil could invade . . . (LM, 183)

The sea takes on an almost mythical strength to protect England from external threats. Once the plague begins to spread, however, references to it gain inimical and apocalyptic connotations. Evoking the humoral logic of balance, the weather turns for the worst: "SOME [sic] disorder had surely crept into the course of the elements, destroying their benignant influence. The wind, prince of air, raged through his kingdom, lashing the sea into fury," writes Lionel. He continues:

> The God sends down his angry plagues from high,
> Famine and pestilence in heaps they die.
> Again in vengeance of his wrath he falls
> On their great hosts, and breaks their tottering walls;
> Arrests their navies on the ocean's plain,
> And whelms their strength with mountains of the main.
>   (LM, 183)

Shelley distills how war operates as a figure of the apocalyptic sublime in her representation of the plague as an arrow fired by a god. Here we see a shift away from Christian revelation to pantheistic nature as the sublime force of the apocalyptic. In conflation of nature, disease, weather, and divine punishment, Shelley describes the combined effects of disease on military forces: the plague "arrests" humankind's naval forces much like a storm. This construction helps her construe nature as an antagonist, as if humankind were fighting against naval forces, to poise her critique against that very figuration. More consistently with the narrative logic of the novel, it reminds readers that fighting against nature, like fighting against an angry deity, is futile.

That futility, however, does not preclude a "politics of possibility."[64] In Shelley's understanding, engaging the slings and arrows of the pestilential sublime could be less a martial act than a means of uniting a population toward a common end, which need not be militaristic—it could be a way of seeking to "make live" without the condition of "letting die." The problem arises when regulatory biopolitics, which takes a statistical view of the population, dilutes the single life into the background of the many. In the wake of the plague, Lionel invokes that affirmative principle, resisting the thanatopolitical inherent in regulatory biopolitics, and holding life above territory and imperial power in a manner that does not follow Foucault's biopolitical model or its historical iterations.[65] Alluding to the statistical technologies deployed in biopolitical regulation and the Malthusian limiting factor of food, Lionel laments, "The hunger of Death was now stung more sharply by the diminution of his food: or was it that before, the survivors being many, the dead were less eagerly counted." Instead, with the new diminution of the population—where, unlike in Malthus's picture, food is abundant—"each life was a gem, each human breathing form of far . . . and the daily, nay, hourly decrease visible in our numbers, visited the heart with sickening misery. This summer extinguished our hopes, the vessel of society was wrecked, and the shattered raft, which carried the few survivors over the sea of misery, was riven and tempest tost" (LM, 254). In defiance of the biopolitical imperative to calculate births, deaths, and mortality and adjust governance accordingly, the plague in Shelley's novel is sublimely incalculable.[66] Shelley's pestilential sublime explodes the biopolitical. The irony is that when the plague was a mere rumor, the danger it posed to England was so small as to be "incalculable;" by the time England is "wrecked," however, the scale of its threat is truly infinite. In a periodic reversal of a biopolitical regulation of the mass, Shelley concludes the novel with the titular, singular last man.

Shelley's response to disease in these ways deviates from many Romantic understandings of human perfectibility. *The Last Man*'s documentation of humankind's slow demise, weathered away by nature, stands in sharp contrast—in an opposing gradualism—to Godwin's and Percy Shelley's belief in the inherent progress of humanity toward utopia, especially in the case of control over disease, and even the transcendent possibilities of "authorial living-giving and textual-world making."[67] Shelley not only challenges this Romantic attitude but also the opposing utilitarian ideology that espoused biopolitical calculation, where the individual matters little against the progress of the whole. Lionel, trying to comfort himself when the plague threatens England, asserts, "We call ourselves lords of the creation, wielders of the elements, masters of life and death, and we allege in excuse of this arrogance, that though the individual is destroyed, man continues forever" (*LM*, 184). Thinking of the unimportance of the single life in the context of the war against disease, he continues: "Thus, losing our identity, that of which we are chiefly conscious, we glory in the continuity of our species, and learn to regard death without terror" (*LM*, 184). But when he looks back on what has already happened, Lionel intimates that the Romantic progressive utopianism is not so assured. What comfort, he asks, can one take in sacrifice? Rather, "When any whole nation becomes the victim of the destructive powers of exterior agents, then indeed man shrinks into insignificance, he feels his tenure of life insecure, his inheritance on earth cut off" (*LM*, 184). Revealing the fiction of anthropocentric egoism, much like that of England's vital superiority, Lionel equates the vitality of all of humanity with that of the nation, invoking the discourse of military invasion, and portraying disease as borne by exterior, inimical agents. As a result, humans are no longer the inheritors of the earth: animals and ecological systems are unaffected by the plague. In opposition to humanity figuring itself as a kind of nation, the plague proves to be the ultimate sovereign.[68]

The plague's sovereignty suggests that humans are subject to the random, incalculable limiting factor of disease. They will not necessarily progress to social control over it, and human suffering should not be understood through a Malthusian or biopolitical calculus. Thus, ethical practice must be focused on empathetic bonds with individuals, with Others.[69] This reading of shipwrecked humanity ushers the ethical imperatives implicit in Burke's account of the sublime experience. The image of the shipwreck intimates the Burkean premise of self-preservation in the sublime experience. Burke argues that "the passions which belong to self-preservation, turn on pain and danger; they are simply painful when their causes immediately affect us; they are delightful when we have an idea of pain and danger, without being actually in such circumstances; this delight I have not called pleasure, because it turns on pain, and because it is different enough from any idea of positive pleasure. Whatever excites this delight, I call sublime. The passions belonging to self-preservation are the strongest of all the passions."[70] Readers of Shelley's novel could perhaps feel Lionel's terror, and their experience would incite Burke's concept of self-preservation; yet, they would feel delight knowing "they are not actually in such circumstances."[71] To this effect, we might attempt to parse the distinction between Lionel's experience—as he is, in the reality of the fictional world, actually facing the disease—and that of the novel's readers. Shelley's novel, however, blurs the distinction between real and fictional experiences on which Burke's critical distance depends. Moreover, the novel not only explicitly references and represents the Burkean sublime in the imagery Lionel presents, as Jennifer Jones suggests, it "re-conceptualizes [Burke's] theory, becoming a sublime text in its own right."[72]

This reaction might seem solipsistic, as the self-preserving response to the sublime appears to be in contrast with "the beautiful which influences social interaction." However, Burke's sublime works through a paradoxical relationship between the individual and the whole: although the sublime experience occurs in the individual, it stimulates the individual toward action and the social. The delight in the sublime strengthens the bond of sympathy, because "during the sublime experience we imagine the experience of . . . victims and our powers of fellow-feeling are strengthened."[73] In Burkean terms, the sublime confronts us with our finitude and limitations, which triggers self-preservation, and through the recognition of the possibility of kindred pain and fragility in others produces sympathy and action—making the sublime experience moral and ethical. But as others have noted, Shelley's views do not map fully onto Burke's political philosophy. For Burke, conservative organicism could foresee a triumph over disease in an ultimate progression of man, rather like Percy and Godwin's.[74] Therefore, Shelley espouses empathetic drive for social action but takes Burke's position to its logical extreme, where it seems at first that "man continues forever," but in fact the sublime force of disease demonstrates that man has no essential inheritance to the earth.

One might argue that the Burkean sympathetic response could trigger collective action against disease, in the vein of the martial metaphor creating a "unified war." This response would be more consistent with a Kantian understanding of the sublime with respect to the natural force of disease,[75] a theoretical grounding less fitting with *The Last Man*'s framing of the sublime. For Kant, the terror and awe invoked by the sublime experience comes from the initial feeling of being overpowered, and that momentary inhibition produces empowerment and strength: "Might is an ability that is superior to great obstacles. It is called dominance if it is superior even to the resistance of something that itself possesses might. When in an aesthetic judgment we consider nature as a might that has no dominance over us, then it is *dynamically sublime*."[76] Read through a Kantian lens, the martial metaphor empowers the self in its ability to impose a narrative order and contain the incomprehensibility of disease, especially at the epidemic scale. The delimiting of disease into an understandable concept is analogous to the boundaries of the cordon. This is the kind of thinking that subtends Adrian's belief that because "the will of man is omnipotent," humans can "blunt . . . the arrows of death, soothing the bed of disease" (*LM*, 60). This is not to say that a Kantian reading excludes an empathetic desire to consider the intersection of social relations and material practices with nature. Percy Shelley, like Godwin, considered disease to be a social problem. As Percy writes in *Queen Mab* (1813) "Kings, priests, and statesmen," create "venomed exhalation [that] spread / Ruin, death, and woe." Or, as Godwin writes in *An Enquiry Concerning Political Justice* (1793), human life will reach a point where there will be a "total extirpation of the infirmities in our nature."[77] In *The Last Man*, Shelley advocates for social action but distances herself from Percy and Godwin, as evidenced by Lionel's acceptance of humankind's ultimate fate. There is no guaranteed progress, so taking a Kantian approach to the pestilential sublime is fallacious and could run contrary to the strengthening of sympathies and "fellow-feeling" by way of xenophobia, nationalism, and military campaigns. Thus, while Shelley supports the revolutionary, reform-seeking aspect of Percy's philosophy of disease and society, she does not seem to follow him to the point of seeing disease purely in social terms, in a way that denies there is anything natural about disease that allows for humans to ultimately forestall it.

The Last Man's treatment of the inevitable sublime submission to disease and the martial metaphor need not lead to totalizing despair, but the novel's self-referentiality does encourage pause, caution, and reflection. Read through the novel's medical discourse, Shelley's very challenge of the human in her reduction of humankind to the animal at the end of the novel allows for new political possibilities.[78] When Lionel remains the last man, he regresses to animal life, not recognizing "the wild-looking, half-naked savage" before him (*LM*, 455). This association intimates Shelley's revisionist strategy of rewriting the idea of community in categories of race, gender, and species; she promotes the material practice of vaccination as a way of embracing the pathologized Other in terms of both racial and special difference.

Lionel's moment of immunization models Romantic disease discourses' affirmative embrace of alterity rather than "coercive and purifying defense."[79] While the episode problematically instrumentalizes the Black body as an immunizing vector, Lionel's recognition of himself in racialized, inhuman terms prompts his wish for the possibility of a revised cultural and social (more than just an immunitary-transactional) exchange with the "[N]egro half clad." Lionel reimagines that earlier encounter, lamenting "the wild and Cruel Caribbee, the merciless Cannibal . . . would have been to me a beloved companion, a treasure dearly prized—his nature would be kin to mine," concluding his parallel subjunctive regrets with the imperative that "a human sympathy must link us forever" (*LM*, 358).[80] These two scenes stand at the intersection of, and in opposition to the pejorative effects of, both contagion and miasma theory's divisive potentials.

Considering Lionel's affirmative communal impulse, in relation to the positive medical effects of inoculation, attests to the possibility that if humankind stops fighting and lives with rather than against disease, then it might remove at least one barrier that drives contentious relationship between self and other; and that, if it stops pathologizing different populations and locations—materialized in social failure like war—and learns to live on equal terms, then it might, likewise, mitigate, though never fully conquer, nature's virulence. And yet, this realization comes at the expense of a possible colonial companion's demise, and at that, only after everyone else is gone. Reading both scenes against themselves expresses the tensions in the martial metaphor's relationship with literary forms and its complicity in biopolitics. As Emily Steinlight suggests, these scenes express the contradictions immanent to biopower: "the transformation of a biological threat lodged within and transmitted by bodies into a racially differentiated human enemy, barred from a supposedly universal humanity; the thanatopolitcal undercurrent of campaigns to protect human life; the immunitary defense of health—of the porous boundaries of the state, home, and body—via a death unleashed on masses of others."[81] Acknowledging this tension, Shelley asks readers to resist the simple, singular impulse of human sympathy and instead face the larger structures of power and representation that forestall the application, permanence, and affirmative contagiousness of such a sympathetic impulse.

While *The Last Man* exposes the fictional construction of the martial metaphor, denaturing its emerging imbrication in British culture, it also provides insight into why it might be so seemingly natural to internalize it. To do this, Shelley touches on an affective dimension of the metaphor at the level of the individual. Midway through the novel, Lionel admits that the production of his narrative serves a medicinal purpose: "I had used this history as an opiate; while it described my beloved friends, fresh with life and glowing with hope, active assistants on the scene, I was soothed" (*LM*, 212). While we could read this as a use of the written word and memory to allay the finality of death, it might also contextualize a similar point the anonymous author-narrator makes when attempting to put together the text of the Sibylline leaves in the Italian cave. At the conclusion of the "Author's Introduction," the narrator writes, "the imagination, painter of tempest and earthquake, or, worse, the stormy and ruin-fraught passions of man, softened my real sorrows and endless regrets, by clothing these fictitious ones in that ideality, which takes the mortal sting from pain" (*LM*, 4). Aligning two moments of authorial isomorphism, where both Lionel and the frame narrator reflect on the acts of writing and narrativization, Shelley shows us that, as a cultural form propagated through literary genres, the martial metaphor itself works as a kind of anodyne. The fact that human nature is responsible for clothing fictions of catastrophe—sublime figures like the tempest consistent with the novel's representation of disease—does not, however, make the martial metaphor natural. Rather, it reveals one of its functions: clothing the existential crisis of death and disease in an "ideality, which takes the mortal sting from pain." In other words, it is natural for us to try to soothe the pain that comes with the realization that disease is not inimical or evil, that it is just a process which need not be understood as a fight. As Shelley would write in an 1845 letter to her stepsister, Claire Clairmont, regarding Percy's death and the persistent presence of disease in her life, "the inevitable must be submitted to."[82] The martial metaphor imbues meaning by idealizing or romanticizing the encounter with, and the always-ultimate surrender to, death. Problematically, however, the militarized narrative constructed by the individual relationship to disease can have dangerous consequences as a technology of biopolitical regulation, as it conducts the individual to fight death and disease as an autonomous liberal subject. It gives a narrative and a meaning to life and health that can be harnessed at the level of the population, becoming politically charged to coerce, conquer, and ultimately produce health differentially.

If culture, as it was for Godwin, is a way to wage war against death, then Shelley articulates both the dangers and hopes associated with that function in terms of the martial metaphor and the progress of humanity that Godwin believed could overcome death. For him the ever-increasing numbers of the dead, and their works, would become an education for the living to improve humankind.[83] For Shelley, history and culture can clearly do the opposite, leading to the detrimental social relations cataloged in the novel. The martial metaphor exacerbates in effect what it served to signify and allay: death and disease.

The novel documents the graduated and analog historical inflections of the metaphor in medical and literary discourse in the early nineteenth century, the sets of military and medical conditions it emerged from, and also draws attention to its own participation in its circulation. We can then read *The Last Man* as a dialectical reflection on the ethics and aesthetics of the martial metaphor. On the one hand, Shelley stresses the literary construction of humankind's assumed bellicose relationship with disease—that parallels the internecine wars within itself—revealing the way military thinking and practice catalyze rather than inhibit disease; on the other hand, she places the martial metaphor prominently in her narration and dialogue, which circulated the language to the reading public. This circulation is especially significant given that less than a decade later the Asiatic cholera did strike England. Thus, *The Last Man* does not unilaterally instruct readers as to what literature can do for the material practices of medicine; rather, it reveals the tension between its martial and revolutionary possibilities.

2

Charles Kingsley Meets Cholera Face-to-Face

Living in an uninfected country while working on *The Last Man* during the first cholera epidemic, Mary Shelley reflected on the martial metaphor as a problematic tool of national identification while also critiquing the effects of war on the spread of disease itself. Three decades later, during the third cholera pandemic, however, Britain's experience with the disease would make Shelley's ambivalence less palatable for other writers. The rise of the sanitary movement during the middle of the nineteenth century pushed Britain toward a more affirmative stance on militarizing medicine.

It was during the sanitary movement that the disciplines of epidemiology and public health first began to take shape through the efforts of such figures as Florence Nightingale, Edwin Chadwick, William Farr, and John Snow. One author, in particular, proved to be a major driving force for the development of those disciplines, in a number of cultural registers, through his circulation of the martial metaphor. Charles Kingsley, a popular writer, Anglican priest, sanitary reformer, and professor of history was a key participant in the medico-scientific, military, literary, religious, and political discourses of the mid-nineteenth century; his social role put him in a unique position to use the martial metaphor to link those various discourses together. Known for his personal interest in social reform and health, and for his association with the masculine strength and energy of "Muscular Christianity," Kingsley was also well-versed in sanitation and natural science in his professional life. Many of his novels, such as *Yeast* (1849), *Alton Locke* (1850), and *The Water Babies* (1863), feature themes of sanitation, health, and evolution in the context of reformist politics, a topic that has occupied much of the recent scholarship on his work.[1] His post-Crimean Condition-of-England novel *Two Years Ago* (1857) is especially relevant to his investment in health. The construction of the martial metaphor is central to the novel. It provides an organizational logic to the deployments of the metaphor across Kingsley's textual corpus.

Like Shelley, Kingsley was writing the martial metaphor at a significant moment in British military and medical history: close to the apex of the anticontagionist sanitary movement, the third cholera pandemic (1846–1860), and the Crimean War. Making direct connections between the sanitary movement's focus on cholera and Crimea, Kingsley develops the material connections between the military and medicine in *The Last Man*; however, instead of critiquing the linkage, he forges the metaphor as a necessary national ethos.

Kingsley is often characterized as having complicated, if not paradoxical, politics. On the one hand, he espoused Carlylean heroics and masculine strength and virtue; on the other hand, he engaged with Chartism and Christian socialism. As I discuss later in this chapter, his ideas for the hygienic management of the population seem at once to empower all people—especially the working classes—to take control of their own health, but emphasized the role of middle-class professionals as expert directors of the battle against epidemic disease. Kingsley's politics, as with his belief in science and his devout Christian faith, however, were not as incongruous as they might appear. He flirted with changes in legislative privilege but remained committed to "an unshaken faith in the rightness of social order," a position that was not uncommon among middle-class liberals and radicals, especially devout Christians who also embraced scientific progress and liberal politics.[2] Kingsley's apparent contradictions allowed him to reconcile material biology and Christian theology and guide them to a productive social end.

The martial metaphor's recurrence in Kingsley's fiction, sermons, pamphlets, and lectures established him as an influential actor in its propagation and contribution. Reading Kingsley in terms of medical and military history reveals how he develops the material nexus of medicine and the military during the emergence of public health. Kingsley drew on his interest in British history, natural history, theology, and the military to write the martial metaphor as a way to define and protect Britain from the pathological infiltration of cultural, biological, and military threats.[3] Exactly how Kingsley mobilized the metaphor varied by genre and venue. *Two Years Ago* garnered the attention of the general public, while other texts provided a medico-military imperative for specific populations: including pamphlets addressed to soldiers in Crimea, sanitary lectures for middle-class women, and religious sermons for churchgoers. Tracking this literary figuration in Kingsley's corpus shows how he weaves the church, the domestic space, the battlefield, and the public sphere through a framework of governmentality, working as a node in the state's larger "conduct of conducts."[4]

Though he was a devout Anglican minister, Kingsley's reconciled the material biology of disease with his religious doctrine; this countered other, outdated religious positions that attributed epidemics to divine castigation. Earlier theocentric understandings of disease were not obviously compatible with the liberal subject's ability to shape the material conditions of his existence. While the "liberal subject" is, of course, a mobile category, Chris Otter's definition is especially useful in this context: the "liberal subject" was the kind of person who was the target and presupposition of minimal state interference who was "free and self-governing," while also "subjected and governed."[5] Kingsley capitalized on religious discourse to make health a moral and political duty of the liberal subject. He claimed that disease was not caused by God in the manner of divine retribution but resulted from original sin and must be fought against constantly, like sin itself. The martial metaphor empowered individuals to resist human, spiritual, and biological frailty while remaining subject to God's natural laws and the state's interest in public health. Meeting the requirements of that empowerment presupposed a middle-class, male individual who was afforded autonomous agency and had an entrepreneurial drive rooted in self-reliance, sobriety, discipline, and the other character traits espoused by figures such as John Stuart Mill and Samuel Smiles,[6] who, not coincidentally, named health as a national trait.[7] The work of individuals in shaping themselves to fight the concupiscent condition of the human soul became the means to forge a conductible and biologically healthy population to mitigate its tendency toward endemicity. Looking to Kingsley reveals how literature helped negotiate that transmuted imperative during the mid-century.

This chapter focuses on how Kingsley specifically mobilized the martial metaphor through various genres throughout his career as a clergyman, scholar, and sanitarian, contextualizing the various iterations as they cohered within his novel *Two Years Ago*. In the novel, Kingsley shifted notably into the Condition-of-England literary genre in order to suture his medical and military politics into a unified nationalist endeavor. Kingsley himself is often discussed in reference to sanitary reform, particularly regarding cholera. *Two Years Ago*, though not often the subject of extensive critical examination, is frequently cited in cholera histories as emblematic of the mid-Victorian sanitary zeitgeist.[8] Tina Young Choi argues that while the disease is clearly represented as miasmic in *Two Years Ago*, contagion structures the narrative, signaling the points of contact between individuals and forward-thinking trajectories of traceable action and effect.[9] But, a novel that inculcated that very reflective connection between self and other, and the solidification between the effect and action of sanitary reform, must also be addressed in terms of its rhetoric of war, as Michael Brown does in his reading of the protagonist, Tom Thurnall, as an emblematic literary example of masculine professionalism in the ethos of war and heroism.[10] Because the unification of self and other worked on the logic of Britishness and citizenry, as both Choi and Pamela Gilbert suggest, we must account for the potentially divisive, violent, and coercive nature of the literary mechanisms that Kingsley uses to suggest each individual (medical professional or not) is a potential actor affecting the bodily lives of others.[11] Attending to this capacity of Kingsley's work, this chapter's reading of his use of the martial metaphor extends the relationship between Kingsley and cholera to the larger epistemic formations that facilitate biopolitical governance. Through the use of military discourse, Kingsley strengthened the connection between the autonomous self and the regulation of the population. In what follows, I focus on Kingsley's participation in the medicalization of British society by uncovering its roots in military medical concerns and showing how his rhetoric drew on this connection to yoke together individual and national health.

To demonstrate this, I begin by describing how cholera metaphorically and materially linked English citizens on the home front with the soldiers fighting in Crimea. Then I show how Kingsley constructed gender to shape his arguments about the way the martial metaphor drives and unifies men and women in their respective, classed social roles. For him, masculinity follows a self-shaping imperative that is tempered by Christian values and a supportive, policing femininity, leaving women as agents of the metaphor but never subjects of it in the same way as men. Kingsley empowers women to follow the disciplinary and militaristic techniques of Florence Nightingale, entreating wives and mothers to tame excesses of masculinity in addition to being vocationally devout agents of sanitary reform.

After addressing Kingsley's construction of gender, I articulate how he saw disease as both a spiritual and a biological battle, first by challenging the notion that God deployed disease in a purely punitive capacity, and second by developing a notion of divine inspiration that acted as an agent against miasma, fortifying individuals against pestilent air. I conclude by suggesting that Kingsley was proposing the metaphor of medical war as a perpetual way of life when he linked his hygienic principles with his theological interpretations of biology, formulating a system of thought in which subjects actively guard against death and disease by producing health. This cultural work had the effect not only of propagating the martial metaphor, but of leading to the very erasure of its construction, specifically its material connections to the military.

Threatening "Us" and "Ours"

Kingsley drew on the unification of time and space between Crimea and London in order to imbue cholera's dramaturgical form with a sense of military urgency; fashioning cholera as a national enemy that threatened the citizens of England and their military forces simultaneously would be a plot similar to the military romance in *Two Years Ago*. I follow Charles Rosenberg in suggesting that disease has a narrative and dramaturgical form that mobilizes communities to perform certain rituals that structure or "reaffirm social values and modes of understanding."[12] The number of deaths due to cholera and the ways they occurred were significant variables in that equation, but it was primarily the way cholera allied Londoners with soldiers in Crimea in the summer of 1854 that unified England's home and Crimean fronts. The connections between medicine and war abroad created the conditions for a culture at home in which militarism came to be an implicit tenet of public health and medicine.

The relationship between the Crimean War and the cholera epidemic shown in *Two Years Ago* demonstrates the metaphor's ability to circulate from military terminology to idiomatic use in the public imagination. Published during the third cholera pandemic (1852–1860) and at the end of the Crimean War, the novel tells the heroic narrative of Tom Thurnall, an adventure-seeking, self-made surgeon who finds himself shipwrecked at the Cornish town of Aberalva. While attempting to make a living and support his father, he notes that the town's poor sanitary conditions make it ripe for disease. The majority of the novel relays Tom's fight against a local cholera epidemic that is concurrent with the Crimean War. In his attempts to overcome local recalcitrance regarding sanitary science, he becomes infatuated with Grace Harvey, a schoolteacher who later tames Tom's obstinate self-reliance and atheism. In the process, Tom also reforms the inept aristocratic landlord and the meek and ineffective curate. The characters' martial heroics occur offstage. Tom returns to war as a spy, while Grace goes to Sebastopol as a nurse with a number of other characters who join the war effort. While the novel does not describe the fighting in Crimea directly, the war remains an underlying narrative force, reflecting how Kingsley obscures the material connections that link war to medicine by metaphor through literary form. By virtue of its plot and setting, *Two Years Ago* emblematizes how the war in Crimea provided a material grounding for the declaration of a figurative war on disease.

Britain's entry into the Crimean War resulted from the indirect threat posed by Russian imperial expansion. Originating in a religious dispute between Catholic and Eastern Orthodox Christians, the conflict that arose between France and Russia was largely a consequence of the decline of the Ottoman Empire. In July of 1853, Russia invaded Moldavia and Wallachia. Britain and France responded by joining forces with the Turks. Britain needed the buffer of an independent Turkey to secure the Mediterranean from Russian expansionism.[13] From the first troop movements, however, it was clear to both sides that this was less a combative conflict than a medical war: as with most earlier wars, the overwhelming majority of casualties in Crimea fell to infectious diseases, including cholera, typhus, and dysentery.[14] In fact, the British sustained devastating losses to cholera before the fighting even began. The *Lancet*'s correspondent in Malta presaged the medical problems in Crimea by saying, "What we have most to fear in an encampment is an enemy that musket and bayonet cannot meet or repel. We have a fearful lesson in the records of the Russo-Turkish campaign of 1828–9, in which 80,000 men perished by 'plague, pestilence, and famine' . . . Let us have an overwhelming army of medical men to combat with the disease."[15] It is no coincidence that the correspondent adopted a militarized rhetoric that resonated with Kingsley's novel. This kind of retrospective rhetorical comparison of deaths in war to that of disease was becoming commonplace during the mid-century sanitary movement.[16] The difference between this writer's usage and Kingsley's deployment of the martial metaphor, however, is that Kingsley's use had a wider circulation and brought the war home to the average citizen in his novels and his religious and sanitary writings. Moreover, Kingsley's recurrent use of the figuration was an ideologically expansive one that brought the British soldier's fight against cholera to bear on the domestic sphere, the Christian's relationship to God, and the citizen's relationship to the state.

The unifying work of the home and battlefront is reflected in the first few lines of *Two Years Ago*, which look back on the novel's events two years after they occurred: "Two years ago, while pestilence was hovering over us and ours; while the battle-roar was ringing in our ears; who had time to think, to ask what all that meant; to seek for the deep lesson which we knew must lie beneath?"[17] The simultaneity of the pestilence and the battle roar imparts a sense of immediacy that connected the war abroad with the medical war in England. The miasmic cloud hovering over "us and ours" alike speaks to those at home and their soldiers. Through a metonymic relationship of contiguity, the two groups remain one social body at the mercy of the same assailing pestilence. Furthermore, through infusion of the past into the present—the novel was published right after the end of the war yet still during the third cholera epidemic—Kingsley's gambit primes readers with the "deep lesson" of the tumultuous period: that life is a perpetual war against disease, sin, and foreign powers.

The move to connect past to the present in terms of war can be better understood by parsing Kingsley's views on historiography. For Kingsley, war was a defining characteristic of what it meant to be a healthy individual, Christian, and nation. It was in the very marrow of the English people. In a review of the first two volumes of James Anthony Froude's *A History of England from the Fall of Wolsey to the Death of Elizabeth* (1856), Kingsley takes issue with trends in scholarship that suggested that England had evolved from its boorish and violent past. He challenges the idea that England's history "is nothing but a string of foolish wars," and that the country's worthiness did not even materialize "before the steam-engine and political economy."[18] Since the Peninsular War (1807–1814), Kingsley argues, "an unexampled peace," had come over England, "from which our ancestors of the sixteenth century were kept, by stern and yet most wholesome lessons; the fancy that peace, and not war, is the normal condition of the world."[19] He counters the claim that England had somehow evolved from a martial nature, interpellating the reader as part of the true English social body and spirit: "We repeat: war, in some shape or other, is the normal condition of the world." He positions the ability to confront enemies and conflicts—be they personified as sin, a foreign army, unsanitary conditions, or socio-economic circumstances—as a foundational requirement of life. He evangelizes: "While the life of the individual and of the universe is one of perpetual self-defence [sic], the life of the nation can be aught else."[20] As a historian, Kingsley understands the martial as one of England's defining characteristics; for him, relegating that history to the distant past, such as "flagellantisms, witch-manias, and other 'popular delusions,'" is not only irreverent, but fallacious.[21] Crimea and cholera, then, become opportunities to learn the normal, bellicose condition of the world and recover the noble essential tradition of what it meant to be English by fighting against disease.

Kingsley's prose on sanitation and Crimea proximate to *Two Years Ago* were part of his larger ideological linkage of the past and the present, the medical and the martial. To help the military side of the effort during the Crimean War, Kingsley wrote pamphlets delivered to soldiers for inspiration and republished sermons given during previous epidemics. The pamphlets were collected and published in 1888 as *True Words for Brave Men*. To the men fighting for their lives against an unseen enemy, Kingsley writes, "Above all, you have felt how difficult it was to die, not fighting sword in hand, but slowly and idly, and helplessly, by cholera or fever."[22] Speaking to them as a social body, he urges individual soldiers to fight against both disease and enemy combatants. While writing the pamphlets, Kingsley also published a collection of his sermons from 1848 and 1849, "Who Causes Pestilence?" (1854). The benefit of publishing sermons was, as Keith A. Francis observes, that clergymen could increase opportunities for further educating and reach an audience that was unable to be present at the original sermon; additionally, they could attempt to authentically recapture and memorialize the sermon's particular historical moment and context, whether it was an event, a series of events, a place, or a person.[23] Kingsley reintroduced the context of the cholera epidemic of the 1830s and late '40s into the epidemic of the late '50s, making the point that cholera had struck before and would strike again. Consequently, his sermons, which otherwise would have been heard only once, had a cumulative effect in shaping public perception of cholera. The redefinition of cholera as a perpetual threat and an endemic of epidemics, codified a mode of epidemiological thinking and governmentality that sought not only to act against epidemics when they struck but also to fight them perpetually by positioning disease as a permanent presence rather than a periodic or singular punishment from God.

During the nineteenth century, Britain had four major outbreaks of cholera (1832, 1841, 1854, and 1866), making it a looming threat to the country throughout the century. As discussed in the previous chapter, the fact that it came from the East in the 1817 epidemic and afflicted British troops was often sufficient reason to identify "Asiatic cholera" with foreign military threats in a number of medical and periodical texts published after the first pandemic. The recurrent use later in the century of the metaphor fostered nationalistic thinking in the wake of the 1831 epidemic that made it conducive to Kingsley's nationalist ideology during the mid-century.

Kingsley was responding to two cholera epidemics from before the mid-century that were instrumental in making disease easily analogous to a military invasion. In that capacity, the non-Britishness of cholera constructed the disease as a foreign enemy that spread globally and did not respect national boundaries. It was a characteristic that Mary Wilson Carpenter identifies with a cosmopolitan nature,[24] giving Kingsley even more ammunition in his campaign to secure England's identity and borders from cholera's diversifying influence.[25] Defending England and its empire from cosmopolitan disease appears in medical texts contemporaneous with Kingsley's use of the metaphor in *Two Years Ago* and the related texts of his medico-military constellation. In *A Treatise on Fever* (1861) by Robert Spencer Dyer Lyons, the former pathologist-in-chief to the British army during Crimea, addresses medical students regarding their imperial mission: "Should your avocations be exercised in other lands, whether as public servants in any of the distant colonies or broad possessions of the British empire, or as adventurers seeking new homes and fortunes in the far west, your knowledge and your skill will be ever taxed in every clime and amongst every race, to stay the destroying hand of this universal enemy of our kind. For in some one or other of its forms, this cosmopolitan disease meets you in both hemispheres, and on either side of the line."[26] Indeed, Kingsley would follow the colonial impulse present in Lyons's address in his 1872 lecture, "The Study of Natural History for Soldiers," where he suggests that studying natural history will make his audience better soldiers and colonizers, citing Alexander the Great as an example. Furthermore, he encourages officers to respect men of science and medicine in the field as "they are soldiers nevertheless, and good soldiers and chivalrous, fighting their nation's battle, often on even less pay than you, and with still less chance of promotion and of fame, against most real and fatal enemies."[27] Working in the same vein as Kingsley's militarization of medical men, Lyons writes, "If you wish to be worthy of your high mission, and equal to the responsibilities of your calling, you must be prepared, with all the resources of your art, to meet this deadly antagonist face to face, and to dispute with him each inch of ground."²⁸ Lyons's call to arms draws on a recurring hypernym of the martial metaphor: the trope of close, face-to-face combat with a disease, a figuration also present in *Two Years Ago*, when Lord Scoutbush, the local aristocrat who develops into a masculine and respectable military leader as a result of an epidemic, wishes to "meet cholera face to face, as one does with those Russians" (*TY*, 35). The protagonist, Tom Thurnall, is an adventurer who has seen the effects of disease, especially cholera, all over the world, much like the medical soldiers Lyons addresses. Even in the context of a call to arms against disease, that qualification identifies war as an instigator of disease along the same lines as *The Last Man*. Lyons also writes, "It is only for the vulgar and the uninformed that war exhibits its greatest terrors on the battle-field [sic]. The medical history of every great campaign that the world has seen, tells us that the most murderous inventions which military science has produced, from the remotest times to the present, reap but a small harvest of death when compared with the long black list of mortality which the rolls of disease furnish in such fatal abundance."²⁹ Lyons's deployment of the metaphor in opposition to an explication of its actual material connections follows Kingsley's own deployment of cholera as a foreign enemy. Cholera's foreignness abetted Kingsley's general rejection of cosmopolitanism, which stood in contrast to his ideal of a pure and developed British national culture.³⁰ Kingsley's propagation of that social construction of the disease helped to occlude Britain's complicity in the pandemic that spread early in the century and redirected attention to cholera as an inimical force, positioning it as something against which both the military and the public had to fight, rather than considering military infrastructure and movement to be one of its vectors.

Live war reporting about the conditions of sanitation on the battlefield allowed the public to make the connections Kingsley drew for them between the cholera epidemic in Crimea and the contemporaneous one in Britain. Crimea was the first war that was reported using both the telegraph and photograph, giving the public access to live and visual information at a speed previously unavailable.³¹ In this vein, Swenson has suggested that conflating the cholera epidemics in Crimea and at home would have felt natural to the Victorians when they looked back on the events of 1854.³² Although the third cholera epidemic had a lower overall mortality rate than the second, the 1850–1862 epidemic included the Broad Street outbreak, which killed more than 500 people in ten days.³³ It was the outbreak that John Snow famously tracked to a water supply that had been contaminated by a nearby cesspool,³⁴ which contradicted the miasmist view that disease was transmitted by foul air emanating from decaying matter and still linked the disease to excrement. Snow speculated that the spread of diseases like cholera and typhoid in Crimea must have been caused by similarly contaminated water supplies.³⁵ Not long afterward, Snow's suspicions were proven correct.³⁶ The deaths caused by cholera in Crimea compounded the public's fear of the disease and came to shape the way medicine would seek not only to ameliorate but actively fight it, which meant searching for its proximate and ultimate causes. After Snow's landmark publication, the Sanitary Commission at the British camp at Sebastopol made a similar find, where it was discovered that the main hospital had been built directly over a cesspool.³⁷ Furthermore, cholera's link to the war fostered the same kinds of anxieties that a major military conflict would have caused. Cholera, like the Crimean war, challenged class configurations within the social order that fostered disease and inhibited national vitality. In response, Kingsley addressed a number of national and military failures that the war brought to light.

In his works, the martial metaphor becomes a tool for correcting those failures as they pertained to national health. One of the most notable was the problematic commissary system in the British military. The primary system of military commissions allowed aristocrats to purchase ranks in the form of promissory bonds. As has been well-documented and argued, that system led to inept and inexperienced officers making catastrophic strategic blunders and prompting events such as the mythologized Charge of the Light Brigade, where Lord Cardigan led an outnumbered and outgunned light cavalry against Russian artillery during the battle of Balaclava.³⁸ Such problems with the ruling class suggested that a redefinition of national heroes was in order. According to Kingsley, the country needed disciplined men who had fashioned themselves in the face of hardship to challenge a system in which indolent aristocrats shaped the nation's military, political, and economic realities and led to problems such as unsanitary conditions for the laboring class, which affected all socioeconomic classes. According to Kingsley, the country needed men like Tom Thurnall. In contrast to the decaying system in which the aristocracy controlled the population through landed privilege, the rise of the middle class would result in strong men who could better their own conditions and, subsequently, the nation's.

In *Two Years Ago*, Kingsley links the mismanagement of enlisted men with the aristocracy's irresponsible sanitary management of the laboring population, framing it through the lens of war and disease. Correcting that problem became a part of the war against disease, being a central aspect of Britain's military reform. Tom, for instance, presages the onset of cholera as soon as he arrives in Aberalva. He tries to preempt the disease by instituting sanitary reforms that entail completely rebuilding the local cottages but the local aristocrat and absentee landlord, Lord Scoutbush, lacks resolve. Tom's attempts to work with him are forestalled by Scoutbush's alcoholic squire Trebooze and his recalcitrant steward Tardew, who aggressively resist Tom's demands that the cottages receive proper drainage and architectural repair. Scoutbush puts on "an air of languid nonchalance which is considered (*or was before the little experiences in Crimea*) proper to a gentleman of his rank and fashion" (*TY*, 135, emphasis added). The parenthetical reference above speaks to the fact that the military failures of the aristocracy were at least partially due to a masculinity that was not tempered by military hardship and self-fashioning. Scoutbush is not an evil man, just weak and full of untapped potential: "And all the while there was a quaint and pathetic consciousness in the little man's heart that he was meant for something better; that he was no fool and was not intended to be one" (*TY*, 131). This is an example of Kingsley's liberal reformist politics working with, rather than against, larger social structures such as class division. Scoutbush requires a model of masculinity in order to better himself and the community: enter Tom Thurnall.

For Kingsley, heroes like Tom could save the nation in the face of foreign and domestic enemies like armies and disease. Surgeons like Tom needed to take political action, to perform scientific work in line with John Snow's in order to better public understanding of the nature of disease, and fight individual cases of cholera in the bodies of the infected. Tom performs all three of these functions by writing to the Poor Law boards, confronting aristocratic landlords, examining water specimens, and performing individual medical interventions. Men like Snow, Chadwick, and Farr helped to ensure the sanitary, sewage, architectural, and legal reforms that gave doctors and the state some control over disease. The policing of the poor was central to the formation of a middle-class authority and the stabilization of its place within the social and political landscape of the mid-nineteenth century, as Priti Joshi suggests in her study of Chadwick's own self-fashioning.[39] Through strength, discipline, and willpower, that subject would deploy medicine to resist the ever-growing threat of disease that accompanied the expansion of Britain's industry, urbanization, and empire.

Related to his male, liberal subjectivity is the affirmation of Tom's socioeconomic status, speaking to the ways the class structures within liberalism were necessary for the martial metaphor to function. Kingsley linked economics and the martial metaphor in his sermon "The Physician's Calling" (1866) at St. George's hospital: "Experience has decided, that in a civilized Christian country . . . the great principle of the division of labour should be carried out: that there should be in the land a body of men whose whole mind and time should be devoted to one part only of our Lord's work—the battle with disease and death. And the effect has not been to lower but to raise the medical profession."[40] While the state of class relations remained a national problem for Kingsley, he nevertheless validated the economic system that allowed medical professionals to develop their expertise and, in effect, better themselves and the nation. That kind of reform within existing class politics is a topic he returned to when discussing the proper role of the woman in society. In the sermon as in *Two Years Ago*, however, Kingsley constructs the middle-class medical professional as a hero of central, national importance. His account of the "rise of the medical profession," certainly concurrent with the passing of the Medical Act of 1858,[41] fits within his characterization of the rise of the middle-class professional expert who would direct the nation in the face of perpetual biological threats. The doctor, in Kingsley's doctrine, not only serves to direct medico-political action, but is a role model for social betterment through self-fashioning, such as when Tom helps Scoutbush perform his upper-class duties in the division of labor. Tom's actions show how Kingsley subscribed to liberalism for the betterment of England in medical and political terms.

Tom epitomizes self-discipline and courage, remaining physically and mentally strong in the face of disease and war, which in the novel function as trials and opportunities for hardening masculine traits. He survives cholera (twice), bullet wounds, bayonetting, shipwrecks (three times), and even hanging; he also frequently advocates for exercise as a corrective measure (*TY*, 96). Tom's intelligence highlights his medical training. His medical credentials appear as a paratactical bombardment of military, colonial, and governmental practices, contrasting him with the local, alcoholic surgeon: "F.R.C.S. London, Paris, and Glasgow. . . . Have been medical officer to a poor-law union, and to a Brazilian man-of-war.

Have seen three choleras, two army fevers, and yellow-jack without end. Have doctored gunshot wounds in the two Texan wars, in one Paris revolution, and in the Schleswig-Holstein row; beside accident practice in every country from California to China, and round the world and back again (*TY*, 89)." Professionally molded by both war and medicine, Tom's background embodies the martial metaphor because his life is dedicated to forestalling death. He literally "never say[s] die" (*TY*, 89). Kingsley's formation of a masculine subject makes Tom an emblem for the intersection of medicine and war. In Kingsley's view, medicine, like war, shapes individuals and nations by making them more resilient against future threats. For a medical practitioner like Tom, part of the resiliency entailed training in the most current and modern forms of medicine.

Tom's medical training speaks to the cutting-edge medical epistemes of the nineteenth century—changes in thought that facilitated the metaphor's emergence in popular and medical discourse. Although Kingsley cites numerous examples in which Tom practices military medicine, the character's history links him with the paradigm of medicine as war in a historical, genealogical, and epistemological capacity. Identifying Tom with Paris connects him, much like *Middlemarch*'s Lydgate, to Bichat's pathological anatomy, wherein emphasis is placed on practical medical training via dissection, and practice is grounded in the body rather than in theoretical nosology. That nosology aligned itself with older medical paradigms like those practiced by the conservative medical professionals of Oxford and Cambridge. Tom's practical training is further highlighted by his title as a fellow from the Royal College of Surgeons (RCS) and his training in Scotland. Scotland was a premier site for surgical training in Britain, especially for surgeons who would perform military service beginning at the turn of the nineteenth century.[42] The fact that Tom is neither an officer nor a gentleman physician but a non-commissioned mercenary surgeon underscores his individualism and his professional and social self-fashioning. He operates under his own imperative to fight and cure wherever he is needed for the purpose of bettering his economic status. Brown argues that Tom's actions mirror a rhetorical move by mid-century surgeons, where they identified themselves with masculine military heroism in public speeches, medical tracts, and eulogies in order to depose medical elitists and win authority and recognition as well as earn the right to regulate their own profession. The appropriation of military heroism by middle-class general practitioners, surgeons, Poor Law physicians, and district medical officers was carried out in opposition to the complacent medical aristocracy and the ineffectual military hierarchy in Crimea.[43] Tom's professional development aligned with the belief that the power to enact social change lies in the middle class, a notion borrowed from the influence of military discourse on the rise of medicine's social standing as a profession. In addition, that professional assignment, which drew from and contributed to the martial metaphor, suggested that militarized, medical masculinity fostered the entrepreneurial relationship between a practitioner's own talents and social mobility while also aiding in medical and social reform.

Tom's cutting-edge medical training links him with the then-prominent liberal medical theories of disease transmission and their respective political stakes. As a sanitarian in alliance with Florence Nightingale, Kingsley frequently furthered the anticontagionist agenda that operated under social reforms based on miasmist understandings of disease. By linking Tom with sanitarians, Kingsley makes him specifically British and liberal. Tom stands in contrast not only with conventional politics but with the literal and overt use of military force on civilian populations through the oppressive quarantines, inspections, and restrictions on freedom that Russia instituted during the 1830s cholera epidemic,[44] following the more conservative contagionist paradigm. *Two Years Ago* reworks the difference between the overt force of quarantine and indirect intervention that limited the restriction of personal autonomy and public health. The novel codes the biopolitics of the emerging institutions of public health into its narrative logic and metaphorical transposition of medicine and war. Militarily, Tom does not partake in direct combat. He goes to the East as a spy and contributes to the war effort with information and surveillance rather than overt force. Medically, he does not expel or contain the sick. Relatedly, sanitary reform operated through informational, surveillant, structural, and political mechanisms rather than direct containment of infected populations, although the militaristic exercise of force was always a possibility. As the following chapter will detail, the coercive and violent logics of quarantine and military medicine worked behind the scenes of public health's regulatory biopolitics, allowing the martial metaphor to operate covertly, occluding its military origins and tactics and its own metaphorical nature. Although the reader isn't privy to Tom's actions in war, they are not left with questions as to its role in masculine and national formation.

Wars and disease serve as trials for Kingsley's masculine men so that they can fashion themselves to greater ends beyond themselves.

Before arriving at Aberalva, however, Tom was purely self-driven, an exemplar of Kinglsey's dictum that "all true manhood exists in defiance of circumstances."[45] Tom is a paradigm of the British man who thrives in a life perpetually at war; yet, he did not recognize a higher power or the limits of his own capabilities: "There were few things he could not invent, and perhaps nothing he could not endure. . . . [A] man who stood alone in and self-poised in the midst of the universe" (*TY*, 46). Although Tom relays that he served as a surgeon for the Poor Law, aligning him with the disciplinary apparatuses that contributed to the medicalization of British society, he lacks the drive to directly serve national interests. The cholera epidemic and Grace's inculcation of a belief in God help Tom maintain his strong self-will, but in a fashion that is productive for the individual and social body.[46] Because of those influences, Tom ends up being more righteous and more capable of fighting disease for the English than he was prior to arriving at Abeverala. Further, the way in which Tom reconciles his secular liberal subjectivity and belief in the material etiology of disease conveys how Kingsley's views on the biological war against disease fit logically into his Christian belief system and nationalist politics.

Moving up the class hierarchy, the only hope for reforming the undisciplined aristocrats' failed masculinity in the novel is proper military service. The local aristocrat, Scoutbush, is in the military as a guardsman but is too meek to do anything really militaristic. It is not until he falls for the American Sabina that his desire for military prowess is enlivened, as he learns that she "will not marry anyone who will not devote himself, and all he has, to some great, chivalrous heroic enterprise" (*TY*, 142). Scoutbush's lack of proper military masculinity emphasizes concerns similar to those of the British medical establishment before and during the Crimean conflict. As the author of the previously cited *Lancet* article writes, "Do not let our soldiers be killed by antiquated imbecility. Do not hand them over to the mercies of ignorant etiquette and *effete* seniority."[47] England needed more masculine military heroes, not weak, untrained aristocrats. After learning of his love interest Sabina's standards, Scoutbush is a changed man: "He read of nothing but sieges and stockades, brigade evolutions, and conical bullets; he drilled his men till he was an abomination in their eyes, and a weariness to their flesh. . . . So in all things he acquitted himself as a model officer, and excited the admiration and respect of Sergeant-Major MacArthur" (*TY*, 144). After he is reformed, the fight against cholera affords Scoutbush an opportunity to become a soldier in the medical war. In addition, Major Campbell, a central mentor figure in the novel who is also self-made through military service,[48] empowers Scoutbush to sever his ties with the lofty, aloof, incapable aristocracy: "Your life has been child's play as of yet. You are now going to see life in earnest—the sort of life average people have been living." Ultimately, Scoutbush becomes "afraid of nothing," only wishing that "one could meet cholera face to face, as one does with those Russians" (*TY*, 351). To this same effect, Scoutbush appropriates the martial metaphor to fashion himself as a proper man and a defender of the nation, both medically and martially.[49]

Scoutbush's militaristic reformation conveys Kingsley's views on gender vis-à-vis self-reliant subjectivity, medicine, and discipline that emerge from the relationship among the three. In Kingsley's paradigm, the militarization of medicine required the distinction of gender roles in order to mobilize the resources under each gender's jurisdiction most effectively. Kingsley defines gender as men tackling the public sphere and possessing the ability to self-fashion, and women taking on the domestic sphere and the role of maternal superintendents and tamers of excessive masculinity.

Mothers, Wives, and Nurses

Kingsley's writing of the female gender associates the martial metaphor's imperative for national health with the domestic, capitalizing on existing gendered narratives to translate military nursing into domestic hygienic management. The Crimean War was the origin of a recurring relationship between women and the military: the repositioning of the supportive wife as nurse. A woman's role as nurse was, of course, literal in many cases as at the end of *Two Years Ago*, but I use the term *supportive wife* to underscore the accommodating nature of women's participation in the production of health for the state through the domestic sphere This intrusion of the state and the medical into the family is not an isolated occurrence, of course. Graham Mooney traces the "intrusive interventions" of public health, seeing their formalization and solidification through the end of the century, with an aim toward "unravel[ing] the perceived dangers and potentialities of home and family life."[50] Mooney notes that much of governing of the population through household worked through women, given their role in the domestic. To that same effect, women figuratively married the paternal directives of public health as instruments of the martial metaphor rather than liberal subjects. Florence Nightingale and Mary Seacole were instrumental in the creation of modern nursing, which is often identified as emerging from the Crimean War.[51] In contrast to the caricature of nurses as drunks in the early Victorian period, perhaps best emblematized by Sarah Gamp in Dickens's *Martin Chuzzlewit* (1842), after the mid-century, nurses' efforts were not just influential in one-on-one patient care and the development of nursing as a revered profession; they were also profoundly influential in the mid-nineteenth century creation of public health through the sanitary movement. Like Farr, Chadwick, and Snow, Nightingale utilized the developing science of statistics to help solidify the field of epidemiology; she also wrote extensively about sanitary conditions. Her *Notes on Matters Affecting the Health, Efficiency and Hospital Administration of the British Army* (1858) had numerous tables and graphical coxcombs, the most notable being her "Diagram of Causes of Mortality of the Army in the East."[52] Moreover, as Louise Penner has suggested, like Kingsley, Nightingale wrote texts with a distinct audience in mind: in addition to her writings on military hospitals and the working class (1858), her *Notes on Hospitals* (1859) focuses on the design and engineering of hospitals, while *Notes on Nursing* (1860) focuses on the sanitary management of the domestic space.[53] To fight the casualties of infectious disease, Nightingale emerged as a domestic, middle-class professional who used military-style discipline and domestic surveillance to police filth and bodies.

For Kingsley, Nightingale served primarily as a model of the female agent on whom the martial metaphor relied for the dissemination of sanitary discourse and its management within the family and the hospital, as the domestic and the hospital were not just metaphorically but also materially and conceptually connected contiguities.[54] Kingsley praised her for emblematizing the role of the female sanitarian. Modeling Grace's vocational passion and discipline after Nightingale allowed Kingsley to solidify the female supportive agent's role in the production of the martial metaphor in his novel. One reviewer praised it for "the sensible way in which [Kingsley] has spoken of marriage life. . . . He uses the story as a means to convey instruction in a popular and impressive form. . . . Mr. Kingsley has a just and delicate appreciation of woman's nature, and has nobly expressed his reverence for her weakness and admiration for strength."[55] In other words, the novel instructed the female agent of the martial metaphor on how to act and showed the male subject what to look for in a wife.

The Nightingale figure that Kingsley adopts functions as a necessary link between military medicine and civilian medicine's adoption of military rhetoric and logic. As a cultural icon,[56] she was the point of articulation for how the idea of medicine as war became a structuring force of discipline in the mid-Victorian period via the intersections of medicine and the family. We can see how the female supportive agent became a vital element of biopolitical regulation by considering Nightingale's military experience, the disciplinary techniques that she inculcated in nurses, and the role that discipline played in the hygienic protocols that allowed liberal subjects to become sanitary. Nightingale does, however, embody a contradiction: she was the normative definition of middle-class domesticity and a self-denying caretaker, yet she also was masculine "like a politician or soldier," encountering opposition only to persevere and overcome it.[57] However contradictory it was, that ideal served as a conduit for Kingsley's introduction of a martial ethos into medicine for a female audience who would come to play an instrumental role in the mobilization of the martial metaphor; it at once empowered, relegated, and regulated them.

Kingsley's ideal woman was necessary to the production of proper individual masculinity and the cohesion of Britain's social body in the face of threats to public health. In a Biblically allegorical description of the unproductive relationships among the socioeconomic classes, Kingsley praises Nightingale as one of the women who could make the laboring classes work symbiotically with the upper classes. Comparing England to the Biblical Jacob and Esau with the former representing the middle and upper classes, and the latter, the working class, Kingsley suggests that a "gulf" lies between them: "Poor Esau," he writes ". . . sails Jacob's ships, digs Jacob's mines, founds Jacob's colonies, pours out his blood for him in those wars which Jacob has stirred up, while his sleeping brother sits at home, enjoying at once the 'means of grace' and the produce of Esau's labor."[58] Kingsley qualifies and suggests attenuation for that inequality:

> Esau has a birthright . . . but it is not . . . any *man* at all, who can tell Esau the whole truth about himself, his powers, his duty, and his God. Woman must do it, and not man. His mother, his sister the maid whom he may love. . . . As long

as England can produce two such woman as Florence Nightingale and Catherine Marsh, there is good hope that Esau will not be defrauded of his birthright; and that by the time that Jacob comes crouching to him, to defend him against the enemies who are here at hand.[59]

In this system of social and labor relations, women served as conduits allowing the upper and middle classes to collaborate with the working class to defend against enemies that, like disease, are in Jacob's midst: the middle-class women must help to clean the homes of the poor and serve as a role model for proper sanitation practices for the middle and working classes. In this paradigm, middle-class women also help men regulate the lower classes and avoid the inefficacy displayed by the aristocracy in *Two Years Ago*. It speaks to the imperative of the middle class to doctor the social body, not only because surgeons like Tom came from the middle class, but because, in the text, the working classes do not actually do much to help themselves. Their cottages are repaired for them, and they tend to blindly follow the Methodist preacher who attributes cholera to God's wrath, a mistake that Tom takes pains to correct. We do not see or hear much from the working class directly in the novel. Their absence reveals the incongruity in Kingsley's reformism with respect to class. The poor are rhetorically constructed as liberal subjects and are included in the abstraction of the whole social body: "We must teach men to mend their own matters, of their own reason, and of their own will."[60] However, in the domestic component of the martial metaphor, the goal, planning, and regulation of that instruction are managed by the middle-class professional and policed by Tom's supportive wife.

Kingsley employs the metaphor in a more complex formulation when calling on women to save the English race by medicalizing the domestic sphere. The domestic woman was often the target audience member of Kingsley's lectures and became an agent through which to propagate his sanitary doctrines. His lectures frequently relied on the martial metaphor's appeal to pathos. In a speech given to the Ladies' Sanitary Association in 1859, "The Massacre of the Innocents," Kingsley calls on women to act in place of and against a stagnant government to protect the English race—beginning with the children—against disease. He hyperbolizes the effects and difficulties of fighting disease in contrast to fighting a military force; disease, represented as "Nature has no protocols, nor any diplomatic advances, whereby she warns her enemy that war is coming . . . she kills, and kills, and kills, and is never tired of killing."[61] He continues: "We talk of the loss of human life in war. We are fools of smoke and noise; because there are cannon-balls forsooth, and swords, and red coats, and because it costs a great deal of money. . . . What [is] so terrible as war? I will tell you what is ten times, and ten thousand times, more terrible than war, and that is outraged Nature" (*MOI*, 152). Kingsley entreats the women in his audience to understand their work in martial terms like Florence Nightingale. The seeming contrast between war and medicine reinscribes the martial metaphor by positioning disease as a much more dangerous threat than any human or national enemy, a recurring rhetorical framing. Disease was more dangerous than a traditional enemy, Kingsley argued, because: "Nature, insidious, inexpensive, silent, sends no roar of the cannon, no glitter of arms to do her work; she gives no warning note of preparation, nor any diplomatic advances, whereby she warns her enemy that she is coming . . . but quietly, by the very same mean by which she makes alive she puts to death; and so avenges herself against those who have rebelled against her" (*MOI*, 152). His lecture draws on and instills anxieties about military conquest by disease, which has no rules. Death by disease thus becomes the mass murder of innocent children, a pervasive trope in Kingsley's speeches, as does the comparison between nature in the form of disease and war. The steps he takes to construct this figuration are quite complex: first, Kingsley uses nature as a metonym for disease, which, as discussed in the concluding section of this chapter, involves its connection to original sin. Next, he structures the conceptual metaphor so that *disease is an enemy* becomes a hypernym of the larger metaphoric system of *medicine is war*. Finally, having equated medicine to war, Kingsley seemingly discounts his original premise by suggesting that a war against disease is more dangerous than a war against humans. This construction, then, further naturalizes the martial metaphor by obscuring the fact that the original equation of medicine and war was, in fact, a metaphor. In the context of a lecture, that naturalization appeals to emotion by heightening the threat of disease. Kingsley plays on the assumed maternal instincts of the audience by saying that they are either a part of or the solution to "the massacre of the innocents" or a part of the problem.

The way Kingsley describes Nature's ferocity and murderousness with respect to gender is not unlike Florence Nightingale's equation of poor ventilation with a crime akin to murder.

> A short time ago a man walked into a back-kitchen in Queen square, and cut the throat of a poor consumptive creature, sitting by the fire. The murderer did not deny the act, but simply said, "It's all right." Of course he was mad. But in our case, the extraordinary thing is that the victim says, "It's all right," and that we are not mad. Yet, although we 'nose' the murderers, in the musty unaired unsunned room, the scarlet fever which is behind the door, or the fever and hospital gangrene which are stalking among the crowded beds of a hospital ward, we say, "It's all right."[62]

On these terms, women are empowered to adopt heroic subjectivities like "soldier" and "doctor" by protecting the innocent against disease. Also drawing on the pathos invoked by murder with respect to infectious disease, Tom indignantly contends that cholera is "always someone's fault: and if death occurs, someone ought to be tried for manslaughter—I had almost said for murder" (*TY*, 281). Kingsley deployed the same appeal to pathos a year after the novel's publication in an anonymous piece for *Frasier's Magazine*, where he chastises hypocrisy, misplaced attention, and the kind of telescopic philanthropy so memorably distilled in the caricature of *Bleak House*'s Mrs. Jellyby, vis-à-vis sanitary reform: "That ten thousand or one thousand innocent people should die, of whom most, not all, might be saved alive, would seem at first sight a matter serious enough for 'philanthropists.'" He continues, arguing that they, "demand mercy for the Sepoy and immunity for Coolie, unsexed by their own shameless and brutal cruelty, would, one fancies, demand mercy also for the British workman, and immunity for his wife and family." Putting this idea in similar terms as Nightingale and Tom's inimicalization and criminalization of disease, he concludes, "One is therefore somewhat startled at finding that the British nation reserves to itself, though it forbids to its armies, the right of putting to death unarmed men, women, and children."[63] In this analogy, the mismanagement of the house doesn't only symbolically stand in for the nation, it synecdochally marks the family as the second organizational tier, one scale up from the individual, that grounds the nation's vitality.[64] Thus, despite empowering women, the analogies made by Kingsley and Nightingale also implicate women as accomplices to murder when they do not practice sanitary principles. This disciplinary function made women responsible agents who could save lives but also facilitate death by making mistakes, not following assigned protocols, or straying too far from the home and the nation.

If, as Foucault writes in *The Birth of the Clinic*, "The struggle against disease begins with a war against bad government,"[65] then, for Kingsley, the war began in the household with the deployments of Nightingalian principles. Women must arrange, inculcate, and police proper sanitary conditions, whether in a battlefield hospital, a civilian hospital, or at home; as such, they support patriarchal medicine's interventions for fighting disease. The relationship between women and medicine, however, was more complicated than simple straightforward support. Kingsley suggests that "The private correspondence, private conversation, private example, above all, of married women, of mothers of families, may do what no legislation can do" (*MOI*, 148). In this paradigm, women must use their influence in the domestic sphere to actualize their "natural share in the sacred office of healer" (*SOH*, 22), and it is through their distributed microcenters of power that they can set sanitary reforms in motion from the ground up.

In *Two Years Ago*, Grace wholeheartedly accepts the selfless vocation of nursing, readying herself to take orders from her superior: "Tell me what to do in this cholera, and I will do it, if I kill myself with work of infection!" (*TY*, 284). Her plea conflates the martial ethos of dying for one's country with that of a natural feminine healer. Kingsley's interpellation of women in a naturalized role as healers, furthermore, follows the mythic narrative of Secretary of War Sidney Herbert's request for Florence Nightingale to go to Crimea to help the sick soldiers being treated in unsanitary conditions. Using the influence that she gained from her work in Crimea, Nightingale finally convinced the government to send a commission to find the nidus of disease. The commission addressed the cesspools in Sebastopol and Scutari, in addition to other hygienic concerns. Not all women would have produced Nightingale's effect, which is not to say that Kingsley's ideals relied solely on women for their enactment. Kingsley empowered women to use their roles as maternal healers to become self-driven cogs powering his medico-military machine. In the military, male physicians needed nurses to do much of the manual patient labor and almost all of the sanitary work while they focused on surgery and physic. The practice carried over into the nursing and sanitary reforms that contributed to the creation of civilian hospitals where the martial residue of the female role became more metaphorical and less literal. The military and civilian nurse in the Nightingale image performs sanitary work and fulfills a supportive role in the home, fighting disease preemptively. Furthermore, by positioning nurses as domestic superintendents, the nursing model empowers women to surveil not only biological but also moral hygiene. The militancy created from a composite of the nurse and the domestic woman was central to the medicalization of the household and its simultaneous extension to the social body. Grace's subjectivity modeled Nightingale's well-known disciplinary and military surveillance practices and attitudes regarding medical care. Nightingale's pedagogy was based on a kind of military fitness. "We shall be poor soldiers indeed, if we don't train ourselves for battle," she instructed.[66] Moreover, Nightingale explicitly linked medicine and disease with national interests through the martial metaphor: "And shall we not fight to save? [sic] to save our homes our country, from disease, from cholera? Let us all fight: every man and woman of us—shoulder to shoulder, every citizen and every countryman and every woman, to our duty and our flag!"[67] Nightingale's domestic ideal fostered the reproduction of that ideology in future generations by modeling and inculcating proper femininity for daughters to emulate and sons to seek out. Kingsley adopted Nightingale's paradigm in order to expound on the kind of femininity that could mend a troubled nation fighting endemic epidemics.

Grace embodies multiple dimensions of proper femininity while emblematizing the martial metaphor in the Nightingalian capacity of being a surveilling and supportive military agent, teacher, and muse. She works as a nurse both in the climatic cholera epidemic in Aberalva and afterward, when she leaves for the war to use her nursing skills to help the British. In Aberalva, Grace acts as a supportive agent for Tom, seeking out cases of cholera and being the only explicitly named woman in the medico-military unit visiting each house: "Headley and Campbell, Grace and old Willis, and last, but not least, Tom Thurnall—these and three or four brave women, organised themselves into a right-gallant and well-disciplined band" (*TY*, 362). She is also identified as the presumed leader of the unnamed brave women following the Nightingalian paradigm. In her position as a schoolteacher, furthermore, she fulfils Kingsley's educational role for women. He argues that health classes should be taught by women to educate young men and women to "not only to take care of themselves, and their families, but to exercise moral influence over their fellow-citizens, as champions in the battle against dirt, drunkenness, disease, and death" (*SOH*, 22).

Grace functions as an intersection between the single household and the nation; she helps alleviate disease in the military, and when she finds Tom, she rehabilitates him, inspiring within him the acceptance of God's grace and guidance.[68] Her role in aiding Tom in his personal evolution aligns with her being likened to Nausicaa (*TY*, 80), just as Kingsley compares Tom to Ulysses. Nausicaa is the Phoenician princess who sees and cleans up the savage-looking, shipwrecked Ulysses to make him presentable. Like Nausicaa, Grace domesticates Tom, making him acceptable to middle-class propriety and tempering the more untamed facets of his masculinity. She reins in the unwieldy aspects of Tom's liberal subjectivity, including his uninhibited masculine self-assertiveness, which, up until the moment he declares his love for Grace, operates without concern for a higher power, namely a Christian God. Tom's activities as a spy and his self-assertiveness land him in a Turkish prison before he reaches Crimea. There he is broken, like the British Army, at the hands of the Russians and cholera. But the defeat of his excessive entrepreneurial individualism allows him to find a new sense of purpose through his wife-to-be's guidance.[69] With respect to actual public health, Kingsley's reliance on the roles of the middle-class male professional hero and the domestic wife and nurse in his novels worked in conjunction with his lectures to mobilize the nation after Crimea. Beyond, but still congruent with his social constructions of gender, Kingsley also relied on theological discourse to make the medico-military war palatable for the nation, rendering war against disease coterminous with the struggle for the Christian soul.

God's Breath: Original Sin, Inimical Nature, and Biopolitics

Kingsley's reconciliation between the material causes of disease and divine intervention in the form of pestilence was a structuring tenet of his deployment of the martial metaphor. By registering with both religious and naturalist worldviews, subjects could gain material agency without letting go of long-held religious beliefs and regulatory apparatuses could draw on religious discourse to produce subjects. Kingsley's ability to operate in both religious and biological discourses gave his use of the martial metaphor extraordinary appeal for a broad audience. The various genres and modes Kingsley utilized magnified this effect. With respect to his fiction, one reviewer of *Two Years Ago* notes that through the novel, Kingsley "obtained a wider audience . . . [M]ultitudes, who would never open an essay of the present state on the world, or the incumbent duties of their generation."[70] For Kingsley, though, the medico-military war had two fronts in the context of Christianity. The first was an affirmative theology and biopolitics that produced health by fighting original sin, the inimical potentiality for disease, and the spiritual analog of the biological seeds of death by infectious disease, miasma, and filth. The second was the battle to undermine the conservative, extremist religious viewpoints that failed to adopt sanitary science and its accompanying agency in producing health.

Read in the context of his 1849 sermon on cholera, Kingsley's novel sutures cholera and war through the intersections of religion and the state. Both the cholera epidemics and the Crimean War proved so socially and politically destabilizing that they prompted national days of humiliation: times of prayer, thanksgiving, and fasting. National fasts and prayers were ordered during the first and second cholera epidemics and during the Crimean War by either the Privy Council or the Queen.[71] In a sermon for the national day of humiliation held at the end of the second cholera epidemic and drafted as part of his pamphlets for Crimean soldiers, Kingsley preached the following: "The Cholera is sent on all those judgments of God [which] are sent, to this life and search men's hearts and set their sins before their face, so they cannot mistake them . . . It will be much better for us then if the Cholera, or Famine, or War, or anything on the face of Earth, however dreadful should come upon us if it did but reach us [to] see what we had done."[72] Kingsley suggests that cholera and war are both entities that show men their sins, allowing men to redeem themselves and, as Gilbert suggests, evolve for the better.[73] As noted by another reviewer, that proposition follows Kingsley's purpose in *Two Years Ago*: to "make known, to all men, his conviction that out of this fiery purgation this noble land has come ennobled, purified, and made stronger, and braver and better."[74] Here, the link between war and medicine speaks to the kind of original sin that leaves an individual prey to disease: the sin of failing to understand that life is war and subsequently taking the appropriate measures to be purged, spiritually and physically. To this effect, the martial metaphor became an instrument to shape the evolution of the self and the nation.

Kingsley's war against disease is, in effect, a war against biological forces. He takes the struggle between life and death beyond Bichat's resistance. Utilizing the figuration of war, Kingsley makes it an active fight by envisioning death, a function of nature, as an enemy that conducts a perpetual siege on life. He posits the figuration of war on a synecdochal relationship between disease and nature, whereby nature is a metonym for disease that acts in martial capacities: "Nature . . . gives no warning note of preparation . . . but quietly, by the very same mean by which she makes alive she puts to death" (*MOI*, 152). Kingsley draws attention, as he did in his lecture to the Ladies' Sanitary Association, to how disease attacks without warning. Nature is contrasted with an implied proper enemy who would signal an impending attack by making a declaration of war. Kingsley unpacks the materialism inherent in humankind's medical war against nature and provides a solution: "Nature is only conquered by obeying her" (*MOI*, 152). He uses similar phrasing in one of his pamphlets for the soldiers in Crimea, aptly titled, "Earthly and Heavenly Wisdom, Or Stoop to Conquer."[75] In his understanding of nature and human agency, Kingsley empowers soldiers and female sanitarians to be on the front lines of the war against disease and to understand their enemy in a material capacity.

In "The Massacre of the Innocents," Kingsley goes on to define the particular kind of war that nature wages, ultimately forging a contradictory image: "Man has his courtesies of war because he spares the unarmed man; he spares the woman and child." Nature, by contrast, is red in tooth and claw, "as fierce when she is offended, as boisterous and kind when she is obeyed. Silently she strikes the sleeping babe, with as little remorse as she would strike the strong man, with the spade or musket in his hand" (*MOI*, 152). This trope of medicine as the ur-war, orders of magnitude greater in terms of mortality when compared to combat itself, is in line with Lyons's contention in *Treatise on Fever*, that deaths in battle "reap but a small harvest of death when compared with the long black list of mortality which the rolls of disease furnish in such fatal abundance."[76] For Kingsley, the war against nature is *worse* than actual warfare because nature uses guerrilla tactics, killing the sleeping child, worker, farmer, and soldier alike rather than following a chivalric military custom between enemies, such as lines fighting face to face on the battlefield or showing respect for civilian life.

One logical implication of medicine being a more terrible military endeavor than traditional war in Kingsley's invocation is that citizens should not use conventional weapons and tactics, and should instead advocate for the new medical model put forth by the sanitarians involving hygiene, infrastructure, statistics, surveillance, and other biopolitical technologies; those methods aim to halt disease at the source rather than relying on brute, overt military tactics like attempting to cordon it once it had already spread. Kingsley's characterization of nature as an inimical force follows a Bichatian logic of resistance but specifies that people must have warlike mind-sets to resist death and disease, as nature both gives and takes life.

Kingsley's feminization of Nature is further indicative of the uneven relationship between male liberal subjects and female sanitary agents. His contentions that Nature gives life only insofar as she is obeyed, and that when obeyed she is conquered, suggest that the male subject's health, and by extension the nation's, very much depends on his ability to understand Kingsley's estimation of the laws of femininity. Women both give birth and conduct the domestic labor and sanitary efforts that allow men to be healthy and productive in the public sphere. Women, in Kingsley's logic, must themselves be conquered medically and religiously, taking their proper places within the social order and the medico-martial infrastructure lest they become enemies of state health in the form of prostitutes or "redundant women," as liberal manufacturer W. R. Greg would say.[77] That uneven relationship is a problem Bram Stoker encounters toward the end of the century in his writing of the martial metaphor, drawing from the consequences of the military medical concerns of Kingsley's epoch.

The relationship between men, women, and Nature is indicative of how Biblical allusion in Kingsley's prose justifies a bellicose definition of life. His conceptualization of life as a war on nature operates within the framework of an Edenic narrative.

> Your bodies are dead by reason of sin, and in the midst of life we are in death. There is a seed of death in you and me and every little child. While we are eating and drinking and going about our business, fancying that we cannot help living, we carry the seeds of disease in our own bodies, which will surely kill us some day, even if we are not cut off before by some sudden accident. That is true, physicians know that it is true. Our bodies carry in them from the very cradle the seeds of death; and therefore it is not because God leaves us alone that we live. We live because God, our merciful heavenly Father, does not leave us alone, but keeps down those seeds of disease and death by His Spirit, who is the Lord and Giver of Life. (*MOI*, 131)

The figuration of the seed of death corresponds to the Fall, which, stemming from the Tree of the Knowledge of Good and Evil, made man and woman mortal and thus susceptible to disease. Kingsley expands on that connection at length in his sermon "The Fall."[78] He equates the failure to fight death and disease with resignation to man's concupiscent condition, the diseased state of the soul tainted by original sin.[79] Disease is Sin's pathogenic progeny. Kingsley's deployment of the martial metaphor reveals how making live entails taking defensive and offensive actions against pathogenic agents that are a reality of nature, rather than simply trying to pray disease away. Yet to help the most people live, the same apparatuses must "let die." As Gilbert suggests in her reading of *Two Years Ago*, through the survival of nations and the human species, "maladaptive 'scar tissue' die[s] and must be sloughed."[80] The novel's narrative closure reflects Gilbert's interpretation: the characters who do not conform to Kingsley's sanitary laws or gender norms, such as the effeminate, opium-addicted Elsey Vavasour, do not survive the cholera epidemic, while the strong characters—like Tom and Grace—marry and reproduce. The seeds of death and disease, as described in Kingsley's lectures, inflect the concept of Bichat's resistance into a war for the production of life. In order to form resistant rather than maladaptive tissue, individuals need guidance in self-fashioning a life against sin and disease.

That specification of resistance into war not only reconciles theology with pathology; it also validates the very work and rhetoric of Kingsley's writings. For if God keeps men alive for the purpose of saving them in the same way that a father protects his children from "danger they cannot see,"[81] then the allusion to God as a father connects to Kingsley and his position as an Anglican clergyman. The role of a clergyman, an analog of God's relationship to all Christians, helped shape conductible, self-driven populations. The reference to a father keeping his children safe and the very mode of Kingsley's address also speaks to the Christian pastoral role and its function in biopolitics. The significance of that connection lies in the Christian pastorate's role as a precursor to governmentality.[82] The postulation of divine support conjoined with taking personal responsibility for health was a way for Kingsley to resist the punitive and unproductive implications of forestalling human agency. The purely punitive model, on which disease was the result of divine agency, operates analogously to Foucault's juridical apparatus: an unproductive exercise of power through which life is not made but simply taken when deployed on its own.

In contrast to the punitive model of the divine taking of life, Kingsley suggests that God forestalls disease through his spirit. God's spirit or breath, which exists in a directly antagonistic relationship to miasmic pestilence, inspires and inculcates a discipline that can produce a subject who fulfills God's desire that humans *make themselves* to "make live."[83] Although the metaphysical dimensions of this argument involve an abstract-seeming notion of causality, the disciplinary model of fighting the seeds of mortality encouraged Christians to actualize hygienically productive subjectivities by grounding them in the material world. Kingsley formulated God's breath as an anti-miasmic agent in the religious allegory of good versus evil within which the human body and the community form a battleground. For this paradigm to operate, however, evil must be represented by an embodied agent like miasma rather than an abstract concept like original sin. Here, miasma is evil, but still a part a nature and of man's own making. Following Nightingale and other sanitarians' focus on air quality, Kingsley uses breath as a conceit to work through the discursive amalgam of disease, miasma, sin, life, and death.

In "The Two Breaths," Kingsley constructs a dialectic of exhalation and inhalation premised on disease and death being already imbricated within life.[84] He writes, "The breath which you give out is an impure air, to which has been added, among other matters which will not support life, an excess of carbonic acid. . . . I beseech you to remember at least these two—oxygen gas and carbonic acid gas; and to remember that, as surely as oxygen feeds the fire of life, so surely does carbonic acid put it out."[85] Basic chemistry and physiology explain the double bind in the life-and-death binary: exhalation, while a natural process, is essentially a gaseous excrement. It is similar to the dialectic of life and death in which life eventually leads to and produces death. Kingsley understood the exchange between life and death via the concept of fire, a symbol of the Holy Spirit and the physical touchstone of God's breath—oxygen. His figuration of fire is one of the clearest examples of his ideological reconciliation of the spiritual and the material in terms of miasmic disease. Fire represents God's spirit but is also a material reality that is emblematic of the life given by God's breath. Like breath, fire resists its own death by consuming oxygen and moves toward death by producing carbon dioxide. Relating the metaphorical life of fire back to material biological life, Kingsley gives an example of an experiment in which a mouse placed in a box will ultimately die by its own breath.

The practical advice Kingsley gives women in "The Two Breaths" reflects his spiritual focus in his village sermon "Life and Death," where he preached: "The [Bible] tells us, God takes away breath, and turns His face from him. In His presence, it is written, is life. The moment

He withdraws his Spirit, the Spirit of life, from any thing [sic], body or soul, then it dies. It was by sin came death—by man's becoming unfit for the Spirit of God. Therefore the body is dead because of sin, says St. Paul, doomed to die, carrying about in it the seeds of death."[86] In this way, death and disease were not a natural state in the prelapsarian world, a contention that Kingsley echoes in numerous other sermons. Accepting God's natural laws is part of a general Christian framework for the production of a viable subjectivity in which the individual is inspired by anti-miasmic agency that provides defense in a fallen world. God offers the material breath of life—oxygen, and the body to metabolize it—and also spiritual breath, the inspiration to live according to natural and hygienic laws.

Ultimately, Kingsley's conceptualization of how individuals should and should not understand their relationship with God is analogous to the different paradigms of state power. Kingsley insists that humans should not conceptualize God in a purely juridical or punitive capacity. God does not only punish and take away life; rather, God's primary aim, and the imperative that individuals should adopt, is viability.

> When we talk of being 'ushered into the presence of God,' we mean dying; as if we were not all in the presence of God at this moment, and all day long. When we say, 'Prepare to meet thy God,' we mean 'Prepare to die'; . . . our notion is this—that this world is a machine, which would go on very well by itself, if God would but leave it alone. . . . Ah! blind that we are; blind to the power and glory of God which is around us, giving life and breath to all things. . . . Because we will not believe in a God of love and order, we grow to believe in a God of anger and disorder. Because we will not fear a God who sends fruitful seasons, we are grown to dread a God who sends famine and pestilence. . . . [W]e believe in Him only as the destroyer. We have forgotten that He is the Giver, the Creator, the Redeemer.[87]

By arguing that people should focus on a god of "love and order" rather than a god of "anger and disorder," and pointing out that the thought of God was tied to the thought of "prepar[ing] to die" rather than continuing to live, Kingsley suggests that Christianity must produce life in the face of death. This is precisely the same kind of paradigm shift that led to the emergence of biogovernance and the change from epidemic to endemic thinking at the end of the eighteenth century, according to Foucault who argues, "Death was no longer something that swooped down on life—an epidemic. Death was now something permanent, something that slips into life, perpetually gnaws at it, diminishes it and weakens it."[88] The institution of hygienic subjectivities and the implementation of sanitary reform were ways to mitigate the permanence of death, working, in Kingsley's logic, as technologies of governmentality. The threat of disease became perpetual but much less spectacular when it was conceptualized as a state of permanent siege rather than a singular event. Consequently, the fight against disease was a matter of everyday conduct, of everyday life.

Two Years Ago links the reconciliation of material biology with Christian doctrine in Kingsley's lectures and sermons. For example, in the chapter "Baalzabub's Banquet," there is a perceptible shift in the narrator's tone while describing the cholera epidemic. After opening with medical facts that portray the exponential growth of the disease, the chapter shifts rapidly to Biblical figurations reminiscent of Revelation: "The next day there were three cholera cases: the day after there were thirteen. He had come at last, Baalzabub, God of flies, and of what flies are bred from; to visit his self-blinded worshippers, and bestow on them his own Cross of the Legion of Dishonour" (*TY*, 258). This metaphor serves two functions: first, it constructs a general image of miasma as a figure of evil through an allusion to disease and putrefaction; second, it vilifies the conservative theology that subscribes to a God of punitive rather than productive biopolitics, a deity who punishes and kills rather than creating and inspiring life and health. Baalzabub is a fitting emblem for cholera, insofar as he is the "the lord of flies," a phrase that connotes evil, disease, and decay. The allusion follows William Farr's model of zymotic disease, in which miasma emanated specifically from putrefying organic material as a kind of fermentation. In this etiology, death is both a cause and an effect of sickness: it produces corruption and decay, leading to corrupt air, which in turn infects the living. This masculine form of Baalzabub is congruent with Kingsley's gendering of Nature. The coupling of Baalzabub and the feminized "Nature" forms a perverse inversion of the ideal hygienic pairing of man and woman. In a configuration similar to Milton's Satan and Sin parenting of Death in *Paradise Lost*, in Kingsley's allegory, filth copulates with the material conditions of Nature's laws (fermentation and decomposition) to breed disease in the human frame. As a miasmic form, Baalzabub, therefore, works in opposition to God's spirit, as the word *spirit* not only evokes breath but carries the meaning of its Latinate root *spirare*: to breathe. Beyond his origins as a fallen angel that rebelled against God, Baalzabub is figured martially. He bestows on his followers military honors: "the Cross of the Legion of Dishonour." Moreover, to personify disease as the Devil is to position it in diametric opposition to God. The idea of God's work as an anti-miasmic, inspirational agent directly contrasts Kingsley's theory of disease with theologies that saw it as an unchallengeable judgment from God, something that could only be accepted in a kind of Jobian capacity.

For Kingsley, then, part of the medico-military war was to be waged against misguided Christian theology. Baalzabub's "self-blinded worshipers" were those who wrongfully interpreted disease as a divine punishment that could be alleviated only by prayer. In the novel, those people appear as a collection of devout and dissident Methodists who become worshipers of Baalzabub insofar as they refuse to help the sick, assuming that sick people deserve the punishment they receive from God.[89] The most explicit example of the religious belief in deserved disease is a Methodist preacher for whom cholera is "God's wrath," and who claims that it is "impious to interfere" (*TY*, 365). He holds that pious Christians can pray to God to end the epidemic but fighting it more directly would be resisting God's will. In the novel, Major Campbell breaks up the preacher's sermon just as Tom notices the symptoms of cholera rapidly taking hold of him; the preacher dies two hours later, becoming a culpable casualty—part of the "tissue that must be sloughed." Whether the "self-blinded" do nothing out of a sense of divine justice or out of blind faith that God will protect them, they neglect the material conditions of existence and allow filth to compound. In an earlier scene, Tom and Major Campbell help the local Anglican curate, Frank, in his "crusade against the Dissenters." Frank had previously failed in his crusade because he was "not overtly manly" and was insufficiently assertive in leading his flock and fighting blasphemy (*TY*, 254). In the Baalzabub passage, the war against disease is cast as a crusade when the enemy is identified as not just filth, but also heathen.

It is important to note that the word *heathen* refers less to divergent sects than to the conservative and extremist Christian clergy who would not take account of modern sanitation science in their theology. Tom confronts those nonbelievers because they are not just harming themselves but spreading their ideas among the townsfolk. Tom's actions link the work of the clergyman with that of the doctor, a position that Kingsley also endorsed in "The Physician's Calling" where he argued that "the clergy should as much as possible be physicians; the physician, as much as possible, a clergyman" (PC, 22). According to Kingsley, physicians and clergymen must work together to produce health and virtue in the general population's bodies and souls. This is precisely why Kingsley used *Two Years Ago*, with its medical protagonist, alongside lectures and sermons, to affirm productive biopolitics and promote the idea that individuals should actively fight death rather than resign themselves to it. This is how Kingsley resolves the seeming contradiction between Christianity's acceptance of death and the reality of infectious disease. His theology was based on humans sharing a biopolitical relationship with God, a relationship that functioned both as humanity's primary weapon in the war against disease and as a productive form of the power to live hygienically. The martial metaphor became, therefore, a way for Kingsley to constitute a Christian, a national, and a biological social body simultaneously; it was an imperative that developed constitutively with England's essential bellicose identity.

Of course, God's breath cannot forestall death permanently. Kingsley believed in the noble efforts of physicians holding the line as long as they could for their dying patients. Of those labors, he writes,

> in all those little efforts [the physician], so wise, so anxious, so tender, so truly chivalrous, to keep the failing breath for a few moments more in the body of one who had no earthly claim upon his care, that doctor was bearing a testimony, unconscious yet most weighty, to that human instinct of which the Bible approves throughout, that death in a human being is an evil, an anomaly, a curse; against which, though he could not rescue the man from the clutch of his foe, he was bound, in duty and honour, to fight until the last, simply because it was death, and death was the enemy of man. (PC, 25)

Nevertheless, biological human frailty would ultimately overcome Kingsley's own good health, and his long battle to produce life would end in defeat. On his deathbed, Kingsley invoked the martial metaphor again. In *Charles Kingsley: His Letters and Memories of His Life*, edited by Kingsley's wife Fanny, she writes, "He promised his wife to 'fight for his life' for his children's sake, and he did so for some time; but the enemy or as he would have said to himself 'kindly Death' was too strong for him, and the battle was over."[90] Though this final resignation was an inevitability that Kingsley had clearly reconciled with his belief system—as evident in his qualification of death as "kindly"—he was ultimately memorialized by a codification of the martial metaphor. The metaphor was contagious, infecting not only the way his wife Fanny and his close friend Fredrick viewed health and sickness, but also, through his textual corpus, various groups of Britons. While knowing that defeat was inevitable—and that eternal life waited for true believers—Kingsley used the martial metaphor to create productive social subjects in one life while keeping an eye on the next.

In Kingsley's iteration, the martial metaphor proved able to draw from and be included in religious discourse while remaining grounded in the materiality of pathology. It could also create a productive form of empowerment, as it gave its subjects not only agency but a duty to the natural and social worlds. Making disease an enemy imposes a kind of order on the belief system, popular in previous centuries, by which fluctuations in human health were explained as divine punishment. Moreover, the martial metaphor imposed an order on disease itself, metaphorizing it as an entity before germ theory could explain and visually present disease through microscopy. This figurative embodiment provided a target for material practices. It gave subjects an object to fight against by adopting disciplinary techniques in the form of middle-class sanitary practices, which were conceptualized by physicians, politicized by prominent social figures, and deployed in the household by women. That fight against death involved not only the empowering right to govern one's own health and life, but also a duty to the larger social body. In these ways, the martial metaphor also appropriated original sin for the purpose of governmentality.

Contextualizing Kingsley within the codification of the martial metaphor changes the stakes of reading *Two Years Ago*. The novel indexes Kingsley's participation in the growth of the martial metaphor as a central conceptual paradigm for medical discourse. Kingsley was thus a prominent actor in the metaphor's emergence. While his novel provided an organizing logic for the larger archive of his deployment of the martial metaphor, it also further naturalized the metaphor, leading to the erasure of its metonymic connections to military medicine—a process reflected in the absence of direct Crimean action in the narrative. As evidenced by the relationship between Tom and Grace, his investment in military and sanitary reform found a mechanism for thriving on gender scripts like those of the domestic ideal and the military hero, all the while reconciling the contradictions between material disease etiology and the notion of divine intervention. By offering subjects a form of empowerment, the martial metaphor fueled an increasingly industrialized nation and expanding empire. His vision for the unification of the two "brothers of the nation" relied on the ruling classes making investments in the laboring population, investments involving infrastructure, public works, regulatory apparatuses for epidemiology such as statistical methods of tracking disease, and political interventions such as the Public Health Acts and the Sanitary Act.[91] The martial underpinnings of that form of self-governance made resignation to death in the everyday material practices of life—the care of the self, the hygiene of the family, and the subjectification of the self under the medical gaze—into a moral and political failure. In this sense, the martial metaphor was simultaneously a mechanism of empowerment and of control.

Kingsley's use of the martial metaphor also helped construct a regulatory apparatus with seemingly contradictory politics. On the one hand, it promoted the middle class's investment in the working class, which entailed seeking political reform, volunteering, and laboring to promote the health of the working class, as well as serving as models for working-class individuals to emulate. On the other hand, it empowered the working class to rely on themselves for their health: according to Kingsley, they should not "comfort [them]selves in [their] carelessness with the thought, 'if [sic] am sick, Parish must doctor me, if I starved Parish must feed me' . . . [for] so long as [they] do so [they] will be miserable."[92] By having it both ways, the system is reinforced from above and below. The subsequent production of working-class health was necessary to the middle class in terms of labor power for economic concerns. Because, after all, if the laboring class was laid low from cholera, who else would sail Jacob's ships and dig his mines?

Beyond concerns for labor power, however, other health economies of the middle class were also at stake in the espousal of the martial metaphor. The ethereal nature of miasma let it penetrate the boundaries of literal cordons and the urban development of class separation,[93] which all of London would experience during the Great Stink of 1858.[94] That event did not actually foster disease, but certainly fostered anxiety. As consequence of interest in sanitary reform, at least minimal health of the working class was required to control everyone's waste, labor performed by nightmen, and later, sewer-builders. As such, disease, whether associated directly with the poor and working class or indirectly with middle-class bodies, became "a problem of all." While still privileging and relying on middle-class male subjects, Kingsley's deployment of the martial metaphor cut across class and gender lines to unify the nation in the perpetual battle against death and disease. In the age of the germ and New Imperialism in the decades following the publication of *Two Years Ago* and the collections of his sanitary lectures, thinking of medicine as war became a way to respond to the ever-more-interconnected world.

PART 2

3

Military Pasts and Medical Futures in Bram Stoker's *Dracula*

The impact of the Crimean War on the medical profession, public health, and the martial metaphor did not end with Kingsley and cholera in the mid-century; it became enmeshed with fin-de-siècle microbial politics and New Imperialism. The British military's interest in the health of its soldiers developed into an emblematic instance of military medicine entering the civilian sphere: the Contagious Diseases Acts (CD Acts) of 1864, 1866, and 1869, passed in response to high rates of syphilis among enlisted men and allowed police to inspect and detain sex workers who were thought to be infected. The detention of suspected sex workers amounted to a quarantine system,[1] a materialization par excellence of the martial metaphor. Contextualizing the visible exercise of military force as a means of medical control allows us to see its influence on seemingly nonviolent yet coercive productions of health in modernity. In its representations of women's sexuality, disease, and the violent exercise of power, Bram Stoker's *Dracula* (1897) expressed, in part, a response to the military's medical politics pertaining to the CD Acts. In this way, though it was published almost four decades after *Two Years Ago*, *Dracula* bridges the martial metaphor from Kingsley to the authors who developed it in the age of germ theory and empire. The novel's representation of quarantine and reflection on the CD Acts highlight their violent, military qualities and signals the punitive and violent practices that underlie the martial metaphor. The entire novel documents the shifting contests between the Crew of Light and Dracula, ranging from weapons to history. *Dracula*'s simultaneous antiquity and modernity, in particular, is one of the dimensions that makes it a unique cultural production for translating medicine into war. In responding to the military and medical discourse of its past and present, *Dracula* helped shape the cultural history of the martial metaphor. Repackaging those histories in a temporally dialectical form, the novel reinforced the metaphor's urgency and rhetorical force at the turn of the century.

Attending to the text's place in the history of metaphorically militarizing medicine brings renewed exigence to the readings of empire, gender, race, and science that have long interested Victorian studies scholars. It asks us to consider how these perspectives might come to bear on the bellicose figuration that continues to structure medical responses to an increasingly globalized, microbial world more than a century later: the anxiety of the primitive, colonized world invading the civilized; degeneration; the decline of women's sexual purity; the colonial logics that drew from and influenced both discourses of race and disease, justifying xenophobic stereotypes; and, how middle-class masculinity and professional expertise created a fantasy of control.[2] In this vein, the novel is, indeed, "an allegory that helps construct a future its own narrative could be seen to reflect."[3] *Dracula* helped fashion a modern medical future by mediating a militant past.

Though chapter 4 deals with germ theory more expansively, it is important to historicize the years leading up to *Dracula*'s publication to see how its use of folklore and national and medical history carries a new symbolic weight when disease qua enemy was reimagined in the form of the microbe. Stoker was well positioned to imbue his Gothic novel with the most up-to-date medical science. He was well-versed in the field, given his family's experience in the medical profession. Most critics believe that he consulted his brothers, both of them medical practitioners—one of them, a military surgeon—while writing the novel.[4] Beyond Stoker's immediate relations, however, during the time of *Dracula*'s composition and publication, germs were certainly in the air, and everywhere else.

A brief survey of medical and popular prose of the late nineteenth to the early twentieth century demonstrates how germ theory gave the metaphor increased traction. The metaphor appeared more often during that era and became a recurring titular frame in the periodical press in articles such as: "The Battle of Life" (1896), "Unseen Enemies" (1899), "The War against Disease" (1899), and "How London Fights the Microbe" (1899).[5] In medical publications, especially printed versions of state-of-the-field addresses given to professional bodies like the Royal College of Surgeons and the London School of Tropical Medicine and Hygiene, the metaphor repeatedly appears as a governing thematic.[6] With Robert

Koch's detection of various pathogenic bacteria and publication of his Postulates with Friedrich August Johannes Loeffler (1884), and Louis Pasteur's research on fermentation, vaccination, and anthrax, it would seem that germ theory exorcized religious and superstitious explanations from disease.[7] Similar to Kingsley's rebukes of theocratic supplication to disease, one bacteriologist writes in his appropriately titled article, "The War against Disease" (1903) that "Until a somewhat recent period many devout persons sincerely believed plagues and pestilences to be a provision on the part of Providence."[8] Likewise, writing in 1887, the year of Koch's discovery of the tuberculosis bacterium, Ernest Wende, a well-known American dermatologist, aptly noted the shift from Bichatian theories of histological inflammation and lesion to the visible identification of pathogens by the microscope: "The day of judging disease solely by signs is past. The cure on general principles, of combating inflammation, of allaying irritation, has given place to the mere sound treatment of the structural alterations of the diseased cutis and its source. The diagnostic value of [a bacterial disease's] disenchantment, is beyond all controversy."[9] If germ theory's evincible causal agent disenchanted medicine from the supernatural, the central role of the martial metaphor reenchanted it with a composite of other narratives. In *Dracula* these narratives are varied but related: the reformulated binarism of good versus evil; the colonial grammars of conquest; the hierarchy of men over women; the differential logics of racial war; and the selective histories of England. Although the novel is clearly informed by the influence of modern germ theory at the fin de siècle, it also carries representations of earlier pregerm disease theories. As part 1 demonstrated, the martial metaphor has a literary, political, and medical history that precedes the age of the germ. Stoker's *Dracula* is no exception.

For a novel medical reading of *Dracula*, it is necessary to consider these preceding and contemporaneous disease theories, along with their ideological and political implications in the late nineteenth century. This chapter continues much of the criticism on the discrete etiologies represented in the novel while offering a more sustained study that integrates the material and metaphorical forms of violence the novel evokes.[10] In doing so, it parses the imposition of social order that scales from cell to nation, traversing through the bodies of women and foreigners by way of illicit sexuality and toxic degeneration. This temporal dialectic in *Dracula* condenses the narrative order imposed by the martial metaphor's aid in the construction of England as anthropocentrically sovereign, reflected in the novel's "triumphant unity" and investment in a reproductively viable futurity at its conclusion.[11] Moreover, given the novel's preoccupation with the act of writing, looking to *Dracula* provides unique insight into the fictionalization and abstraction of material violence and militarism into metaphor. Indeed, that simultaneous textual exposition and erasure of violence takes the form of a "transtemporal . . . entity that ruptures reproductive futurity, the basic foundation of the contemporary social structure."[12] Reading the blurring of conceptual and bodily boundaries that the Gothic does so well in these terms shows that while *Dracula* stoked the fire of militarizing medicine for nationalist, gendered, and colonial ends, it also laid bare the contradictions in this process—how late Victorian England failed to live up to the salubrity, identity, and hygienic progress on which the metaphor was constructed. In effect, tracking the martial metaphor in *Dracula* unearths the fallout wrought by Kingsley's *Two Years Ago* and the sanitary zeitgeist it embodied.

Considering that *Dracula* looks back to the earlier part of the century and before, we can understand the novel's dialectical relationship to time on three levels—the military, medical, and biopolitical—all of which form the conflict between the Crew of Light and the vampire. The Count is an archaic military antagonist, hailing from an ancient race of warriors, who infiltrates England as a pathogenic threat: a disease that threatens the reproduction of the middle class by infecting women's bodies while revealing the fragility of the Englishman's. In response, the Crew of Light employs violent and, ostensibly, medical means to stop the vampire, all while deploying both the language of war and the language of medicine to author their narrative supremacy. These medical and military discourses converge in the novel's representation of biopolitical governance and sovereign power. Stoker's articulation of the use of force in a medical and juridical capacity exposes the residual coercive sovereignty in late British modernity's sexual politics. In an idealized grand narrative of political progression, this "transtemporal incursion" intimates a regression from Kingsley's, who promoted the positive, productive exercise of governmentality for the formation of disciplined, hygienic subjectivities. However, understanding the history of the martial metaphor that *Dracula* narrates, and is itself part of, suggests that the violence of the *ancien régime* was never really gone but remained an underlying logic of public health's relation to the state, latently supported by thinking of medicine as war. By making the vampire and the struggle against him a metaphor, Stoker provided Victorian readers with conceptual distance from the very military histories and way of thinking he invokes. Thus, he effectively occludes the material history of the martial metaphor by sublimating the fear of the foreign and the sexually illicit along with infectious microbial disease and theories of degeneration into a single enemy.

I begin this chapter by showing how the Crew of Light self-identify as a military force, constructing their identity as heroes from a mythic British past. The novel's use of military language solidifies the discursive infrastructure of medical war, conflating biological and territorial invasion through the pathologization of the vampiric threat in specific, racial terms. The foreigner becomes an assailant to blood and soil. Next, I consider the representation of women's bodies as sites of contest. Accounting for the male protagonists' fight against a pathologized view of women's sexuality, I show how the history of the CD Acts transmute the incursion of military medicine in the civilian world into a metaphorical abstraction. In the third section, I discuss the overdetermined nature of Dracula's etiology, showing how old and modern conceptualizations of disease come together to agentify it, in the novel alone and in conversation with contemporaneous debates surrounding quarantine measures and smallpox. Following a discussion of the novel's references to bacteriology, I conclude by articulating how *Dracula* invokes the imperatives of tropical medicine through its representations of parasitology, laying the groundwork for how Conan Doyle and Conrad develop and respond to the martial metaphor in the wake of germ theory, the Boer War, and the Scramble for Africa.

Consecrating Blood and Soil

As an overdetermined anxiogenic figure, an amalgam of all that is Other, the vampire has a particular affinity with the mobilization of the martial metaphor. The male protagonists and their anxieties about reverse colonization and degeneration frame *Dracula* as a military medical narrative. Allusions to national histories for both Dracula and the Crew of Light are written in religious, military, and imperial terms. In contrast, the medical techniques and knowledge the protagonists employ represent the modern aspect of their work against the microbial and epidemic pathogenicity of vampirism. Examining the tension between the ancient and military and the modern and medical, exposes how the metaphor codes imperial threats into biology.

The male protagonists write of their undertaking as a medical war in their various letters, diaries, and communiques, praising each other as soldiers. When Dr. James Seward is unable to diagnose Lucy Westenra, he calls on his mentor Van Helsing, whom he espouses in an adornment of militaristic qualifiers. The Dutch physician has "an iron-nerve, a temper of the ice-brook, an indomitable resolution, [and] self-command."[13] "Temper of the ice-brook" is a misquotation of the description of the sword Othello uses to commit suicide: "A sword of Spain, the ice-brooks temper . . . a better never did itself sustain upon a soldier's thigh."[14] The reference to a military commander signals Van Helsing's leading role in the Crew of Light and imbues the iatric work with the connotations of combat. The play on *temper* suggests that Van Helsing's affect is cold and hard, that his mettle is as strong as tempered steel. These are ideal qualities for both the physician and the soldier who must make hard choices about life and death. In Lucy's case, it is whether to perform an experimental blood transfusion and, later, whether to decapitate her undead corpse. The framing of Van Helsing as a stoic, courageous soldier prefigures his ability to prescribe Lucy's posthumous mutilation with callous, clinical efficiency. After diagnosing vampirism, Van Helsing reaffirms that martial profile: "We shall all be informed as to [the] facts, and can arrange our plan of battle with this terrible and mysterious enemy" (*D*, 208). The scientific "facts" and logistical "plan," are narrativized through a crusading leitmotif. The martial self-identification of the doctors and professional men working against Dracula draws on military history, medieval romance, and the mythos of knighthood. Van Helsing likens the group specifically to Crusaders: "The old knights of the Cross. Like them we shall travel towards the sunrise; and like them, if we fall, we fall in good cause" (*D*, 278). Such an identification enfolds their contest in a nationalist cultural history. The cross referenced is St. George's flag, a component of the Union Jack adopted during the Third Crusade when St. George was exalted as a warrior saint. George, as the patron saint of England, is also a fitting military reference. He was a Roman soldier martyred for refusing to deny his Christianity and was mythologized in medieval romance for slaying a dragon—a clear analog for Dracula. The use of the red cross in the context of the spiritual and military rhetoric framing the Crew's "campaign," moreover, alludes to the Crusaders' retaking of the Holy Land from Islamic rule. In this vein, John Twyning suggests that "*Dracula* becomes the occasion for the characters to forge their own associations with history through the re-enactment of a popularly circulated version of the ancient or mythic past."[15] The past the Crew invokes, then, is religious, cultural, and territorial, giving symbolic weight to their mission.

Reviewers of the novel were also keen to point to its anachronistic dimensions, such as its references to the Crusades. One contributor from the *Spectator* contended that Stoker's story "would have been more effective if he had chosen an earlier period. The up-to-dateness of the book—the phonograph, typewriters, and so on—hardly fits with the medieval methods which ultimately secure victory for Count Dracula's foes."[16] This reviewer's appeal to contemporaneousness notwithstanding, the novel's anachronisms are quite suited to the cultural work of the martial metaphor. Mapping the temporal onto the spatial, the novel progresses toward reenacting the Crusading narrative as they track Dracula back to his homeland. While Dracula leaves London by ship on the *Czarina Catherine*, the Crew of Light travel by modern rail, following the route of the Orient Express, which opened in 1883 and became a popular tourist attraction of the "mysterious East." Centuries earlier, Northern European crusaders took the same route to reclaim the Holy Land.[17] The conclusion to their mythic narrative reinscribes the story of the Anglo-British colonizers overtaking the threat of reverse colonization, this time instigated by Dracula.[18] They chase the vampire home and invade his territory. By doing so, they take Mina's body back from foreign telepathic control and parasitic colonization, purging English territory and identity from vampiric infection.

The military discourse subtending the territorial and corporeal fight against Dracula is largely linguistic, but it is also logistical. The novel documents an assemblage of tracking—tracing the vampire's past to project his present and future actions. These practices are indicative of the British military's surveys and epidemiological cartography preceding and contemporaneous with Stoker. In the very beginning of the novel, Harker recounts his preliminary research on Transylvania conducted at the British Museum. He notes that he is "not able to light on any map or work giving the exact locality of the Castle Dracula, as there are no maps of this country as yet to compare with [British] Ordnance Survey maps" (*D*, 10). Like the Count's lineage and ties to his land, the Ordnance Survey has a long military history in the physical and imaginative constructions of Britain and its empire. The impetus behind the Ordnance Survey can be traced back the Jacobite Rebellion (1745–1755), when Lieutenant Colonel George discovered an inadequate cartographical survey of Scotland, leading to the creation of a topographical form for military intelligence. In 1791, the British Ordnance survey was established as a governmental agency to map England's southern coast in the face of French Invasion during the Napoleonic Wars. As the maps became a popular item and point of pride, the Ordnance survey remains a cultural icon of British identity into the twenty-first century.[19] The Ordnance Survey exemplifies how survey maps became central to the imagined community and development of empire in its post-Enlightenment aspiration for precision and "national power."[20]

Harker's seemingly minor reference to military maps, then, reflects both ideological and material connections between mapping, medicine, and war. Within the scope of the novel itself, it marks the epistemological site of contest between Dracula and the Crew of Light. In terms of the history of Victorian culture, the fact that a military technology, used for national defense and emerging from the strategic need to suppress rebellion, was translated into a widely circulated civilian text and became an icon of national identity follows the very same trajectory of the martial metaphor's movement from the military to the everyday. The survey and the martial metaphor, however, are not solely connected by way of analogy. The Ordnance Survey influenced a medical dimension of national protection, as the survey maps were utilized by sanitary reformers like Chadwick to plot London's topography over the developing drainage and sewage infrastructure.[21] Similarly, Charles Booth would use statistics from the 1881 census to map the "general condition of inhabitants" in certain neighborhoods.[22] The medical dimension of the maps speaks to the fact that while the maps served as tools for defense, they also exposed the nation's contours. For instance, in 1811 after an influx of tourism because of the maps' publication, they were withdrawn from sale as their circulation provoked concerns about national security.[23] The anxieties of exposing the nation's boundaries materialize in *Dracula*, as the contest between the foreign and the national and as a resonance of cholera's demonstrated social leveling. Dracula utilizes atlases of London to plan his biological reverse colonization, foreshadowed by Harker's observation that the Count's atlases "had been much used" (*D*, 29). Using maps, Dracula traverses sectional boundaries—from East to West, from Whitechapel to "fashionable London" in Piccadilly. These boundaries were believed to be cordons that delimited disease to certain neighborhoods in the mid-to-late-nineteenth century. The dissolution of preconceived boundaries previously justified through biological and social taxonomy aligns Dracula with cholera, a disease, as part 1 outlined, with military resonance in Victorian culture, and which itself spurred modern epidemiological mapping. Indeed, in a fitting parallel to Snow's discoveries during the 1854 Broad Street Epidemic, Dracula, like cholera, does not respect the social and classed borders that were imagined to be physical boundaries of disease. As the Crew collates their archive of information, they take to cartography to track his various safe houses.

Just as the map is a site of contests between Dracula and the Crew, so too are their histories and self-identification. As the target of the Crew's military campaign and epidemiological investigation, Dracula is a formidable antagonist. The representation of the Crew's mission as a crusade serves as a counterbalance to the Count's centuries-long maturation in *militares artes*. Analogous—and consequently then standing in opposition—to Seward's description of Van Helsing, the Count is "hard and warlike . . . [having] *more iron nerve*, more subtle brain, more braver heart, than any man" (*D*, 278, emphasis added). He also has considerable experience with political and military strategy: "in life" he was a "soldier [and a] statesman" (*D*, 263). Moreover, the Count's family history informs his martial prowess. Dracula's country had been a battleground for centuries.

> We Szekelys have a right to be proud, for in our veins flows the blood of many brave races who fought, as the lion fights, for lordship. . . . Here, in the whirlpool of European races, the Ugric tribe bore down from Iceland the fighting spirit which Thor and Wodin gave them, which their Berserkers displayed to such fell intent on the seaboards of Europe, ay, and of Asia and Africa too, till the peoples thought that the were-wolves themselves had come. Here, too, when they came, they found the Huns, whose warlike fury had swept the earth like a living flame, till the dying peoples held that in their veins ran the blood of those old witches, who, expelled from Scythia had mated with the devils in the desert. . . . What devil or what witch was ever so great as Attila, whose blood flows in these veins?" He held up his arms. "Is it a wonder we are the conquering race?" (*D*, 34)

Harker recounts pages of Dracula's genealogy in which the Count expounds further, giving away the secret of his age: "Was it not this

Dracula, indeed, who inspired that other of his race . . . who, when he was beaten back came again, and again, and again though he had come alone from the bloody field where his troops were being slaughtered?" (*D*, 35). Related to Attila, compared to the Norse Berserkers, and single-handedly taking down an army, Dracula is, indeed, a seemingly unstoppable military antagonist. Stoker's notes for the novel indicate that in addition to folklore and vampires, a significant portion of his research for the novel were the histories of war and invasion.[24] The Count's martial prowess and vampirism are related, entangled with his blood as a metonym for his lineage and pathogenesis. The combination makes him a dual threat: "Dracula's twin status as vampire and Szekely warrior suggests that for Stoker the Count's aggressions against the body are also aggressions against the body politic."[25] In other words, Dracula is a biopolitical threat both to the individual woman's body, as in the cases of Lucy and Mina, and to the greater population in precisely the manner of an infectious disease, as vampires "go on age after age, adding new victims and multiplying the evils of the world" (*D*, 190). Dracula threatens the nation not simply through direct destruction or the taking of life, but through a contagious, reproducible degradation that he fosters from within the nation itself. Consequently, he threatens England and Englishness. The Count himself uses a biological metaphor to describe his lineage's conquest: "The Szekelys—and the Dracula as their heart's blood, their brains, and their sword—can boast a record that mushrooms the Hapsburgs and the Romanoffs" (*D*, 35). Dracula's race dwarfs families whose long histories and rule would have been well known to the average Victorian reader. The mycological metaphor bespeaks the stamping out of one group over another through propagation and continuity in two dimensions. The Dracula supersede other races vertically, dominating and becoming the higher ruling order; they also outgrow them horizontally, through territorial conquest. Compounding these spatial metaphors, Dracula also overwrites the conquered race's history, rendering insignificant the English self-written plot in the face of his own.[26]

Dracula's military history, then, informs the viability of his racial invasion, one that codes Victorian anti-Semitic stereotypes and related xenophobic narratives. His military origins have been made resilient through generations of battle. As an inimical force, with morbid vampirism as his weapon, Dracula is a "technology of monstrosity," a conflation of all forms of otherness in his transgressions against English racial, sexual, class, and gender norms.²⁷ As Dracula comes from the East, it is no surprise that he colonizes the body of the aptly named Lucy Westenra. In attacking the middle-class woman's body, Dracula parasitizes the primary site of reproduction of the British race, compromising the stock of future generations.²⁸ The framing of Dracula as invasion, pollutant, and parasite stems in part from the anti-Semitic association of vampires with the East in the novel. Metaphors of blood and Jews as social parasites were prevalent in Victorian culture, especially in the 1890s. There are numerous references to stereotypes and cultural myths associated with Jews in Victorian culture, such as Dracula's hooked nose, hairy palms, and other "villainous" features, many of which were also associated with venereal disease.²⁹ Those phenotypic features of race drew on the contemporary rise of eugenic science. Eugenics was closely aligned with anti-Semitism, as physical traits were taken as signs of criminality on the basis of the pseudosciences of physiognomy and phrenology; the Jew was, in Sander Gilman's words, "medicalized."³⁰ *Dracula* borrowed from narratives describing the mixing of immigrants—specifically Eastern European Jews—in the East End of London. Like the foreigner—especially the Jew, and unlike the true Brit—the vampire emerges from a "whirlpool" of race. The Jew was often a stand-in for hereditary—reproducible—corruption, in the form of parasitism, criminality, weak constitution, sexual perversity, and other atavistic qualities that stood in contrast to the narrative of the British as the pinnacle of evolution.

Dracula mobilized the representation of racial difference as a medical disease. Eugenics, and the medicalization of race more broadly, drew on two of the most prominent narratives of decline in the nineteenth century: degeneration and reverse colonization. By the fin de siècle, the threat of degeneration of the "imperial race" loomed over Victorian culture.³¹ Degeneration denoted the deterioration or devolution of the human species. It was a prominent cultural and medical concern at the end of the century, following the publication of texts such as Max Nordau's *Degeneration* in 1892 and the work of Cesare Lombroso, Herbert Spencer, and Francis Galton. In *Dracula*, the Count, consistent with the novel's temporal ambiguity and blurring of conceptual boundaries, is both evolved and degenerate. He is "a brute" (D, 208) associated with animality—lions, bats, and rats—and, alluding to the popularity of anthropometrics, "is a criminal [that] has not a full man brain" (D, 296) but a "child brain"; yet, Van Helsing also acknowledges his cunning to "be the growth of ages" (*D*, 209), suggesting that Dracula's criminal and primitive acumen has been cultivated over time, making his evolved degeneration even more threatening.

Like Dracula's degeneracy and evolution, England is touted as being the pinnacle of modernity while at the same time suffering imperial decay. The fear of the civilized world falling to an incursion of primitive forces was expressed in terms of actual invasion, cultural decline, biological disease, and heredity. *Dracula* links all four of those registers through the figure of blood because it wasn't just that foreigners would bring disease; it was that by mixing with the population, they would pollute the British race itself, leading to its degeneration. For instance, Van Helsing claims that Dracula invades in the "wake of imperial decay" suggesting that vampires are associated with eroding national defense, "linked to military conquest and to the rise and fall of empires."[32] Thus, as in Shelley's *The Last Man*, militarism and imperialism play a role in disease. At the same time, that conflation in *Dracula* produces a vicious cycle: empire must be defended in the face of its own decay, conditions which the empire itself creates and exacerbates. By highlighting the biological weakness of the British race through narratives of invasion, the novel encourages a nationalistic urgency for medical protection, and offers the martial metaphor as a response.

The battle over racially appropriate blood is waged between the Crew of Light and Count Dracula on two main fronts: London and the middle-class woman's body. The battle evokes the connection between territorial and biological invasions—a consecration of blood and soil. The population, and more specifically women's fertility as the resource for reproductive futurity, is at stake. While Dracula wins the battle for Lucy's body, he ultimately leaves London and retreats to Transylvania. Similarly, when the protagonists invade his home territory and eradicate the Count, he loses control of Mina's body and she falls back under Seward and Van Helsing's medical control. The overdetermination of blood, or its functions of a nexus of anxieties regarding sex, race, and medicine,[33] provides Stoker the medium through which to amalgamate the orders of the body, the population, and national territory in a way that encodes seemingly temporally distinct forms of power and governance.

The first mode of contest between the Crew and Dracula is fought over and in women's bodies. The Crew's attack takes the form of the modern, still-experimental medical procedure of blood transfusion, conceptually linked to weaponry in the form of Seward's lancet—an icon of pre-twentieth-century medicine. Etymologically, that instrument of medical armamentarium has martial connotations as well. *Lancet* is the diminutive of *lance*, denoting both the weapon and the act of its use.³⁴ The lancet counters Dracula's fangs as well: both are piercing instruments; both have the function of breaking the skin and aiding in the transfer of blood—albeit in different directions. Dracula and the lancet are, in effect, pinned against each other in a fight over Lucy's body. While Dracula draws blood and introduces the vampirical agent, the lancet restores racially appropriate blood to counteract the vampire's corrupting infection. Early in the novel, Seward's nervous fiddling with the medical instrument foreshadows Lucy's execution. In a letter to Mina, Lucy foreshadows her impalement by the magnified lance—the stake: "[Seward] was very cool outwardly, but was nervous all the same . . . and then when he wanted to appear at ease he kept playing with a lancet in a way that made me nearly scream" (*D*, 58). Before the male protagonists enlist the violent "medieval" methods that "ultimately secure victory," as one reviewer noted, it is significant that they try to diagnose and treat vampirism in a medical capacity. Medical technologies, such as chloral hydrate, the hypodermic needle, and blood transfusion, are part of the larger "up-to-dateness" of the novel, like the typewriter, the phonograph, and the Kodak camera. The Crew's medical work complements the exceptional work of violence they exercise to ultimately treat the untreatable, undead Lucy and exterminate Dracula. However, the Crew's work is also narrative, insofar as they make legible the Count's movements, characteristics, and stratagems; they map and "arrange [their] plan of battle" (*D*, 208) through archiving and writing. In Choi's words, "Narrative serves as a crucial means by which these characters attempt to resist being engulfed by Dracula's counternarrative, and to insist upon the dominance of their own telling."³⁵ Understanding the Crew's work as narrative, medical, and violent, provides insight into how the martial metaphor worked in similar dimensions during the late-Victorian era.

The relationship between women's bodies and the nation, then, reflects the violent underpinnings of the martial metaphor's biopolitical function. *Dracula* presents the battle against vampirism in the form of both poles of biopower: the disciplinary techniques applied to individual bodies and the regulatory biopolitics of population, which together constitute race, nationhood, and security in the wake of the nineteenth century's endemicity. On the one hand, Mina is emblematic of the disciplinary apparatus in her attempt to maintain normative Victorian femininity.

She appropriately "confesses" the signs of Dracula's control over her and self-surveils under the auspices of hygiene when she denounces herself as "unclean," lamenting "that it should be that it is I who is now his worst enemy" (D, 248). On the larger scale of biopolitics, Van Helsing and the others work to regulate the population at large by preventing the spread of vampirism. The two levels of biopower converge on Lucy's and Mina's bodies as they become metonyms for the nation itself. The blood transfusion scenes entangle discourses of medical practice, racial purity, and sexuality in the form of war. Transfusion becomes an occasion for militarizing masculinity beyond the casting of a mere medical gaze; it allows for an exercise of force. The language of blood loss and sacrifice identifies the medical procedure in martial terms, as when Arthur valiantly declares that he "would give every last drop of blood in [his] body" to save Lucy (D, 113). The descriptions surrounding blood, and Arthur's in particular, are especially telling of the broader historical resonances of the violent exercises of force that scaffold modern biopolitical relations.

Arthur's blood retains the residue of older societal caste structures and power. As an aristocrat, his blood carries vestiges of the premodern era before the birth of biopolitics, carrying the symbolic value of a society in which power lay in the ability to spill blood through "the honor of war," in the "sovereign with his sword," and in the willingness to "risk one's blood."[36] The entire scene is subtended by the vocabulary of courage and violence, which imbues the action with the symbolic function of blood in the premodern world. The vampire is a figure of the feudal order and the old world in the cultural imaginary, as reflected in the genealogy Harker recounts early in the novel. By way of Lucy's infection and attempted treatment, Arthur risks his blood through a relatively new medical procedure.[37] Blood transfusions were not safe until the beginning of the twentieth century, making the scene with Arthur martially and medically heroic, heightening the risk and courage involved.

Because of Dracula's nightly feeding, Lucy needs multiple transfusions from the entire group of men, including the foreigners Quincy and Van Helsing. Although Arthur's blood is prioritized because it is aristocratic, it is worth noting that Quincy, Van Helsing, and Seward still fall into the Foucauldian model of an appropriate race through their bourgeois status and Anglo-Saxon origins—marking a shift from aristocratic blood superstition to bourgeois techniques of science and management. The transfusions' inefficacy suggests that British and even Anglo-European blood is not enough to keep Lucy alive; moreover, Dracula and Lucy's physical strength and resistance to common injury and disease foil the declining biological viability of the British. The abating national strength testifies to the accumulation of specific anxieties about degeneration related to military viability at the turn of the century. Not but two years after the novel's publication, the onset of the Boer War revealed the insalubrious constitutions of the working class that filled the ranks, an anxiety also evident in Conan Doyle's prose and fiction, which is explored in depth in chapter 4. The seeming contradiction in the blood's simultaneous association with older forms of societal order and modern medical techniques betrays the metaphor's role in not only moving from a society of aristocratic lineage to one of middle-class hereditary and hygiene, but also in masking how previous forms of power linked to the older order do not concomitantly disappear. Moreover, if we account for the connotations and scientific discourse of blood, and its ontological status, at the fin de siècle, it becomes clear that *Dracula* deploys the fluid in a dynamic temporality. Jessica Howell contends that by the late 1800s blood's biological value was overshadowed by its chemical value—rather than a privileged substance per se, it became a fluid medium for analysis. Thus, while Dracula harkens back to blood's older caste structures and good versus evil binary, at the same time, its multiple associations, particularly the biochemical resonance of its becoming a medium for something else—like parasites—reinforces the narrative of reverse colonization.[38]

Lucy herself visibly becomes a threat to English blood by way of her sexuality. While Lucy's sexual impropriety becomes vividly apparent postinfection, however, there are several indications that Lucy is a "fallen woman" and a product of degeneration even before being corrupted by Dracula. This contradiction contextualizes the contemporary inflection of the kinds of imperial decay in which Dracula thrives. Lucy's behavior suggests a hint of promiscuity before she is hypersexualized as a vampire: she confesses to Mina that she wishes she could marry all three of her suitors, and this informs Van Helsing's later joke that this "sweet maid is a polyandarist" (D, 158). Moreover, her sleepwalking is a hereditary taint that makes her susceptible to Dracula.[39] Mina appeals to eugenic purity when she notes that Lucy's father also suffered from somnambulism. Mina is so concerned that she manifests physical unease over the impropriety of Lucy's somnambulism: "My heart beat so loud all the time that sometimes I thought I should faint. I was filled with anxiety about Lucy, not only for her health, lest she should suffer from the exposure, but for her reputation in case the story should get wind" (D, 89), suggesting that

Lucy's nocturnal ambulation hints at indecent sexual encounters. Lucy's medical and moral qualities before she becomes a vampire intimate that she is corruptible by Dracula because she is already corrupt, a condition that the novel maps onto England itself.

Lucy's sexual transformation into a vampire resonates with patriarchal medicine's attempt to control and discipline women's illicit sexuality for the sake of purity of the race. It was a shift from a question of morality in Christian terms to a duty for race and nation—that is, to retain sex for appropriate bourgeois reproduction. Lucy's affliction, then, can be read as a transformation from a necessarily virginal to a sexually transgressive woman; her illness parallels venereal disease in its "illicit nature of transmission and degenerative effect on her health."[40] Numerous passages highlight Lucy's corruption, such as when Arthur recoils in horror when she suggestively calls for him (D, 188). As heredity was increasingly medicalized as a concern at the fin de siècle under the influence of evolutionary theories, particularly with respect to disease and degeneration, illicit sexuality was one nexus between the two that emblematized that conflation. Of course, the irony here lies in the fact that Stoker intimated Lucy's compromised sexuality even before her infection. Moreover, within their very ideology of monogamy, the transfusion itself, Van Helsing admits, is debasing by Victorian norms. Once Lucy becomes undead, it is no longer just Arthur's bloodline that is at stake. There is a danger of vampirism compromising the entire population. Lucy enacts that threat by feeding on children in an inversion of appropriate Victorian motherhood. Medical control of women's sexuality, then, becomes another iteration that establishes how moral and physical disease can be constructed as an enemy of the population. She has become a "nightmare" with a "whole carnal and unspiritual appearance, seeming like a devilish mockery of Lucy's sweet purity" (D, 190). Van Helsing urges Arthur to let him perform her decapitation and impalement under the aegis of "a duty to others" (D, 184), as vampires "go on age after age, adding new victims and multiplying the evils of the world" (D, 190).

Part of the medical war in *Dracula*, then, is the war between women's sexuality and the medical establishment, a rhetorical construction used by then-contemporary feminists like Josephine Butler. Van Helsing's duty to prevent the spread of vampirism justifies the vehement spectacle that allows for both strict surveillance and violent, punitive treatment, especially in the case of Lucy's inability to be cured though medical means. That form of power reveals the juridical qualities of the martial metaphor underwriting public health legislation in the decades leading up to *Dracula*'s publication and informs the violent dimensions of the Crew's medical treatment of women.

The "Stimulating" and "Bracing" Work of the Contagious Diseases Acts

The representation of women's sexuality in *Dracula* was informed by the CD Acts, which answered a military need to control venereal disease. Lucy's aberrant sexuality as a vampire can be read as a form of rebellion against patriarchal medical control of women's bodies. Hers was a pathological rebellion that the Crew of Light aggressively suppressed, her "wantonness" coding a sexual autonomy that Lucy gains in lieu of her proper middle-class domestic reproductive function.[41] On Van Helsing's orders, the Crew secures weaponry: knives and a sharpened wooden stake. Their work involves driving the stake through Lucy's heart. It is a return to the piercing image of the lancet, reimagined as a punishment. But while their action is bellicose in form, as they enter Lucy's tomb, Seward reminds the reader their work is a medical endeavor: "To me a doctor's preparations for work of any kind are stimulating and bracing" (*D*, 190). Traces of military medicine in the medical policing of women's sexuality are ritualized in the violent attack on Lucy. In the fictional reference to the CD Acts, the vocabulary and grammar of war made its way into gendered medical politics.

The CD Acts were possibly the most emblematic material connections between military medicine and civilian public health during the nineteenth century. They are especially relevant to the larger argument of this book, that the martial metaphor developed from military medical practices. The Acts' origin lay in protecting the health of enlisted men, the raw bodies needed to expand and defend empire. The targets, however, were civilian women, and as many scholars have suggested, the acts were tied to long-developed anxieties and obsessions over women's sexuality.[42] In 1857, after the Crimean War, the Royal Commission on the Health of the Army noted an extremely high rate of venereal disease, most notably syphilis, in the armed forces. Their concern was investigated by the Committee to Inquire into the Prevalence of Venereal Disease in the Army and Navy in 1864. The Commission did not initially call for anything like the CD Acts, but it did spur continued interest from surgeons and military and bureaucratic officials. By 1864, however, venereal disease was the cause of one-third of all cases of illness in the army, which prompted more direct medical action beyond gathering statistics. That year, the CD Acts were passed. The 1864 act applied to eleven garrisons and dock towns across Ireland and England. In an entanglement between military officials, medical practitioners, police officers, and local and national bureaucracies, a regulationist system was enacted to control the spread of venereal disease by stopping it at its assumed source. The acts allowed for the compulsory examination, arrest, and detention of suspected sex workers. Plainclothes police officers would identify women and require them to be examined by a military surgeon. If a woman was found to be infected, she would be placed in a lock hospital for up to three months.[43]

The 1866 act introduced a more overt system of surveillance and medical policing, instituting periodic examinations of all known sex workers. The 1869 act then increased the length of detention, extended the system to five more districts, and increased its physical jurisdiction to a fifteen-mile radius outside each of the explicitly defined dock ports and garrison towns. By 1869, the acts were extended well beyond the "defined limits of exceptional legislation for the military."[44] Beyond concerns about venereal disease and sex work, the CD Acts represented an extension of medical, legislative, and moral intervention into the lives of the poor—a continued development of the kind of middle-class-led sanitary reform that drew from the epidemiological concerns of the British military. In that capacity, the CD Acts continued to foster the medicalization of the social body relative to the military.

The CD Acts operated on the precedent of the continental and colonial system already implemented in Hong Kong and India and later brought to Malta.[45] The use of lock hospitals and CD Act–like policies in the colonies predated their domestic deployment, starting as early as the 1850s.[46] In 1861 in the British-controlled Ionian Islands, Lord Henry Storks secretly introduced a requirement that every prostitute submit to an examination by an army surgeon or face three months imprisonment. This was an initial testing of biopolitical technologies in the colonies that would later be deployed in the homeland, a practice that David Arnold and Ann Stoler have characterized as creating "labs of modernity," also evident in Conan Doyle's writings on the Boer War. Such a practice was contingent on military-supported colonial structures, and that genealogy signals one of the many colonial legacies of the martial metaphor's military history. Read in tandem with the proclivity for racializing the poor in colonial terms as if they were a distinct race from the English middle class reflects how the struggle for the purity of the English race is turned inward on the population as an internal war. The war for purity from "foreign" pollution developed from and reinscribed biological racism associated with classist and xenophobic anxieties of contagion, filth, and degeneration.

The direct control, arrest, and spectacularization of diseased sex workers by medico-military authorities under the CD Acts was juridical in nature, signaling the violent and military forms of power attached to the figurative language of the martial metaphor. The use of military surgeons, local police, and government organs to expose the hidden signs of venereal disease through medical examination translated those hidden medical signs into spectacle through registration, court proceedings, and incarceration. In mandating the detention of women suspected of sex work, the CD Acts amounted to a quarantine-like measure. As Léopold Lambert has argued, "spaces of precaution" such as the military quarantine, operate much like "spaces of punishment." Sovereign power suspends individual freedom, and any space can become a carceral quarantine.[47] The lock hospitals were in effect quarantines, keeping infected sex workers away from civil society. The very qualification of the word *hospital* with *lock* implied a social evil that put normative society in peril.[48] The lock hospital dates to early modern and medieval times, when it was used to confine lepers and prevent the spread of the disease and social panic.[49] In the nineteenth century, sex workers supplanted the lepers of the eighteenth century, as syphilis became "the dreaded symbol of social contagion."[50] In their militaristic logic and material practices, the CD Acts waged an internecine war on selections of the civilian population. If, for Agamben, the concentration camp is the "hidden matrix" of modern sovereignty, then the martial quarantine is, if more conceptually, a hidden matrix of public health. The use of force and state of exception structured by military control is always operative. There is an invisible war on the population, only occasionally emerging to openly display its violence but always containing that possibility—the state of exception that defines sovereignty.

Dracula offers the rhetorical contribution of affording martial language for the metaphorical portrayal of governmental intervention as a potentiality for war against elements of the population, making coercive actions like quarantine and isolation thinkable and actionable. The physical division of the quarantine forms the principle racism at the core of biopolitical regulation and its imperative to make live and let die, creating racial boundaries that neutralize polluting infiltration. Although the quarantine remains a material possibility in public health, in the Victorian era as now, the boundaries it creates still shape the productive power of regulatory biopolitics. This premodern form of power continued to reside in the Victorian era's present. The martial metaphor subtends the relation between war, sovereignty, and medicine by translating it from a material linkage to a figure of speech. For modern biopower, discipline and regulation are understood as nonviolent and nonrepressive; they are productive. It is precisely under this aegis that the metaphor functions as a mechanism of control. Fiction like *Dracula* that frames disease as a monstrous military enemy inculcates this obfuscation in the form of a literary abstraction.

In the military's war against syphilis, sex workers were the casualties. Thus, the ill health of the enlisted man and the British social body were projected onto women's bodies. Stoker writes about that fear of an epidemic of venereal disease and, by treating Lucy as the conduit of it, illustrates the punishing dynamic of the CD Acts.[51] In the discussions that led to the development of the CD Acts, the idea of introducing the compulsory examination of enlisted men as the primary intervention was quickly dismissed as detrimental to morale.[52] Their rationale had been to promote the health of enlisted men—not even for their own sake but for that of the expansion and defense of empire—at the expense of working-class and impoverished women. The Acts ignored the economic conditions that often drove women to sex work and fostered the social determinants, such as poverty, that negatively affected their health beyond venereal disease.

In the logic and practice of the CD Acts, women's bodies became, as Walkowitz suggests, a national enemy within.[53] Josephine Butler discusses this projection of men's ill health onto sex workers via the CD Acts, and war as such, onto women in her 1871 extended essay, "The Constitution Violated." Regarding the CD Acts, Butler writes, "Until war be waged against impure men, as well as against impure women, it will remain impossible to define prostitution. It is amazing to see in this unequal war waged against the weaker sex only. . . ."[54] Tabitha Sparks suggest that the repeal movement, which succeeded in 1886, represented middle-class women taking control of their bodies and sexuality from the medical establishment.⁵⁵ While the CD Acts in execution most directly affected the bodies of working-class and impoverished women, this repeal was a political cause that occasioned the intervention of middle-class feminists to demand legal and physical autonomy as a broader issue. *Dracula* shows patriarchal medicine's response to this repossession: the reinstitution of quarantine and explicit juridical punishment. The extension from the impoverished and working- to middle-class feminists comes to bear on the infected women in the novel.

Lucy's vampirism is a threat because of her sexuality and because she embodies feminist movements that resisted medical military control of women's bodies. As a vampire with sexual agency, Lucy breaks free of medico-legal disciplinary control and flouts the self-regulatory behaviors imposed by medicalized norms. That sort of feminist activism was absorbed in the 1880s and '90s into the character of the "New Woman," a figure distinctly modern in her involvement in public issues and her effort to reform social, educational, political, and medical inequities prompted by the sexual double standard exemplified by the CD Acts.⁵⁶ The weakening masculine control over women's bodies and gender scripts came to be defined in a medical capacity that demanded a military-like response. Unlike Mina's treatment in her hygienic and confessional discipline, the military's punitive response to Lucy's perverse sexuality ends in her impalement and decapitation. If Mina is the model of discipline, hygiene, and confession, the correlative image associated with Lucy is less the discipline of the military drill than the spectacle of violence, the state of exception, and the show of force associated with her eternal quarantine and punishment.

Though Lucy's ritualistic mutilation has been read as sexual penetration, gang rape, and a reassertion of heteronormative masculinity,⁵⁷ reading it in a medical idiom situates the older violence of juridical power and quarantine as coextensive, yet occluded, with biopower; it links martial violence with the racial imperative of public health that was narrated in Lucy's convalescence. The symbolism of penetration, in medical terms, echoes the opposition of Dracula's fangs by Seward's lancet and Van Helsing's hypodermic needle. Seward records the "stimulating and bracing" medical "work." Following the tenor of Van Helsing's "ice brook" martial temper, "Arthur took the stake and the hammer, and when once his mind was set on action his hands never trembled nor even quivered. . . . [He] placed the point over the heart, and as [Seward] looked I could see its dint in the white flesh. Then he struck with all his might" (D, 191). In this scene, the lancet and needle are rewritten as the material weapon of the stake. The suggestion is that the underlying violence of the martial metaphor becomes necessary when medical procedures like transfusion fails, reflecting how coercive control is necessary and available when discipline fails. The ritual concludes with the simultaneous spectacle of purgation, following "the Thing's" transmuting back into "Lucy as [they] had seen her in life," and her quarantine. Seward recounts how they "cut off the head and filled it with garlic . . . soldered up the leaden coffin, screwed on the coffin lid," noting, too, that "when the professor locked the door, he gave the key to Arthur" (D, 193). The soldering, screwing, and locking all function as containment; her head severed, her thoracic cavity punctured, Lucy is sequestered under eternally enforced detention.

If, as Sparks suggests, Stoker's novel narrates the medical establishment's "seizing (back) control" of women's bodies following the 1886 repeal of the CD Acts, then in terms of the martial metaphor, the novel also reflects the way literature aided that process. While the repeal had rescinded medical control of venereal disease through legal mechanisms by the time *Dracula* was published, the martial metaphor remained a way to perpetuate the same conflation of public health with national defense. In its reflection and response to the CD Acts, the novel attests to how the martial metaphor sustained the linkages among national defense, degeneration, medicine, and the control of women's sexuality.

Opportunistic Infections, Polyvalent Etiologies

In terms of disease, thus far this chapter has attended to the relevance to syphilis and the broader but not-unrelated rubric of degeneration. To fully appreciate the expansive, ramified cultural work of the novel in narrativizing the metaphorical militarization of medicine—and archiving the longer history of this very process in its own narrative—we must essentially perform a kind of nosology of *Dracula*. This entails delineating the distinct etiologies and other discrete pathologies that the novel incarnates in the vampiric form: the broader rubrics of contagion, miasma, germ, and parasite, along with animal vectors; and the specific diseases of cholera, smallpox, rinderpest, plague, and malaria. If Dracula is, in Van Helsing's words, "a whirlpool of race," likewise, he is a whirlpool of disease. Following the preceding discussion of the CD Acts, the contagionist logics of quarantine provide a useful point of departure for this nosological exploration.

Dracula is replete with quarantine and isolation. One reviewer of the novel specifically noted the pathogenicity of the vampire's contact: "Count Dracula is a vampire of the most malignant kind. The worst of it is he carries contagion with him."[58] Van Helsing invokes the language of defense and contagion when he warns the other protagonists to "guard [them]selves from his touch" (*D*, 219). The reference to cleanliness when Mina vilifies her own person after intimate contact with Dracula speaks to the dangerous transmissions between bodies: "I must touch and kiss [Jonathan] no more" (*D*, 248). And, the conclusion of Lucy's second death narrates the containment of sexuality—in addition to juridical punishment—resonating with the history of the CD Acts. But in addition to its symbolic function, the stake can be read as an apparatus of quarantine. Its function is not to destroy the undead but to immobilize them, which, in conjunction with the hermetic sealing of the coffin prevents further movement and spread of the disease.[59]

The image of quarantine appears more explicitly toward the end of the novel. In Transylvania, Van Helsing, with the complicity of the rest of the Crew, quarantines Mina after she displays signs of infection that are potentially injurious to the group. He creates a visible barrier to confine her, outlined with a Eucharist wafer, and not only does it seem to protect Mina from Dracula, it provides a measure of security to the crew as well. That circle of protection, however, makes her, in effect, a prisoner to it: "She could not [leave], none of those that we dreaded could [enter]. Though there might be a danger to the body, the soul was safe" (*D*, 316). Like governmental quarantines, that measure of protection requires a willingness to sacrifice the infected for the sake of the greater good. And yet, by doing so, Mina's soul is protected at the expense of her body, because though she is becoming a vampire, she will not be able to perform the unnatural acts associated with it—drinking blood and spreading the contagion. The quarantine operates as a counter to vampirism, another medical element in the oppositional narratives between the Count and the Crew. The quarantine delimits Dracula's expansive "ever widening circle of semi-demons [that] batten on the helpless" (*D*, 52–53).

But beyond the Crew's actions that delimit the spread of vampirism, the two doctors voice a particular medical idiom that distills a convergence of violence, medicine, and writing by alluding to a specific history of contagion in Victorian England. Van Helsing pledges that they "find out the *author* of all [their] sorrow and to *stamp* him out" (*D*, 193, emphasis added). Later, Seward reiterates, "I have studied, over and over again since they came into my hands, all the papers relating to this monster; and the more I have studied, the greater seems the necessity to utterly *stamp him out*" (*D*, 263, emphasis added). This is a key phrase to understanding *Dracula*'s role in representing and naturalizing the martial metaphor. The characterization of Dracula as the "author" and the framing of the Crew's response to that authorship as "stamping" evokes the narrative contests between both parties. Macy Todd suggests that the violence in Van Helsing's words is expressed through the act of writing itself: as evidenced by the composition of narrative timelines; the detailed character descriptions and archiving of records the Crew manages so that they can "arrange [their] plan of battle with this terrible and mysterious enemy"; and by how at the end of the novel Harker, in reference to Dracula's death, celebrates that "the very trace of all that had been was blotted out." The shift between metaphors betrays the relationship between writing and violence, where violence eradicates not only the signs the agent wishes to target but also aims at erasing the signs of its own production.[60] When considered in conversation with medical prose and debates that predated Stoker's use of the phrase, Van Helsing and Seward's use of "stamping out" sheds light on how physicians were carefully using the martial metaphor to navigate the politically anathematized practice of quarantine in the form of isolation. The phrase *stamping out* emerged from the British government's policies to stem the spread of rinderpest, specifically denoting the practice of culling whole herds of cattle during the 1865–1867 rinderpest epizootic. By the 1880s, the continued risk of smallpox provided medical practitioners and researchers a means to reframe extreme but effective measures that had been used against the cattle plague.[61]

When working through the symptoms of Renfield's zoöphagy, Seward's commentary alludes to rinderpest in a subtle reference to one of the most prominent authorities on the subject, Dr. John Burdon-Sanderson. "I might advance my own branch of science to a pitch compared with which Burdon-Sanderson's physiology or Ferrier's brain-knowledge would be as nothing," Seward writes (*D*, 71). This reference to Burdon-Sanderson has tended to be overshadowed by interest in brain science and vivisectionist discourse surrounding Seward's espousal of David Ferrier.[62] Apropos of *Dracula*, stamping out justifies the use of physical force by virtue of superiority, through the metaphor of differential heights and the need for epidemiological security. The work of Sir James Simpson and Sir William Budd, in particular, provide insight into how Van Helsing and Seward's framing of Dracula's extirpation relates to medical researchers and practitioners of adoption of the martial metaphor in a manner that follows a similar process of violence that erases the evidence of its production.

Sir James Young Simpson, a Scottish obstetrician best known for his introduction of chloroform to obstetrics, drew on the discourse of stamping out rinderpest when proposing isolation measures to stem the spread of smallpox. In a widely discussed 1868 pamphlet, Simpson writes, "The public mind has, during the last two or three years, become familiarised with the idea of '*stamping out*' a disease, in the instance of Rinderpest . . . I believe the same principle of stamping out could be as successfully applied to the extirpation of small-pox." Simpson acknowledges, however, that stamping out smallpox should not follow precisely the same method as rinderpest, which entailed "killing all animals labouring under the disease; and in many instances all those which had been exposed to the contagion of it, but were not yet attacked."[63] Simpson seeks to enact quarantine-like measures through practicing isolation and extending the emergency jurisdiction of intrusive government powers to suppress disease.[64] This was the ideological obstacle in the way of Simpson pushing the practice forward. He had to argumentatively maneuver around the coercive nature of contagionist measures and their incursion on free will. The rhetorical ploy Simpson conducts in the language of "stamping out" not only capitalizes on the martial metaphor, it also contributes to the very conceptual process of occluding the violence attached to the metaphor's metonymic linkage with militarism.

Also worth noting is the figuration and elision of violence into medical writing through the metaphor's presence in William Budd and James Simpson's prose. In the same way that Simpson translates the violent process of killing cattle to the peaceful process of isolation in humans with smallpox, Budd advocates for "State Medicine" and legal surveillance and isolation measures to eliminate smallpox from England in his widely discussed lecture "Can the Government, Further, Beneficially Interfere in the Prevention of Infectious Disease?" (1870). Discussing the eradication of cattle plague, he questions if "Men are prompt enough to see and act upon this when their flocks and herds are threatened: why are they slow to see and act upon it, when their own lives are at stake?"[65] In other words, he asks why the government will intervene to protect cattle but not the population. The relevance of Budd and Simpson's texts to *Dracula* extends beyond their explicit reference to rinderpest and stamping out disease, as both Budd and Simpson utilize the metaphor of war to frame their arguments for legally enforcing isolation measures in response to infectious disease. While Simpson's use primarily takes the form of using the verb *attack*, Budd's use of military discourse pervades his lecture: "Of all the legions which make up the great army of death, that of the infectious diseases is, with one doubtful exception, at once the most active and the most deadly," he writes. Advocating for more aggressive governmental measures, Budd concludes: "By beating down these plagues wherever they appear, by crushing them in their small beginnings, by pursuing them into their strongholds, and rooting them out, by making every advantage gained the ground of new reprisals, by carrying on incessant, implacable, internecine war against them, against our direst enemies, which in sober truth they are—we should soon see a great falling off in the number of their victims, and gradually pave the way to their extermination."[66] Of all the soldierly words and constructions in this elaborate declaration, *internecine* is especially telling, as it denotes destruction of the human and the microbial, but more significantly, is also defined as the war within an organization or group, not unlike how the martial metaphor justifies war not only against foreign but internal threats. Budd adds exigency to his argument for repressive isolation measures because of a permanent infiltration of bacterial life within the human and social body. This suggests, though doesn't explicitly state, that those infected populations—like infected cattle—are enemies. While like Simpson he overtly negates the connection between culling cattle and people, the resonance of the necessity for such logic—as opposed to the literal practice of culling—remains embedded in the argument. The urgency and danger of smallpox justifies the extremity of coercive warlike emergency measures, such as the restriction of individual freedom and aggressive state intervention.

The influence of Budd's use of the martial metaphor is evidenced when following references to his speech in the medical and periodical press. There are a number of reprintings and responses to his speech, most of which replicate Budd's various implementations and general rhetorical framing of the martial metaphor. In a version printed in the *Lancet*, the author writes, "Dr. Budd commented on the universal presence of infection, and the inadequacy of the existing sanitary machinery to cope with it. We have a small board of able men, largely occupied, among other things, with writing very excellent reports. *But we want a standing army, well-trained, and ably commanded to garrison the land.*"⁶⁷ The reference is an accurate abstract of the entire speech, imbuing the article's military exigency in a single quotation. But the exact wording from Budd's speech with respect to the Privy Council's reports and the recommendation for public officers does not use the metaphor in the original version of his speech.⁶⁸ In other words, the *Lancet*'s commentator rewrites two of Budd's specific proposals with the metaphor pervading most other parts of his speech. An editorial in the *Times* takes this a step further when it challenges the "summary power" of extirpation measures. The author argues that, "When Mr. Budd calls of a '*standing army*, well trained and ably commanded to *garrison the land*,' he will too certainly alarm all but the soldiers, in other words, our doctors, themselves."⁶⁹ Given just these few examples, published just a few days after the speech, it is clear how the violent, extreme measures of rinderpest get translated into the arguments put forth by Budd and Simpson. As a relevant medical historical context to Stoker's novel, these writings show how Van Helsing and Seward's desire to stamp out Dracula resonates not only with the political debates of aggressive responses to contagion, but also the compositional process of figuring medicine as war to appropriate the exigency of militarism while eliding negative connotations associated with its violence. Reading the novel with this medical and periodical prose, then, reflects on the fictional and rhetorical qualities of the martial metaphor as shaped through the written word. With the discussion of the context of political crossover between human and animal already established via the history of rinderpest, one final reference to contagion should also be considered: plague.

In *Dracula*, plague amalgamates foreign and temporal threats to modernity according to their colonial projects, and functions as a point of contrast with English national identity and history. Dracula's antiquated and feudal origins juxtaposed with the mythic narrativization of the Crew is fitting plague's connotations of foreignness and antiquity. By the late nineteenth century, plague was mostly confined to colonial and tropical locations such as India and connoted medieval epidemics; yet it proved to be a useful point of reference for medicalized war like that against malaria. In the same year as *Dracula*'s publication, colonial medical officers declared a "war on plague" where it was the most significant threat that "India has had to face since the Mutiny," in the words of Bombay Surgeon General George Bainbridge in 1899.⁷⁰ The plague campaign for the British was, indeed, one where warfare and medicine were metaphorically and materially aligned in defense of empire.[71] Commenting on its invasiveness from the East in *All The Year Round*, one contributor notes that an 1878 plague epidemic made its way from China and "threatened to progress through Russia westwards,"[72] not unlike the march of the first cholera pandemic. Acknowledging its racialized history, the article further details the plague's historical linkage with Jewish populations and their persecution.[73] As such, we can infer that *Dracula*'s anti-Semitic valences similarly follow the anxiety of the incursion of the old world into the new. Indeed, the medieval blaming of plague on the Jews coincides with folkloric appearances of supposed vampirism that were concurrent with plague outbreaks.[74] Given the xenophobic association of the foreign, racialized Other with disease, it is hardly surprising that Stoker would amplify Dracula's objectionable corporeality with the ability to turn into a rat, a fitting creature to more literally "stamp out." It is important to underscore how this ideological temporality marks an analogical opposition to the Crew of Light's self-authored characterization. While they, too, link their project to English history in the Middle Ages, their story is one of triumph, Christian virtue, and the restoration of order, rather than strife, where the lack of control and explanation over material conditions of the plague afforded only projection by way of blaming the Other rather than encouraging amelioration.

The plague, moreover, expresses another contradiction in the novel's subscription to the martial metaphor. Like the bacterium that inhabits the parasitic fleas supping the blood of the rodents on which they travel, the disease remains embedded in the novel's rats, despite not being specifically referenced. In tracing the arrival of Dracula's boxes via ship at Carfax, the male protagonists encounter a swarm of rats that Van Helsing identifies as under the Count's control. The Crew finds that the house suddenly "become[s] alive with rats . . . multiplying by the thousands" (*D*, 222). The propagation of the rats and the spread of "the mass," mirrors the rapid expandability of contagious disease in the industrial, urban, and global nineteenth century, a transmission determined by person-to-person contact as well as the self-replicating capability of contagious disease under the germ model. Much like the contagionist idea of quarantine in the late nineteenth century, *Dracula* signals "the incursion of the past into the present," as Maud Ellman contends in her study of modernist networks.[75] The relationship between rats and vampires is one of primitivism. But though they are both images of the archaic and less-evolved, they also both thrive in the festering conditions of modern industrial England. Thus, Dracula exercises his "primeval power with the modern know-how of the modern rat," infiltrating contemporary transportation networks.[76] Rats, like Jews, were specifically associated with medieval plague, and while that connection with germs—specifically *yersinia pestis*, the plague bacterium—does not fit precisely into the history behind Stoker's publication of the novel in 1897, the link does resonate with mythologies that persisted in the cultural imaginary at the fin de siècle.[77] Of course, rats had been associated with plague in ancient medicine and in folklore for centuries; closer to the time of *Dracula*, the notion recurs in Goethe's short poem about the Pied Piper (1803) clearing the rats from a town, later retold in Robert Browning's "The Pied Piper of Hamelin," and in a number of fairy tales in the 1890s. In their polyvalent connotations regarding the old and the new, rats, then, signal the ironies of British industrial modernity, as the filth associated with rats is symptomatic of an environment that they thrive in.

Intimately bound with the novel's contagionist narrative device, Dracula, too, has a number of characteristics that align him with miasma. The presence of rats suggests that Dracula is not only a contagion but also a miasmic infection, as rats in Victorian England emblematized dirt and filth with environment.[78] The dimension of the vampiric pathology materializes reverse colonization by way of soil—the invasion by previously colonizable territory—showing how the side effects of modernity kindle the very threats that the modern state and science proposed to defend against. Stoker himself would have been quite aware of the discourse on miasma given his mother's experience with cholera, which as part 1 demonstrated was a disease at the center of early nineteenth-century etiological debates. Stoker's mother, Charlotte, told her children "horror stories" about the cholera outbreak in Sligo, Ireland, which while detailing both contagionist (quarantine) and miasmic interventions, had a number of pestilential figurations of the order of miasma. Describing what reads like a post-apocalyptic wasteland, she mentions the urgency to fumigate and notably describes the visibility of the miasma: "On some days the Cholera was more fatal than others, and on those days, we could see a heavy sulphurous looking cloyd [sic] hang over the town."[79] Stoker later suggested that such stories influenced his conceptualization of vampiric pestilence.[80] Charlotte Stoker describes cholera as a cloud that "comes from the East" by way of the sea,[81] in a associative logic similar to the figuration of the plague's continuity with the ocean in *The Last Man*.

While *Dracula* also retains resonances of the pestilential cloud, especially evident in the storm that arrives with the ship carrying Dracula and his boxes (*D*, 77), the novel's representation of the vampire as miasma condenses Charlotte's sulfurous cloud from the East into the density of polluted, foreign soil. The dirt travels by sea and protects Dracula. Fostered by interring himself in his native, portable land, he emanates from the environment like a noxious putrefaction erupting from decaying matter.

The Count's salient miasmic characteristic and his protean ability to shift into a mist are grounded in his boxes of dirt. There are numerous instances of Dracula as a mist-miasma, noxious odor, and pathogenic particulate floating through the air. In Harker's journal, specks of matter in the air announce the vampire's arrival.[82] Similarly, Lucy is infected by a "whole myriad of little specks." Mina sees "a thin streak of white mist" creeping toward their lodging (*D*, 226), and after Seward and Van Helsing see the illicit contact between Dracula and Mina, they light a match but see "nothing but a faint vapour" (*D*, 247). Beyond the visual signs of miasma, the telltale olfactory offense emanating from putrefaction and filth characterizes Dracula as a pathogenic air, following the Chadwickian logic that "all smell is disease," and more so if taken into Harker's specific mention of the Count's "rank" breath early in his journal account of their meeting (*D*, 24). Seward mentions that the Carfax Abbey house, in particular, emits an "earthly smell, as of some dry miasma" (*D*, 221). In these descriptions, vampirism is linked to insalubrious environments. Harker magnifies that association when he says that the odor "was composed of all the ills of mortality and with the pungent, acrid smell of blood, but it seemed as though corruption had itself become corrupt" (*D*, 221). That final qualification implies that Dracula emerged from corruption already in England. On the one hand, this allows for the sanitization, the elimination of the foreign and internal elements that would make for a degrading environment (like Lucy). On the other hand, it fosters the idea of a productive power through discipline and regulatory biopolitics in the form of sanitation. In other words, it encodes both modes of defense for the sake of national purity.

While blood remains in the subtext of the entire novel, its mention in the context of Dracula's miasma relates penetration and pollution of the interior of the body to that of a corrupt and putrefied environment. Like the rats, this figure dissolves the boundaries between the primitive and the civilized in modernity. Dracula's miasmic form motivates the disciplinary and biopolitical regulation of the population through sanitation, following Laura Croley's contention that reform literature's "rhetoric of colonization and miscegenation" helps shape the Count's persona.[83] Recalling the martial through-line of Kingsley's work, the middle-class sanitary movement promoted cleaning drills and hygiene protocols among the working class, which instilled individual discipline in, and surveillance of, subjects. The Crew of Light is associated with the social reforms of the sanitary movement, yet unlike Kingsley's characters, they retain the juridical and coercive force of contagionism. We see the protagonists work with the curative means of ventilation, for instance, when they open the chapel door at Carfax and feel "the purifying of the atmosphere" (D, 223). This locale is characteristic of a "low lodging house" or rank slum reminiscent of places visited by social reformers, staining the Count's lodgings with the modern entropic processes of urbanization, industrialization, and empire.[84] The circuits of capital and international trade across the empire allow Dracula and his boxes of dirt to make their way to England. London provides a breeding ground for the noxious atmosphere he exudes; the boxes of his filth filled with premodern dirt and "mould" thrive (D, 79), his nidus maturing in London's ecology of urban and insalubrious filth. Dracula's invasion, then, can be understood as what today we might call an opportunistic infection. Gestures to this ambiguity are evident as early as *The Last Man*; however, Stoker's use of horror and spectacle channels fin-de-siècle anxieties less as critique of the modern empire and more as promoters of the martial metaphor for its protection. As with the invocation of contagionism, the discourse of miasma in *Dracula* invokes the temporal disjunction and points to how modern germ theory hadn't disproven contagion and miasma theory. Rather, Stoker shows how germ theory conceptually brought contagionism and miasma theory together in terms of medical science and biopolitics. Theories about race and xenophobia can explain why Stoker holds on to earlier idioms of contagion and pollution as they combine into a disease agent that is both alive and can reproduce. They foster fear to promote defense.

Contextualizing contagionist and miasmic valances of the Count sheds light on how Stoker was working with germ theory by making Dracula a parasitic disease. The vampire represents infectious disease as "an active, intelligent agent that attacks the body."[85] The idea that diseases are caused by living organisms rather than inanimate chemicals or vapors made disease a living agent that penetrated the boundaries of the hermetic, liberal subject.[86] When figuratively mapped onto the national body, bacteria became a prominent expression of reverse colonization, and in many tropical medicine texts, for instance, descriptions of bacteria and native populations are conflated.[87] The images of polluted environments, metonymically linked to the people occupying them, helped create the us-versus-them divide that was and remains so conducive to military thinking, applied both in the colony and the homeland. Given the countless images of boundaries being penetrated in the novel, pollution should be read as an intrusion into the demarcation of what was worth defending in Victorian Britain: the middle class. Stoker animates such intrusions with microbiology. For instance, Mina's dream, in which Dracula appears as a miasmic "white mist," includes an additional construction that signals vital agency: "Not a thing seemed to be stirring, but all to be grim and fixed as death or fate; so that a thin streak of white mist, that crept with almost imperceptible slowness across the grass towards the house, seemed to have a sentience and a vitality of its own" (*D*, 266). The fact that the vampiric miasma possesses self-awareness and is an ontologically discrete life gives a shape to inimical malevolence that fiction like *Dracula* attributed to infectious disease and foreign bodies. When Harker is disturbed by the idea of bringing Mina with them as they chase Dracula back to his castle in Transylvania, he voices an objection underwritten by the rearrangement of the ontological order of things wrought by germ theory: "Have you seen that awful den of hellish infamy—with the very moonlight alive with grisly shapes, and every speck of dust that whirls in the wind a devouring monster in embryo?" (*D*, 307). The embryological metaphor personifies the particulate matter of filth and miasma, but also, given the embryo's association with growth, the figuration evokes the danger of vampirism's capacity for perverse, mass reproduction.

The connotations of birth and growth cultivate the Victorian preoccupations about microbes because, like other organisms, microbes reproduce themselves. The sheer incomprehensibility of their numbers adds an entirely new order of magnitude to the abstract conception of disease as an object external to the body. Van Helsing alludes to the problem of microbial reproduction when warning the Crew of the apocalyptic potential of leaving Dracula unchecked: the vampires will multiply and "create a new and ever-widening circle of semi-demons" (*D*, 52–53). The "ever-widening circle," and the discourse of multiplicity imbue a statistical, epidemiological quality to vampirism that equates microbes with entire populations. Microbial—or vampiric—reproduction is, as Susan Zieger suggests, "geometrical" and outstrips the rate of human reproduction.[88] The militarized discourse of parasitology, its resonances with miasma, contagion, bacteria, and colonization coalesces the threads that Budd initially brought together in his 1869 speech on governmental intervention to stamp out smallpox. His metaphoric use of the human body as a soil, of disease as a seed, and his definition of infection in terms of a disease's "spread," "scattering," "multiplication," and "propagation" conceptually converge in *Dracula*.[89] In the form of the vampire, the novel expounds the multiplicity of the germ, its use of the body as its growth medium, and its parasitic infection of empire.

Parasitology provided Stoker with a resonant vocabulary to articulate the anxieties of reverse colonization through a modern scientific understanding of a primitive life-form emerging from imperial encounters. This medical grammar grounded the abstraction of the martial metaphor in the materiality of the military. This subfield of microbiology grew out of tropical medicine, especially during the Scramble for Africa, the late-nineteenth-century zeitgeist whereby European powers sought to occupy and divide the entire continent, as I discuss at length in the concluding chapter. Tropical medicine was intimately entangled with military infrastructure, providing biomedical support for the military's presence in India, Malay, and parts of Africa. It is thus the second instance of military medicine to which Stoker responds and allegorizes in the anachronistic medico-military war against the Count. Stoker developed the logics of invasion, colonization, and racialization as he drew from contagion and miasma to understand the living germ, and ultimately into the more specific threat of the parasite. Tropical parasites were understood as one of the most formidable obstacles to European colonization, especially malaria. As such, the disease functions as a consonant opposition to the Crew of Lights defense against reverse colonization.

The sanguine transmission of malaria certainly resonates with the way blood operates in *Dracula*. Indeed, the disease most relevant to both tropical medicine specialists and the public's perception of the field was, arguably, malaria. While the malarial parasite's life cycle was not discovered until 1897 by Ronald Ross—the year of *Dracula*'s publication—the association among the insect, blood, and malarial fever was already circulating in the public imaginary. Patrick Manson connected the mosquito to malaria in 1877, and in 1887, Albert King published an article in the American *Popular Science Monthly* on Charles Laveran and Patrick Manson's 1884 work on mosquito vectors and malaria.[90]

Therefore, Dracula's actions, such as feeding on the human organism would have been funneled through the popular understanding of parasitism. Van Helsing's observation that "he can flourish when . . . he can fatten on the blood of the living," parallels the mosquito's noticeable growth when feeding. Even before Van Helsing explains the pathology of vampirism, Harker notes that Dracula is "gorged with blood" and that "[h]e lay like a filthy leech" (D, 52) after feeding, analogizing him as the most emblematic of parasitic organisms.

Several similarities between the vampire and malaria link the fight against Dracula with the military narratives of tropical medicine specialists. On the side of the protagonists, the self-descriptions of the Crew as knights follow the same literary imagination parasitologists like Ross and Manson used to curate their public images.[91] In the periodical press, they would facilitate their associations with national defense, imperial expansion, and knighthood.[92] As one twentieth-century commentator recalled, the history of Ross's contribution "against the malaria-carrying mosquito has been truly described as more romantic than any story of knight against huge dragon [. . .] this kindly knight was to show himself possessed of patience, imagination, determined and highly-developed reasoning power, and above all faith and courage."[93] In terms of the antagonist pathogen, Taylor-Brown notes the pathological and physiological connections between malaria and the Count's mechanisms of infection. The vampire's fangs work like a mosquito's proboscis; its elongated, needle-like mouth is a mechanism that King theorized as a possible explanation for how germs infect the cells.[94] This figuration works as a naturalized opposition to the Crew's use of the lancet and hypodermic needle for transfusion. Moreover, the Count's power to transform into animals resembles the vector-borne transmission of parasites that pass through intermediate hosts, just as the malarial parasite uses the mosquito to infect humans. Finally, vampirism, in its blood transmission and association with foreign infiltration, would have resonated with British travelers, soldiers, and sailors returning from the colonies infected with malaria.[95] This is what makes vampirism specifically a metaphorical parasitism, where the body stands in for the nation, and not just a disease brought by foreigners. The introduction of foreign elements and disease would change the very nature of the nation and its internal ecology, much like the body. Vampirism incubates and replicates inside the social body—like the material pathology of vampirism, which needs human blood, and the metaphoric parasitism that Dracula enacts when he drains and colonizes England at the site of its reproductive futurism. The fear the vampire inculcates is that the future lineage and nature of Englishness would mutate, degenerate into a primitive, composite Other. But Dracula did not so much create something entirely new. Instead, he proved to be an evolution of something already diseased. As with the question of Lucy's predisposition to a metaphorical and material diseased state, the placement of foreign soil in filthy English environments collapses the boundaries between the foreign and the English; between the sick, and the presumably healthy. Dialectically, however, in disclosing the indistinct fissures in the grand narrative of English progressive victory over disease, the novel ultimately posits perpetual defense as a means to achieve a social correlative to the novel's triumphant unity, its normative closure.

Understanding the bacteriological and parasitological qualities of the vampire in *Dracula*'s engagement with a constellation of diseases and a history of etiology more broadly helps us recognize the way literature shaped the martial metaphor, as it oscillated between metaphorical and material reality. A central part of the anxiety that germ theory provoked was the realization that microbial life could be everywhere and anywhere due to its infinitesimal size, which resonates with one of Dracula's metamorphic abilities: "He became so small—we ourselves saw Miss Lucy, ere she was at peace, slip through a hairbreadth space at the tomb door" (D, 211). Willis suggests that disease objects as germs become "Gothic specters," anthropomorphized as agents while remaining hard to see even through a microscope.[96] This spectral agentification was the next phase in the development of the martial metaphor, and one, as we have seen, that is inseparable from the discourses of colonialism. The metaphor at once rationalized and secularized disease to the point that it was no longer a magical, divine, or unintelligible force, yet when aided by the literary form, the metaphor allowed modern etiologies like germ theory to retain this fictional, or as Willis puts it, "phantasmagoric," aspect. Reading *Dracula* in this context uncovers how the fictionalization of the martial metaphor has been obfuscated and imbued with inimical agency, hiding the very process by which the material histories of military medicine informed that metaphoric transformation. This reshaping made thinkable the translation of social and cultural threats into biological ones, imputing the political into the medical only to use the resulting figuration to do the reverse: to use medicine as politics by other means.

Dracula is a self-conscious product of mass culture reflecting on technologies like the typewriter that allowed for the mass reproduction of narrative, not unlike the hidden world of microbial life with its reproducible, agentive pathogenesis. In its mass circulation, *Dracula* replicated and mutated the martial metaphor, encoding—from the accumulation of medical, literary, and military history—the fin-de-siècle zeitgeist of insecurity: fear of microbes, racial anxieties of degeneration, reverse colonization, women's sexual freedom, and the fragility of British men. But what is really horrifying is not the vampire itself. Rather, it is the way in which *Dracula* propagated the thinking of medicine as war and increased the reach of medicine's jurisdiction into so many facets of modern life, spreading and respawning the nationalist and colonial ideology that affected the production of differential health in dehumanized populations deemed to be threats.

4

Arthur Conan Doyle's Imperial Armamentarium

In moving from the miasmic specter to the minute germ, the front line of medicine's fight against morbidity and mortality assumed a microscopic order in the final decades of the nineteenth century. While Kingsley led the charge against inimical miasma during the middle of the century, the soldiers of the martial metaphor—both medical and literary—faced a radical reconceptualization of the way this war would be fought and what the enemy actually was. Stoker introduced the vampire, human-sized but informed by microbial life—in particular parasitic—and reenchanted medicine in the fictional frame of war. Stoker's invocation of the Gothic and monstrous relied on a highly visible and abject inimical disease. As a Gothic novel, *Dracula*'s use of the martial metaphor relies on excess, on tableau and spectacle. Just as literature like *Dracula* circulated the metaphor while occluding its material military origins, Arthur Conan Doyle's detective fiction and medical and historical prose gave exigency to the martial metaphor through the discourse of scientific visibility. Doyle provides a grammar for the threatening phenomena of the microscopic invisible world, mapping bacteria and parasites onto the larger scale of empire.

Doyle circulates the metaphor through two paradigms: detection and immunity, both of which are informed by the medical sciences of bacteriology and toxicology. In *A Study in Scarlet* (1887), the narrator John Watson, a military surgeon just returned from the Second Anglo-Afghan War (1878–1880), famously writes that he "gravitated to London, that great cesspool into which all the loungers and idlers of the Empire are irresistibly drained."[1] In Doyle's fiction, imperial structures often figure as producers of infectious and polluting detritus. Watson and Holmes serve as the empire's "immune system," according to Laura Otis, because they recognize and disarm pathogenic others.[2] Indeed, Holmes upholds the biopolitical tenet that English society "must be defended." In the Holmes stories medicine is war, but this war is less explicit than the one in Crimea, nearly indiscernible in fact, at least until the early twentieth century, after Britain's war in South Africa. Unlike the police and the military, Holmes and Watson work in unofficial capacities. In maintaining the system by differentiating and eliminating the threats of the modern imperial age, but not being official repressive organs of the state, they keep the disease-producing social order intact. In other words, they identify and fight infections but don't treat the root of the problem, maintaining the exclusionary and differential way of producing Englishness. This is a vicious cycle much like the martial metaphor's tendency to exacerbate the conditions and anxieties that require it. Holmes defends society by seeing the invisible traces of social pathologies in everyday bourgeois life, in the same way bacteriologists find their subject matter anywhere and everywhere. In this era, medicine could identify threats and allay symptoms but rarely cure, even though it was promoted as a perpetual war, as we have seen. Detection in Doyle's writing works similarly.

The logic of immunity in the individual body is also apparent in Doyle's writings, appearing just as it was gaining purchase as a physiological theory toward the end of the century. Filth, bacteria, and poison are conflated in this picture, inasmuch as they all represent toxic infiltrations of the self by the Other, and immunity becomes a discourse for understanding how the body parses this distinction. Immunity thus naturalizes the martial metaphor by grounding it in the body. In this chapter, I consider the contradictions between Doyle's espousals of Englishness and empire across his corpus and his portrayal in his fiction of England's complicity in its own physical and societal sickness.

When placed in conversation, Doyle's fiction and medical writings reveal a fraught relationship between the physician-author and the martial metaphor. Whereas his medical-journalistic and historical writings espouse the martial metaphor as a way to understand the relationship between humans and disease, his fiction troubles the validity of the same metaphor and exposes its contradictions. Empire must be defended even though doing so continually opens the door to new physical disease through the expansion of territory and military infrastructure, as Shelley's *The Last Man* reflected in the case of cholera, and to new and inherent modes of corruption of the English race, as Stoker's *Dracula* intimates.

The scholarship on Arthur Conan Doyle with respect to medicine and metaphor has made this connection rhetorically, that is, as a way to write about Doyle's fiction and its relation to Victorian medical discourse.[3] Laura Otis's characterization of Holmes and Watson as an "imperial immune system" makes sense to modern readers, although Doyle himself does not use this construction to describe Watson and Holmes's work in defense of the empire. However, rather than serving as an argument against Doyle's use of the metaphor, this absence reveals how Doyle framed medicine and war before and after the turn of the century in a mode logically congruent with the viability of, but not explicitly citing, immunity. The fact that the metaphor is not overtly visible but is presented through the discourse of detection, as it is informed by bacteriology and immunity, suggests that it becomes an invisible structure for social order. Later, after an accumulation of concerns regarding Britain's military fitness beginning in the 1870s and exacerbated by the failure of the Boer War[4] in large part due to bacterial epidemics, Doyle deploys the metaphor explicitly in the face of a declining race and inability to control foreign territories.

Beyond infectious disease and immunity, it is also crucial to consider how poison plays a role in shaping the metaphor of medicine as war and the nation as a body in the milieu of the larger empire. Different threats to the individual and the national body—contagious, toxic, polluted, degenerate—come to be embodied in colonial and internally corrupt, others while remaining immanent in the system that wants to rid itself of them. The role of the pathogenic and the toxic speaks to how national identity works in Doyle's Holmes fiction. England defines itself militarily in terms of imperial expansion and conquest, and Englishness is strongest after exposure to contamination: "Only against foreignness can England show its true mettle," as Joe Childers suggests.[5] Doyle presents the martial metaphor as a way of testing and strengthening Englishness, not unlike the relationship between vaccination and immunity. Thus, Englishness operates much like masculinity and nation do for Kingsley, with war and disease making men, and their assemblage into a nation, stronger through a kind of purging.[6] Reading Kingsley's fiction and prose in terms of medicine and war reveals how Crimea and cholera prompted middle-class men to forge strong masculinity while supported by wife-nurses in the war against miasma. By the time Doyle's work becomes popular, the martial metaphor's role in this middle-class health index had become embedded in social order; however, cultural productions like fiction also begin to show this had not lived up to produce the hygienic resiliency Kingsley proselytized.

Considering how medical readings signal the contradictory logic of health and Englishness in the Holmes fiction, I examine the ways bacteriology, immunology, and toxicology are not only related through detection and medicine but are also conceptualized and linked by a military ethos across Doyle's writings; they converge within the framework of the martial metaphor. The logic of the immune system as bodily defense reflects that of the military as national defense by way of the martial metaphor, a structuring concept in Doyle's medical prose and fiction. Recalling Bichat's definition of life, the health of the individual is inherently pathologized: life is always engaged in the process of death, and consequently it is diseased in its mortal capacity. If life is a war to forestall disease, a life is productive only insofar as it makes itself not-diseased. For Doyle, Englishness functions the same way. As Doyle defines Englishness and national health in the face of imperial and internal threats, it is an interminable process of exposure, identification, and resistance—a process much like the activity of the immune system. Examining these associations lets us see how Holmes's immunological detection and Doyle's own investment in militarism in his prose come to be incorporated into the contemporaneous medical discourse, in which the body defends itself internally, systemically, cellularly.

This chapter takes a two-part structure because tracking the martial metaphor across Doyle's fiction and prose reveals a stark change at the turn of the century. In section 1, I show that bacteria do not appear overtly in Holmes stories before 1899, and the martial metaphor is visible only in Watson's role as a military physician. Given that Doyle trained as a physician during the development of bacteriology, immunology, and toxicology, it is necessary to determine how these developing specialties influenced his understanding of medicine in military terms. I offer an extended reading of Doyle's medical prose and the related scientific conversations of the period. I begin by discussing the literary techniques in Doyle's article "Life and Death in Blood" (1883), as they operate in the contemporaneous theories of cellular immunity. I follow this with a reading of the significance of toxicology and Claude Bernard's experimental medicine, as they appear in the Holmes stories such as *A Study in Scarlet*, *The Sign of Four* (1888), and "The Adventure of the Speckled Band" (1892). I show that while Doyle's prose affirms the martial metaphor more overtly here, its subtle presence as a structuring logic in his fiction before the Boer War is rhetorically aligned with differentiating self and other, poison and cure, and the English and the foreign. I conclude by showing how Doyle's article on Robert Koch's failed cure for tuberculosis primed the idea of pharmacological "torpedoes" as a way to supplement the body's internal immunity with medical technology. In section 2, I show how Doyle drew from military medicine during his personal experiences in the Boer War as a military surgeon to assert the martial metaphor more explicitly in his writing after 1899. I then trace Doyle's expressions of distress both at the military's inability to support its troops medically and at the declining vitality of the British as a physically robust military force in *The Great Boer War* (1900), *The War in South Africa: Its Causes and Conduct* (1902), and other works on the war and its medical complications. I then discuss how Doyle's defense of British concentration camps shows how military practices at the end of the nineteenth century were transmuting the shape of modern biopolitical governance. I conclude by examining the appearance of infectious disease in inimical constructions in "The Adventure of the Dying Detective" (1913) and "The Adventure of the Blanched Soldier" (1926). Doyle uses bacteriological threats in his later fiction to simultaneously spur and allay the anxieties of a weakening British race and empire. Although Doyle, an avid supporter of British imperialism, uses the martial metaphor to support its imperatives, reading them against the grain in the context of their military history and their facile resolutions suggests that imperial structures and military actions were not only sick but exacerbating rather than dispelling disease.

Across Doyle's corpus, the promotion of the militarism and its power to destabilize the equation of Englishness with health ultimately reinscribe the martial metaphor. That is, they either reproduce the intellectual formation itself or they foster the conditions to require the metaphor's narrative order. Ultimately, however, Doyle's overmobilization does the cultural work of circulating it as a necessary and accessible language to understand infectious disease, anomic disruptions, and the medicalization of social difference.

I

Detecting Microbial and Imperial Threats

If bacteriology, and medical science more broadly, sought to make the invisible visible, then the literary representations of the martial metaphor worked in the opposite direction. They occluded the military history of the figurative war against germs by replacing the repressive, overt representations of the law and power with the science of detection and the disciplinary social ordering it fosters.[7] Detection was the key to the metaphorical militarization of medicine because of the then-evolving public interest in bacteriology and, more broadly, the gain in cultural purchase of medical visuality. Both of these were linked with the anxieties of empire and its defense. Literature like Doyle's Holmes fiction, in tandem with essays in popular periodicals and the medical press, spurred the public's adoption of these intersections. As Jennifer Tucker suggests, "Journalistic images of the war against germs produced for mass audiences during the 1890s bear witness to the intensifying scientific and popular interest in bacteria and to the readiness of many scientists to exploit military and imperialist iconography and racial stereotypes to show germs as unruly tribes of deadly microorganisms."[8] To understand how this military, imperialist, and racial iconography works in Doyle, we must look at how his journalistic writings on medicine informed the martial metaphor qua detection.

Doyle, training as a medical student from 1876 to 1881, was at the center of this epistemological shift. Joseph Bell, a medical school professor of Doyle's, served as the model for Sherlock Holmes with his uncanny observation and deduction skills. Bell himself suggested in an 1893 introduction to *A Study in Scarlet* that "Dr. Conan Doyle's education as a student of medicine taught him how to observe. . . . Eyes and ears which can see and hear, memory to record at once and to recall at pleasure the impressions of the senses, and an imagination capable of weaving a theory or piecing together a broken chain, or unravelling a tangled clue, such are implements of his trade to a successful diagnostician."[9] Linking this kind of observation to bacteriology, he continues, "The greatest stride that has been made of late years in preventive and diagnostic medicine consists in the recognition and differentiation by bacteriological research of those minute organisms which disseminate cholera and fever, tubercle and anthrax. The importance of the infinitely little is incalculable."[10]

If Bichat's medical gaze enabled pathological anatomists to observe lesions in tissue, then by the 1860s the medical gaze was increasingly a microscopic one. In this new era, cells rather than tissues were the objects of medical knowledge. Moreover, in contrast to pathological anatomy, which studied disease postmortem, research could focus on living cells in tissues and fluids, and the gaze could investigate disease processes as they occurred rather than just through their ultimate effects.[11] Bichat's assemblage of functions that resist death, then, came to be known at the cellular and chemical levels. Doyle's writing reflects this shift, evident in his use of imagery, plot devices, and narration.

As a consequence of the new granular focus of medical research and disease etiology, immunity and bacteriological discourse became the two central scientific systems of thought that subtended the martial metaphor. Together, they linked the internal, "natural" defenses of the body with medical technologies for the same end. Both of these concepts were fundamentally entangled with nationalist and military technologies and imperatives. The martial metaphor, however, occluded this material association by naturalizing the logic of defense. With the emergence and acceptance of new medical technologies came a new kind of medical gaze, one that viewed disease and its physiological counterparts in the body, the components of the immune system, and demonstrated an organic correlative of the martial metaphor at the microbial and microscopic scale.

The emergence of bacteriology in the 1880s led medical scientists to start thinking in immunological terms,[12] investigating the mechanisms by which bodies themselves fought off disease. By the 1890s a number of articles in the *British Medical Journal* and the *Lancet* cited Elie Metchnikoff's theory of cellular immunity, and did so through the martial metaphor.[13] John Burdon-Sanderson, a physiologist and histologist discussed in the previous chapter for his work on cattle plague, responds to this development, contending that "the vast accumulation of exact knowledge as to the morphological characters and physiological endowments of microbes is not valued for its own sake, but because it enables us to understand the reactions they invoke in the living body," particularly reactions that signaled when "invaders are in possession and that disease has begun."[14] Before Metchnikoff's theory, it was believed that what made one immune was the lack of some component or quality that predisposed one to disease, a conceptual remnant of humoral theory. Doctors and scientists began to move beyond general characterizations of immunity that framed certain inherent constitutions as more vulnerable to disease than others. As microscopy and bacteriology matured and scientists began observing pathogens in the body fluids and tissue in vivo, scientists like Metchnikoff and Koch began to consider how the body actively engaged foreign microbes and, as Burdon-Sanderson puts it, the "weapon by which [pathogens] exercise their power of injury."[15]

Apart from representations of the body as a site of battles against disease, the concept of immunity has a long biopolitical history. Originating in a legal etymology from *munus*, meaning both gift and obligation, the term is linked to the political and legal status of the municipal. *Immunity* originally singled out individuals as not subject to municipal obligations while still included within the legal system that made that determination: it created exceptions to the law by demonstrating that the law exists without exception.[16] The martial metaphor performs correlative imaginary work with respect to disease: it creates a "disorder" in the form of war—a pathological state of human relations—inviting an ideological ordering on death and disease. In other words, the only way to understand disease in an age that was moving away from theological accounts was through an imposed discourse of disorder, namely war, that required an antithetical yet equally bellicose response. Although Ed Cohen has traced the idea of immunity as self-defense through the political philosophy of the Enlightenment and the biopolitical practices of the nineteenth century, the way this political focus linked public health with military practices has not been fully explored. Moreover, it was not until the 1880s that immunity materialized in the body and came to be associated with military medicine and public health by way of the martial metaphor. Doyle's writings help us see how war, bacteriology, and immunology converged in this period.

Doyle was aware of Koch's work from its inception, and he deployed the martial metaphor to explain the implications of bacteriology to a lay audience. In March of 1883, a year after Koch's discovery of the tuberculosis bacterium, Doyle published "Life and Death in Blood" in the popular periodical *Good Words*. The essay's title polarizes life and death as the surrogates for health and disease, humans contra microbes. Although Doyle doesn't mention Metchnikoff's immunity explicitly, he does prefigure it in his discussion of leukocytes as the agents of life.[17] The titular and ordering logic of Doyle's essay were invoked in an image accompanying a 1912 article in *Harmsworth Popular Science* (fig. 4.1).[18] The illustration's caption informs the reader that "the facts of health in its most important aspect can be actually seen under the Microscope . . . [Microbes] seek to multiply in the blood, and there we can see health and disease in visible forms," health and disease, recalling Kingsley's masculine assertion against cholera in *Two Years Ago*, are "face to face—nay, locked in deadly embrace . . . Health and Disease are realities henceforth for the rest of the spectator's life."[19] This visual

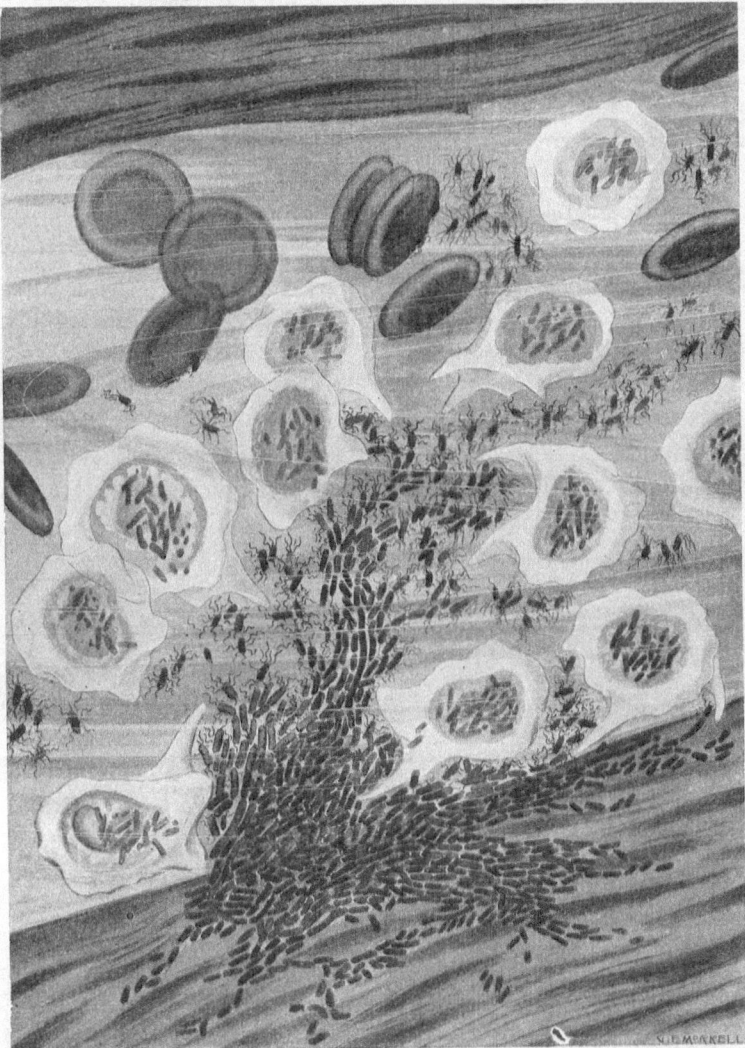

Figure 4.1. George F. Morrell, *Health and Disease in Deadly Combat*, 1912, print. Courtesy of the Wellcome Collection, https://wellcomecollection.org/works/ngc7gs94. Originally published in *Harmsworth Popular Science*. Used under CC BY 4.0 license.

representation, along with its text, bears an uncanny resemblance to Doyle's 1883 essay, and indeed marks a trajectory for the martial metaphor's continuity into the twentieth century.

Doyle interpolates readers into the martial metaphor with inviting language that unites individuals with their physicians against microbial invaders. He achieves this enlistment through the discourse of microscopy. Working in the spirit of a scientific romance and prefiguring his science-fiction work,[20] Doyle invites the reader to shrink down to the size of blood cells to watch the inner battle on the microscopic order: "Had a man the power of reducing himself to the size of less than the one-thousandth part of an inch, and should he, while of this microscopic stature, convey himself through the coats of a living artery, how strange the sight that would meet his eye."[21] Showing his shrunken reader the healthy life of the blood, Doyle identifies red blood cells, which carry oxygen, and the living creatures in the blood, the leukocytes, which "[hurry] away into the blood stream as an independent organism[s]" (*LD*, 178). Though Doyle remarks that leukocytes increase in number in diseased states, he would not have known exactly how these "bodies" work against disease. What is important to note here, however, is that the leukocyte is "the creature possessing the attributes commonly associated with life, which is found in healthy human blood" (*LD*, 178). These are the very cells Metchnikoff characterized in more aggressive language only two years later, suggesting that "when one accepts the concept that phagocytes fight directly against pathogens, it becomes understandable that inflammation is a defensive mechanism against bacterial invasion."[22] Doyle goes on to describe the forces that oppose the leukocytes: "In diseased conditions numerous others appear, differing from each other as widely as the flounder does from the eel, and presenting an even greater contrast in the effects which they produce" (*LD*, 178). And in forecasting the remainder of his essay, he proposes "to glance at some of the work done of late in this direction—work which has opened up a romance world of living creatures so minute as to be hardly detected by our highest lenses, yet many of them endowed with such fearful properties that the savage tiger or venomous cobra have not inflicted one fiftieth part of the damage upon the human race" (*LD*, 179). Worth nothing is that the body is at once protagonist and setting (their blood as medium), following what Emilie Taylor-Brown characterizes as the "microscopic rhetoric dovetail[ing] with the conflation of body and landscape (common to medical cartography and imperial romance) that was increasingly used by parasitologists to visualise and communicate the movement of parasites within the body."[23] The construction of the microbial world suggests a journey—in genre terms, the narrative is a romance—that is both military and imperial, as the creatures described are linked to savage colonial animals like the tiger and the cobra. The latter, indeed, is reimagined in the Holmes fiction as an imperial biocontaminant, a way for those subjugated by empire to retaliate with natural and developed biomedical weapons, as I explain in the next subsection.

These lower-order creatures are pitted against the human race, a significant concept in Doyle's work in terms of Englishness, as a number of scholars have suggested.[24] In the same way, colonized races are often opposed to the English, who are frequently characterized as degenerating. Koch uses the language of racism and colonization when he writes of bacteria in terms of "cultures" and "colonies."[25] Doyle characterizes the contest between humans and microbes in the same way, informed by the Darwinian struggle for existence, a struggle in which bacteria invade and die but leave their progeny in the human blood: "The horrible process goes on until either the race dies away, or their victim is exhausted" (*LD*, 179). While we don't get any description in this scene of leukocytes "battling" bacteria, the contest is clear, in that it is one life or another; either the bacterial "race" is not strong enough to live in the human blood, for reasons that were at that point not fully understood, or the victim succumbs to the infection. In this way, Doyle's essay primes the episteme of immune-defense in British readers, an idea as anxiogenic as it was exciting.

Where Kingsley and other sanitarians viewed the invading enemy as a visible filth or an olfactorily perceptible miasma, the advent of modern germ theory created a paradigm in which inimical bodies were everywhere and anywhere. Doyle's "strange sight" frames the interaction between the healthy body's agents and microbes as an inimical one by simultaneously speaking of the smallness, even invisibility, of the microbes and rhetorically figuring them as life-sized enemies fighting in the human order of the world. When Doyle invokes the discourse of microscopy to explain life and death in the blood, he speaks to one of the foundational shifts in the way medicine was understood through the conceptual domain of war. Although bacteriology gave the doctors, readers, and general public of the nineteenth century a new way to look at the world, it was not an entirely reassuring one.[26] On the one hand, inimical pathogenic agents could be seen through specialized equipment by medical specialists who now knew what to look for. This shift was also significant for understanding the discourse of expertise that appeared in the Holmes stories.[27] On the other hand, these foreign bodies were imperceptible to the naked eye or the sensitive nose and could at any moment penetrate the boundaries of the porous subject. The way to allay preoccupation with this was to give these agents visibility. Only what can't be defined is truly threatening; as Holmes puts it, a threat would "cease to be dangerous if we could define it."[28]

Drawing on the visuality of the microscope, Doyle invites readers to watch the battle between life in the body and the death in the invading bacteria. The effect is to scale the abstract battle between life and death down to the microscopic level and put the relationship between the microbial agent and the human—and the perception of their encounter—on level footing: "Let us go to the bedside of some poor fellow suffering from this complaint, and having once more assumed our microscopic proportions, let us inspect personally the condition of his circulation. We see again the transparent serum, the busy yellow discs, the languid omnivorous pieces of jelly; but what is this? Writhing their way among the legitimate corpuscles there are countless creatures, thin and long, with snake-like body and spiral motion" (*LD*, 178). Doyle's invitation to shrink down and observe the leukocytes shifts back to a more expository mode when he gives his forecasts for the latest work he discusses in his essay. However, the cohortative mood—"let us"—encourages the reader to take part in the romance. This is the very technique he uses in his essay on Koch's cure to describe his laboratory in Vienna. By shifting back and forth between the external, human world and the microscopic, Doyle puts his readers in the position of the doctor examining a patient's signs before embodying them in the microscopic medical gaze, letting the readers internalize this visual narrative by imagining it in their own bodies.

This invitation to imagine, however, operates beyond the realm of the rhetorical. The narrative mode Doyle deploys resonates with what Meegan Kennedy has called "speculative insight," the use of imagination and speculation for hypothesis to supplement the objectivity of the clinical gaze. For physicians, it worked as a form of exploratory reasoning and for physiologists like Claude Bernard, a mode of active experimentation.[29] In this passage, Doyle encourages the reader to reason and experiment with guided speculation from the perspective of the microbial and human level. In doing so, he prompts the reader to do the imaginative work and internalize the martial metaphor in their own visions of cellular battle. On this line of writing science and medicine Martin Willis similarly makes the case that observation through the microscope occurs in a space between the real and the imagined. The job of the imagination, when joined with the microscope, is to construct an image of what lies *beyond* the eye and the lens's limits. This is a clear departure from "objective" viewing.[30] The linkage between the imaginative and the empirical in the use of the microscope became a central element of the fictional examination of infectious disease's influence on Victorian society.[31] While Willis links this effect to the Gothic mode, and to *Dracula* in particular, I suggest that it is also operative in Doyle's "Life and Death" and in his Holmes fiction. In each case, what is needed is a technology for identifying the pathogenic, be it the trace of a criminal or a bacterium. In Doyle's detective fiction, the foreign threat is small and invisible to the nonexpert, like the bacteria in blood. Holmes's work is analogous to that of the bacteriologist in that both trace the links between people: Holmes follows the criminal through his malevolent activities, while the bacteriologist follows the microbe from carrier to victim.[32]

Even while inspiring anxiety in terms of microbial smallness, "Life and Death" works to be uplifting, supporting its reader's faith in the progress of biomedical science toward victory in a battle the human race had long been losing: "Given that a single disease, proved to depend upon a parasitic organism, can be effectually and certainly stamped out, why should not all diseases depending upon similar causes be also done away with? That is the great question which the scientific world is striving to solve; and in the face of it how paltry do war and statecraft appear, and everything which fascinates the attention of the multitude!" (*LD*, 180). Recalling Kingsley's and other writers' use of the device from the mid-century forward—the suggestion that war and its casualties are insignificant in comparison with the ravages of disease—Doyle reinscribes the martial metaphor by creating a disjunction between war and disease. When he suggests that nation-on-nation war is of "paltry" interest beside bacteriology, he rhetorically figures medicine as *the* war. If human wars are so inconsequential, the war of medicine is the ur-war. This is not just a philosophical abstraction; it is demonstrated time and again throughout history in the power of disease to curtail military force.

With his ur-war construction, Doyle also offers another comparison to statecraft. By suggesting that medicine-as-war is the primary concern of the state, guided by the development of science, he obscures the actual military and political history involved in making medicine into this metaphor, eliding the material points of contact between medicine and war, even more so if we consider his use of the phrase *stamping out*, discussed in the previous chapter with respect to William Budd and James Simpson. In Doyle's pre–Boer War fiction, this leads to the hidden disciplinary structures that the martial metaphor bolsters; in these works, rather than bacterial or parasitological infections, "disease" takes the form of poisons, corrupted Englishmen, and foreign others, and "medicine" becomes detection and forensic science.

Toxicology and "Experiments of Destruction"

Toxicology is a recurring element in Doyle's writing that links detection, medicine, and the martial metaphor. His conflation of contagious microbes and toxins shapes both his own and Holmes's relationship to empire. The discourse of toxicology, furthermore, as it relates to the experimental medicine of Claude Bernard, informs how war structures the forensic sciences in Holmes's detection. Doyle himself had more than a passing knowledge of poisons; training at Edinburg in 1876, he would have studied under Sir Robert Christianson, one of the founders of modern toxicology.[33]

Conceptually speaking, the essence of medico-military war is the imperative to keep out that which is toxic to the individual or national body. We see this in the operant logic of "Life and Death," in which leukocytes are characterized as "legitimate" in contrast with the spiral, "snake-like" bacteria—a description that imbues the microbial with a malevolent and colonial quality by recalling the earlier mention of the "venomous cobra." This language also resembles Doyle's recurrent use of the poison trope in the Holmes stories, where it works as a pathogenic agent through not only toxicity but contagion: these works of detective fiction exemplify a rhetorical trend of conflating organic toxins, drugs, and infectious agents as "foreign-born biocontaminants"—the chemical and biological weapons with which the people subjugated by the empire fight back.[34]

Contagions figure in Doyle's use of poison in that he writes poisoners who either originate in or have recently returned from colonial, tropical areas. In "The Adventure of the Speckled Band," for instance, Dr. Grimesby Roylott, the impoverished and sole remaining member of a noble family, travels to India, gains a medical license, and returns looking ill, behaving cantankerously, and bearing a poisonous swamp adder with which to kill his stepdaughters for their estate. The antagonist of *The Sign of the Four* is Jonathan Small, who served as a soldier in India after spending time in jail for murder. He returns to England seeking stolen treasures and brings with him a native of the Andaman Islands, Tonga, who is armed with poisonous darts. Poisoning is figured as a contagious vice spreading from the colonies and infecting corruptible Englishman, metonymically linked to their corrupt Englishness and also physically brought back to England by them. Doyle also associates poisons with bacterial infections in his medical writings. In "Life and Death," he solidifies this connection when he describes Koch's ability "to cultivate the infection [*Bacillus anthracis*], as he might grow monkshood or any vegetable poison in the soil of his back garden" (*LD*, 179).[35] Holmes and Watson, too, frequently encounter foreign figures who have been "cultivated" by exotic colonized cultures to deploy poisonous biocontaminants, and to this extent their work is to identify and neutralize the effects of such agents, like Roylott and Small.

Doyle's use of the poison trope is structured by the militarization of medicine not just in its conflation of foreign contagion and contamination but also by way of Claude Bernard's experimental methods and their relation to pathology. Bernard, one of the most significant figures in nineteenth-century medical history, was best known for *An Introduction to the Study of Experimental Medicine* (1865). A vivisectionist, he explored pathologies in live animals, often introducing them himself to see their effects, be it an anatomical aberration or a foreign substance. The discourse of toxins in Doyle and Bernard further links the two figures, by way of the martial metaphor, in terms of experimentation. As a physician training in the 1860s and '70s, it would have been difficult for Doyle to be unaware of Bernard's work; even though he does not mention him in the Holmes stories, he refers to him in passing in "The Parasite: A Story."[36]

Holmes' detection skills are due not only to his keen powers of observation but, like Bernard's, to his vast experience with experimental science. This is abundantly evident in Holmes's first appearance in *A Study in Scarlet*, when Watson enters Holmes's lab: "This was a lofty chamber, lined and littered with countless bottles. Broad, low tables were scattered about, which bristled with retorts, test-tubes, and little Bunsen lamps, with their blue flickering flames. There was only one student in the room, who was bending over a distant table absorbed in his work"

(SS, 7). Holmes informs Watson that he is working on a hemoglobin reagent to detect occult blood for forensic purposes; he is studying "the scarlet thread of murder" (SS, 37). He also admits that he "dabble[s] in poisons" (SS, 9). In this introduction, we learn that Holmes performs work not unlike Bichat's pathological anatomy, when he tries to time the process of postmortem bruising: "When it comes to beating subjects in the dissecting rooms," Holmes contends, "it is certainly taking a bizarre shape" (SS, 6). Finally, Holmes does his own "experiment of destruction," when he tests the mysterious pill found at the crime scene on a live terrier (SS, 58).

Holmes's work is aligned with Bernard's through their common training and technologies. Holmes and Koch, in their observation and detection skills, exemplify Bernard's ideal experimental scientist, who "forces nature to reveal herself by attacking her with all manner of questions."[37] For Bernard, the experimental method is the central weapon in the fight against disease. In making his case for experimental medicine, Bernard writes, "the experimental physician . . . possess[es] weapons with which he must act . . . [and] in wishing to determine with the aid of modification (poisons) the laws of the phenomena of life, we attack the problem of therapeutics directly."[38] As Ed Cohen notes, Bernard challenges Hippocratic medicine for its passivity by reconfiguring medicine, in the name of health, as war.[39] If war is politics by other means, then for Bernard, war on the animal body is medicine by other means. One method that emerges from this bellicose reconfiguration is the direct provocation of disease and death in experiments. It is thus no surprise that he characterizes many of his techniques as "experiments of destruction,"[40] in which the investigator impedes or "destroys" a physiological function in order to reverse engineer a pathological process. In terms of the broader connections between war and medicine, the pursuit of destructive activities as a means for the ultimate goal of healing follows the same logic as killing to make live.

One of Bernard's best-known experiments of destruction was the use of poison, making him further relevant to the toxicological trope in Doyle's writing. According to Cohen, Bernard may have been the first to deploy poison medically as a part of medicine's developing armamentaria, using toxic substances to develop therapeutic ones.[41] For example, Bernard experimented with curare—an umbrella term for a number of South American plant-based alkaloid toxins—to immobilize animals while he experimented on them.[42] He famously demonstrated that curare causes paralysis by affecting the motor nerves while leaving the sensory nerves unaffected. Curare appears explicitly in Doyle's "The Vampire of Sussex" (1924) and, though it is not named, the poison in *A Study in Scarlet* is often read as curare.

This is only one of the many exotic toxins in the Holmes stories; others are Tonga's blow dart, which is "certainly not" an "English thorn" but a dart tainted with a powerful "vegetable alkaloid";[43] and the poisonous snake in "The Adventure of the Speckled Band" (1892), which kills Roylott, the maddened physician who used it as a murder weapon previously. In both of these stories, Englishmen are infected by empire and bring the contaminants back. In the latter, Holmes claims that the use of an exotic toxin would occur to "a clever and ruthless man who had had an Eastern training,"[44] one contaminated by empire. "The Speckled Band" is particularly anxiety provoking in terms of colonial contamination, in that it is a doctor who brings the snake back as a murder weapon. This inverts the martial metaphor by having an English medical man deploy biomedical knowledge for personal gain rather than the promotion of health. In neutralizing villains like Roylott, however, Holmes doesn't outright pathologize and cure what is plaguing the empire, the system that is producing the imperial detritus; he regulates its toxic, contagious waste. This indeterminacy, the way Holmes both upholds empire and displays its inherent pathogenicity, speaks to the way poison works in a dialectical fashion with respect to health and disease.

"Poison" can be used as a weapon for or against health. In toxicology, it is often difficult to define poison qualitatively; consequently, it is a tenet of toxicology that it is the dose that makes the poison.[45] Doyle understood this, discussing it in his published response to one Colonel S. B. Wintle, an unapologetic antivaccinationist: "Anti-vaccinationists harp upon vaccine being a poison. Of course it is a poison. So is opium, digitalis, and arsenic, though they are three of the most valuable drugs in the pharmacopoeia. The whole science of medicine is by the use of a mild poison to counteract a deadly one. The virus of rabies is a poison, but Pasteur has managed to turn it to account in the treatment of hydrophobia."[46] Doyle acknowledges that medicine operates through the dialectic of the *pharmakon*. The etymology of *pharma* reflects the fact that a drug can be at once poison and remedy. This shares a similar paradox to the biopolitics of the martial metaphor: medicine that heals but that also draws on metaphors of killing and violence; medicine that both makes live and lets die. I discuss an example of the way medical knowledge, in a broader biopolitical sense, was used to lay siege to the colonial population during the Boer War in the second section of this chapter. This indeterminacy follows Childers's suggestion insofar as the tension between remedy and poison reveals how concepts of foreign filth, others, and contagions from the empire worked to reaffirm Englishness, which defined itself by resisting the incursions of the foreign and the other even while requiring the Other to define itself.

In this way, the trials of corrupt Englishman and savage foreign invaders worked as a kind of "vaccine" much like Holmes's drug use, strengthening Englishness by exposing it to what it was not. Doyle's embodied metaphor of military medicine, John Watson, works the same way: he is damaged goods, poor and disabled from his time on the outskirts of empire, injured by a bullet wound, yet he works with Holmes to give a narrative shape to his crime detection. Moreover, he acts as a touchstone of Englishness, keeping Holmes in check with the proprieties of middle-class English life, as Holmes is good at his job precisely because he can identify with what falls outside normal Englishness through his contacts in the lower class and his ability to disguise himself as one of them. Holmes is in a sense immune, exempt both from the law and from social inclusion by his identification with the poor, the degenerate, and other undesirables overlooked by the proper British subject. These disguises would endanger Holmes's very identity without Watson serving as a touchstone.[47]

Watson polices not only Holmes's behavior but also his health, most notably in chastising him for using cocaine in *The Sign of the Four*: "Remember I speak not only as one comrade to another, but as a medical man to one for whose constitution he is to some extent answerable" (SOF, 124). Cocaine works as a kind of *pharmakon*, stimulating and sharpening Holmes's skills while also causing tissue damage. The drug also signals the pathological qualities inherent in both Watson and Holmes. Watson cannot take the drug because "[his] constitution has not got over the Afghan campaign yet. He cannot afford to throw any extra strain upon it" (SOF, 123); that is, his body is corrupted, a product of the cesspool of empire. But he also suggests that habitual cocaine use is a "pathological and morbid process which involves increased tissue change and may induce permanent weakness" (SOF, 124). Thus, even Holmes and Watson fall into this ambivalent position between poison and cure. In Childers's words, Holmes's drug use works like a "vaccination, allowing him to push the limits of Englishness, to move about the

London cesspool with relative immunity, to explore ambiguity in his own identity, and still be able to return, and to help define what Englishness is and how it should function."[48] The drug functions as ergogenic aid, helping him work at full capacity by artificially stimulating his mind as if it were performing its usual work of observation and detection. Much like the discussion of Otis's use of immunity as a metaphor to describe Holmes above, we should likewise evaluate Childers's reading in relation to Doyle's own understanding of vaccination.

The strengthening-by-exposure quality of actual, rather than metaphorical, vaccinations is evident in the fact that they are, per Doyle's definition, "poisons." At scale, vaccination practices do incur "losses," as some people can get sick from the prophylaxis. Doyle called vaccination "one of the greatest victories ever won by science over disease," invoking the martial metaphor again and characterizing antivaccinationists as degenerates: their notion of progress was to "revert to the condition of things as they existed in the dark ages before the dawn of medical science."[49] Through its connections to contagion, foreign contaminants, vaccination, and Bernard, "poison," as a discourse and a technological actant, plays a significant role in the history of the martial metaphor. This is because not only are poisons tied to the development of more effective pharmacological weapons, as I show in the final chapter, and a common metaphor for framing internal and foreign threats, but the compounds are associated with foreign contaminants that threaten the national body in the same discursive formations as infectious diseases from abroad.

Bernard and Doyle are "blood-related" beyond their toxicological connections, too. For both, blood serves as an organizing principle for health and disease. In Doyle's essay on microbes and leukocytes, it is the medium of life and death, and in his fiction, it is a trace of crime and contamination that the detective puts under a medico-forensic gaze. Doyle describes how Koch theorized that bacteria live in blood and proved it by transferring blood from an infected animal to a healthy one, which then became ill. For Doyle, blood is, then, the life-giving medium, carrying oxygen—recalling Kingsley's identification of oxygen with life that resists death—and leukocytes, the only creature "in healthy human blood" with vital qualities. This medium can be infiltrated by foreign agents, and consequently biologic battles with infection are thus fought in the blood, evoking Stoker's use of the fluid, and the illustration in *Harmsworth Popular Science*.

A *Study in Scarlet* eponymously characterizes the work of detection in terms of blood: "There's the scarlet thread of murder running through the colorless skein of life," Holmes instructs Watson, "and our duty is to unravel it, and isolate it, and expose every inch of it" (SS, 37). Blood becomes not that which sustains life but that which gives evidence of its being compromised. Nonetheless, the medico-scientific technique to be applied is characterized in the discourse of microscopy, as much of the work of detection entails blood and learning where it came from and how it was spilled. The "scarlet thread" is the fabric of life that is tainted, a stain that needs to be isolated and examined. This figure evokes a groundbreaking technique developed during the advent of germ theory that was used extensively. In order to be made visible, bacteria needed to be chemically stained; to see tuberculosis, Koch used the methylene-blue staining technique developed by Paul Ehrlich.[50] While we can indeed read Holmes as identifying systemic structures that create corruption—insofar as his stories leave those structures open to critique by the reader—Holmes and Watson find the discrete pathogens and "isolate them," but they ignore the cultural medium that allows them to thrive. In other words, they allay symptoms rather than curing the social disease.

Bernard theorized that the *milieu intérieur* held the blood, as a sealed-off interior environment of the individual body. This biopolitically affirmed the individual as the locus of the medical battle against death. He writes, "The stability of the internal environment [*milieu intérieur*] is the condition for the free and independent life."[51] While this has often been taken as a theorization of homeostasis, and even seems to point back toward humoral theory, the role of the blood in cordoning off the self and providing an internal protective environment for the vital tissues prefigures the role of immunity as natural self-defense, and also makes a cellular parallax of Kinglsey's war against disease and the universe. Bernard takes the earlier sanitary discourse and humoral theories, which focused on individuals within a milieu, and *incorporates* that milieu into the individual. Moreover, Bernard's focus on "independence" performs significant biopolitical work—through, for example, his belief that the more independent a warm-blooded animal is, the more it is contingent on a protective environment. Bernard's metaphorization of the individual as "naturally autonomous" in its environment naturalizes the individual as a biological monad.[52] His theory of physiology thus reaffirms liberal subjectivity, a subjectivity based on bounded, walled individual sovereignty. The regulation of public health through intervention on a single individual works as a disciplinary technology, but like the panopticon and the military genealogy of the martial metaphor, its operation remains partly invisible in order to create the imaginary boundaries of the liberal subject.

At this intersection, the different orders through which the martial metaphor permeates become clear: the nation, the military, the public, the individual, even the milieu interior, where it embodies national sovereignty at a cellular level. Metchnikoff accounted for Bernard's "free and independent" quality, the sine qua non of an organism's sovereignty, through the theory of immunity, an activity by which the organism continually produces its own "localized integrity."[53] What is significant about this bodily incorporation of agency is that it provides a physiological naturalization of the individual, as a "free and independent" life responsible for its own health, while still allowing a site for state intervention. This intervention often took the form of public health operating through the social body by shaping the conditions for the individual's body and their internalization of disciplinary techniques—a tension, as we have seen, as early as Shelley through Stoker, that practitioners, politicians, and authors constantly worked through.

Both Doyle and Bernard, while recognizing that infectious disease affects populations, narrow the scope of the medical down into the interior of the individual at a cellular level. On the one hand, this heralds Metchnikoff's picture of immunity as organismal self-defense.[54] On the other hand, it highlights the martial metaphor as an individualizing technique. Under the paradigm of germ theory, post-Koch, diseases like cholera don't invade nations as ghostly miasmas or essentialized figures themselves; infected individuals do. This becomes a crucial point of contention for Doyle and for British society after the turn of the century, as the individual body becomes the node at which the nation defends itself against infection, specifically through vaccination, in both military and public health. This is a new stage in the development of empire, one where the concern is not only about what soldiers might encounter "out there," but about what colonized subjects might bring back to England. This is not to say that bacteriology was necessarily a "liberating" discourse, however. As Latour suggests, the developments of microbiology redefined the idea of individual liberty, insofar as the government appropriated the right to investigate and surveil individual citizens and limit their movements, on the grounds that no one had the right to infect anyone else.⁵⁵ To this effect, the martial metaphor naturalizes the desire and the imperative of the liberal subject to accept this individual intervention, once it has been developed, in order to secure his or her body—to make it, in Cohen's words, "a body worth defending." This in turn makes individuals into subjects of the state as a protective and defensive force.

What Doyle and Bernard share, moreover, in terms of the martial metaphor, is a complication of the division between health and sickness that is not unlike that between poison and remedy. This is less apparent in Doyle's medical writings than in his Holmes stories, in which the source of the foreign biocontaminant is often revealed to be an Englishman corrupted by empire, like Roylott or like Jonathan Small, who brings the subhuman Tonga with his poisonous darts. These contrast with characters like Neville St. Claire from "The Man with the Twisted Lip" (1891), who steps out of bourgeoisie norms but does not undergo a constitutional change because of his foreign contact; his pathology can be simply washed off the surface, as Holmes does to reveal St. Claire's disguise. In this way, Holmes disciplines without involving the repressive state apparatus of the police; he and Watson handle society's corruption internally.

The blurriness here maps onto conceptual theories of health and disease. For Bernard, health and sickness are not so much opposites as points on a spectrum. As Georges Canguilhem observes, Bernard identifies the ontological status of disease less in terms of its proximate invading cause—a microorganism, for instance—than in terms of the dysfunction of bodily operations that causes damage to tissue.⁵⁶ The essence of tuberculosis, for instance, is not *Mycobacterium tuberculosis*, nor the blood and sputum that collects in the lungs and causes suffocation. Rather, it is the body's own "normal" mechanisms causing the inflammatory response that yields the blood and sputum that cause hypoxia.⁵⁷ This kind of chain of events mirrors Bernard's weapon of choice in the medical war, his experiments of destruction, in which the researcher provokes the normal physiological mechanisms into becoming pathological.

What is significant about this ambiguity between health and sickness in terms of a martial spectrum—and which is present in Doyle's fiction but not in his medical writings—is that it bespeaks the invisibility of the martial metaphor. Not unlike Stoker, Doyle's fiction wrote the metaphor's very erasure. What makes Doyle's pre-1899 fiction different is that the construction itself isn't present in any of the dialogue or narration; yet it thematically and narratively governs many of his stories. While Doyle's medical prose affirms this binary distinction along with the martial metaphor, his fiction destabilizes its validity insofar as it maps onto nation and empire—England, and even Englishness itself, is always already pathogenic. Immunity operates in a similar paradigm.

Metchnikoff linked the juridical concept of immunity to the body's natural biology through the metaphor of war. Before Metchnikoff's cellular immunity, immunity in the body was understood either as a constitutional predisposition to disease or as *vis medicatrix naturae*, the way individuals harmonize themselves with the environment. Metchnikoff reimagined "the healing power of nature" inside the body in the form of phagocytes, construed as cellular agents of the body in a martial capacity: "It is evident that [pathogenic] spores are attacked by blood cells and probably killed or disintegrated. Thus the function of blood cells is to protect the body against infectious agents"; consequently, the phagocyte "represents the healing power of nature."[58] Metchnikoff's model also fits into Bernard's theory of the pathological where, when one understands that "phagocytes fight directly against pathogens," inflammation then evidences the defensive mechanism against bacterial infections.[59] It is important to note that at this point, Koch and Metchnikoff focused on different specific physiological mechanisms that might marshal natural defense, the former on the blood serum's capacity to circulate antibodies, and the latter attributing it to the phagocytes' digestion of microbes themselves.[60] Burdon-Sanderson summed up the different perspectives on the specific mechanism of bodily reactions to disease and its by-products: "We have learned to-day that the organism of man and of the higher animals possesses a self-protecting power, which it can exercise either in arresting the development of the living excitors of disease or counteracting their poisonous products."[61] What is significant here is that both Koch and Metchnikoff belonged to the same system of thought that invoked the martial metaphor at the cellular and molecular levels of the body; the same system that Doyle reproduces in "Life and Death." Burdon-Sanderson, moreover, refines the martial metaphor in a way that focuses less on the organism and the invader at the level of an ecological struggle for existence; and, more specifically at the even more granular level of each corresponding combatant. He writes, "We have further seen that the contest which takes place in the organism between invading microphytes and the living elements of the living territory is not a hand to hand fight between tissue elements and microphytes, but one in which both at (so to speak) a certain distance, and in which the weapons are poisons and counter-poisons, toxines and anti-toxines [sic]—words which imply that the pathological endowments of these bodies are antagonistic."[62] This specification materializes and in a certain capacity reassembles Doyle's conceptual confluence between microbe and poison. It not only follows the embodiment of the martial metaphor at the morphological level of immunity and its cellular components; it also accounts for the instrumental means of bacterial agency in a way that correlates to the larger scale of criminal toxicology in his detective fiction.

This work on immunity, pathology, bacteriology, and biochemistry would lead directly to the technological developments of exogenous medical agents for aiding or supplanting immune defense. Public hygiene would no longer be the only weapon against disease; the new wave of defenses included drugs, vaccines, and antitoxins—technologies that are also plot devices and logics informing Holmes and Watson's detection. Doyle suggested that this new mode of medico-military warfare—the use of "weapons"—"represents an entirely new departure in medicine."[63]

Conan Doyle and Robert Koch's Battle with Tuberculosis

As early as 1881, Thomas Huxley foresaw this "new departure," characterizing the future of medications as "pharmacological torpedoes" and citing potentially toxic yet curative substances like strychnine. Having brought the etiologies of many infectious diseases under the gaze of the microscope, the next step in medical science was to materialize a chemical cure that targeted microbial agents rather than symptoms. Furthermore, Huxley's vision included the targeting of specific diseases and compromised tissues, heralding the drug-receptor theory and antimicrobial chemotherapy of the early twentieth century.[64] Doyle and Koch converged on the realization of this dream in 1890, marking a significant moment for the martial metaphor in the development of weapons against diseases that had already intruded into the patient's body, in contrast to inoculation, which worked prophylactically.

After "Life and Death," Doyle's next major publication on bacteriology in the periodical press was an essay for the *Review of Reviews* in which he detailed Koch's claim of developing the first pharmacological weapon against bacteria. By the late 1880s, Koch had demonstrated the bacterial etiology of a number of diseases, including anthrax and typhoid, all of which he described in martial terms, but what brought Doyle and Koch together was tuberculosis. In 1882, Koch demonstrated the existence and pathogenicity of *Mycobacterium tuberculosis*. Only eight years later, he announced a cure for it. A number of scholars and Doyle himself have indicated that Koch was pressured by the government, in the competitive atmosphere between France, Germany, and England, to discover new microorganisms and find a way to cure one rather than merely inoculate against it. Koch suggested that his cure, tuberculin, would be the first demonstrated chemotherapy. Doctors and patients alike flocked to Germany to see it. In November of 1890, Doyle, whose wife suffered from consumption, joined them.

There are a number of telling parallels between Doyle's essays "Koch's Cure" and "Life and Death," particularly in their shared language of colonialism and the military. For instance, the comparison between cultivating infections, as Koch was doing, and growing the monkshood vegetable poison is replicated verbatim. The reader is also given the same image of being guided through Koch's laboratory.

> Here, too, under the microscope may be seen the prepared slides which contain specimens of those bacilli of disease which have already been isolated. This one, stained with logwood, where little purple dots, like grains of pepper, are sprinkled thickly over the field, is a demonstration of that deadly tubercle-bacillus which has harassed mankind from the dawn of time, and yet has become visible to him only during the last eight years. Here, under the next object glass, are little pink curved creatures, so minute as to be hardly visible under the power of 700 diameters which we are using. Yet these pretty and infinitely fragile things are the accursed comma-bacilli of cholera, the most terrible scourge which has ever devastated the microbe-ridden earth. Here, too, is the little rod-shaped filament of the Bacillus anthracis, the curving tendrils of the Obermeyer spirillus, the eat spores of Bacillus prodigiosus, and the jointed ranches of Aspergillus. It is a strange thing to look upon these utterly insignificant creatures, and to realize that in one year they would claim more victims from the human race than all the tigers who have ever trod a jungle. A satire, indeed, it is upon the majesty of man when we look at these infinitesimal and contemptible creatures which have it in their power to overthrow the strongest intellect and to shatter the most robust frame. (KC, 552)

Here, too, the perspective is on the human scale, highlighting the seeming contradiction between the physical smallness of microbes and the magnitude of their war against humans. The bacteria threaten the sovereignty of humankind in the great chain of being. If, in colonial settings, humans are threatened by savage beasts—the mention of tigers echoes their appearance in Doyle's earlier essay—then nowhere on the "microbe-ridden earth" are they safe from these "utterly insignificant creatures." Man's "majesty"—his sovereignty in physical health and intellect—is under siege and is readily "overthrow[n]" by "infinitesimal and contemptible creatures." The political metaphors are not accidental. Doyle challenges the physicality of material strength in number and size. In contrast to his approach in "Life and Death," he doesn't conflate the microscopic with the human-sized; instead, he makes the same suggestion as Holmes in *The Sign of the Four*: "Man's greatness lies his perception of his own smallness" (SF, 176).

Doyle was not resigned to the microbe; quite the opposite. His underscoring of man's susceptibility is a rhetorical strategy for inculcating the martial metaphor and its regulatory practices. He invited Victorian readers to grasp a completely new paradigm of medicine and health, one in which doctors, public health politicians, and Poor Law guardians were not enough. Before bacteriology, humankind had no idea of the extent to which it was at war with disease. The situation was much worse than the sanitarians thought: microbial threats could be present even without visible filth or noisome miasma. What readers internalized from "Life and Death in Blood" was that the power to defend against microbes lay not with hygienically productive subjects, as Kingsley thought, but with specialized professionals: bacteriologists, pharmacologists, and immunologists were the wave of the future.

Doyle made Koch a hero for his microscopic vision and his ability to translate colonial imperatives into biomedical practices. Humankind needed medico-scientific experts like Koch who thought and worked like Sherlock Holmes: "Koch is the great master mind . . . which is rapidly bringing under subjection those unruly tribes of deadly micro-organisms which are the last creatures in the organic world to submit to the sway of man" (KC, 552). While Holmes can hunt down and bring under control the imperial lumpenproletariat and colonial others that invade the metropole, Koch subjects the inferior races—codified as "tribes"—of microbes that have yet to submit to humankind's rule. Here the work of bacteriology is analogized to colonial occupation and subjugation. It is also no coincidence that Koch's research in Germany is framed as a military, imperial project: this was its function. Doyle cites Koch's government-initiated investigations into the 1883 cholera epidemic in Egypt. The same offensive, expansionist rhetoric is present in Koch's own reflections on medical progress. In 1898, Koch wrote, "In the past one took a more defensive attitude . . . We have now moved away from this defensive point of view and have seized the offensive. We must be prepared, first, to detect the infectious material easily and with certainty, and second, destroy it."[65] Koch's vision of creating a compound, a kind of internal antiseptic,[66] to fight a disease already acquired represents this mode of offensive medico-military war.

Koch's weapon, even in Doyle's characterization, embodies the biopolitical tenet of making live and letting die at a histological and cellular level. When Doyle saw the means of destroying infectious tubercular material in Koch's laboratory, he realized that it was not the weapon people had hoped for—what was already being called "The Remedy" and "Koch's Lymph." Tuberculin's actual nature and composition were still a secret, although it would later be revealed that it was composed of a dead culture of the bacteria, extracted from lymph, mixed with water and glycerin. But Doyle clarified the matter when it became sensationalized in the press: "It must never be lost sight of that Koch has never claimed that his fluid kills the tubercle. On the contrary, it has no effect upon it, but destroys the low form of tissue in the meshes of which the bacilli lie" (*KC*, 556). It does not kill the bacteria but causes necrosis of the infected tissue, the hope being that the bacteria would die along with it; in other words, it lets it die.

The hope, however, proved false. In one of his most compelling—and probably disappointing—uses of the martial metaphor, Doyle asserted that tuberculin "continually removes the traces of the enemy, but it still leaves him deep in the invaded country" (*KC*, 556). If we read this in terms of Holmes and Watson's work, we can see how tuberculosis operates like a foreign invader and imperial lumpenproletariat. The detective and the military doctor work to eliminate or, in an appropriately biopolitical description, "slough" England's native corruption first: if they destroy the weak and diseased Englishmen, they neutralize the foreign invaders.[67] By eliminating people like Jonathan Small and Roylott, they can keep out the likes of Tonga and the swamp adder. They cannot, however, remove all of the enemies "deep in the invaded country."

Tuberculin itself occupies a notable place in the history of the martial metaphor. On one level, it was a crucial actant in bringing Doyle and Koch together and giving Doyle the opportunity to propagate the metaphor through a widely circulated story. On another level, even though it was a disappointment, it was productive in the fight against tuberculosis in other ways. Doyle saw early on its significant diagnostic potential, and it is still used for this in contemporary medical practice. In addition, the initial uncertainty over the drug's efficacy led to more systematic protocols and methods for evaluating therapeutic interventions and contributed to what is known as scientific or evidence-based medicine. Although Koch was searching for a kind of internal antiseptic rather than a vaccination, his ineffective cure seemed closer to the latter. In either case, and accounting for its spectacular failure, tuberculin anticipated Paul Ehlrich's "magic bullet," the first successfully synthesized materialization of Huxley's torpedo, which I discuss in the concluding chapter. What we see here, at the intersection of immunology, bacteriology, toxicology, and pharmacology is not only how the martial metaphor came to be naturalized inside the body, but also how medicine worked with in a new epistemology to create a supplementary, exogenous way of bolstering or in some cases seemingly supplanting the body's natural defenses against infectious disease.

II

On the Front Lines of the Boer War

So far I have discussed the explicit operation of the martial metaphor in Doyle's medical writings and its subtler, nearly invisible deployment in the Sherlock Holmes stories before the end of the century. I showed how the metaphor underpins Holmes and Watson's defense of Englishness, this guiding imperative being informed by bacteriology, toxicology, and immunology. I have articulated how it works as an invisible metaphor guiding Doyle's fiction while appearing as an explicit one in his medical writings.

Before 1899, there were few material connections between medicine and war in Doyle's writings. With the outbreak of the Boer War, however, Doyle came to be personally invested in the martial metaphor in a unique way. Unlike the previous authors to deploy the metaphor, Doyle's connection to the military was in firsthand experience. In this section, I argue that Doyle himself embodied the martial metaphor through his service in the Boer War, a conflict that exacerbated anxieties over the degeneration of the British race. Doyle's experiences with disease in South Africa led him not only to continue deploying the metaphor in his medical writings, but to use it as a plot device and a conceit in two Holmes stories in the early twentieth century. Facing a weakening social body, Doyle reaffirmed medicine-as-war in the popular imaginary in a more explicit and threatening capacity, rather than letting it do its biopolitical work below the surface and under the guise of detection, as he had before 1899.

Doyle embodied the martial metaphor during the Boer War, adopting in a fitting irony a defining characteristic of John Watson: he practiced military medicine. After being rejected as a soldier because of his age, he signed on to take command of a hospital. The rejection itself has significance as part of a trend the British would have to come to terms with after the war. Nearly two-thirds of recruits were turned away from enlistment for poor health.[68] These recruits came primarily from the working class, who formed the mass of the army as enlisted men. The conditions of the war tested the health of the British social body, and in 1899 it seemed to have failed miserably.[69] The fin-de-siècle anxieties over degeneration that appeared in Doyle's earlier fiction and in Stoker's *Dracula* seemed to have been realized. It was no longer just the loungers and idlers of empire who were contaminating England. The very stock of bodies that sustained the country's labor and military force was diseased.

The Boer War was the sequel to an earlier campaign in South Africa against the Boers, who were Calvinist Dutch farmers. The first conflict began after Britain tried to assert full control over South Africa and forced the Boers out of their settled coastal regions to more inland territories, the Orange Free State and Transvaal. In 1877, the British annexed Transvaal and set off the first Boer War, which led to the Boers gaining independence. In 1885, gold was discovered in Transvaal, and the British found an economic incentive for taking the territory, adding to their already festering anxieties over possible intervention by Germany. The local Afrikaner government was not amenable to British interests, however, which led to a revolt by British occupants against the Boers. When this failed, Britain began increasing its military presence. When the Afrikaner president, Paul Krauger, demanded they withdraw, the British refused and war was declared. This was the bloodiest and most costly war fought by the Victorian army, who was plagued with long sieges.[70] Moreover, due to the British invention of concentration camps, the war proved highly unpopular in England and abroad.

The war posed two challenges to the health and fitness of the British as a race, which highlighted the inextricable imbrication of medicine with military imperatives. The first was the vitality of the Boers pitted against the British soldiers; the second was the typhoid bacillus, *Salmonella typhi*, also known as enteric fever—the same ailment Watson is recovering from when he first returns to England in *A Study in Scarlet*. Doyle compounds typhoid into the mass of munitions dealt by the Boers in his telling: "On the morning of February 5th the army sallied forth once more to have another try to win a way to Ladysmith. It was known that enteric was rife in the town, that shell and bullet and typhoid germ had struck down a terrible proportion of the garrison."[71] The metaphor here is thus solidified in the conflation of the bullet and the bacillus, this construction itself becoming a recurring trope in early to mid-twentieth century medical writing.

In terms of the first enemy, the Boers themselves, the British were not fighting ill-equipped and poorly conditioned natives. Doyle portrays the Boers as a race more evolved in martial prowess. He opens his 552-page tract *The Great Boer War* by foregrounding the connections between biology, evolution, and martial prowess of the enemy, imperating the reader to once again imaginatively experiment as he does in "Life and Death in Blood."

> Take a community of Dutchmen of the type of those who defended themselves for fifty years against all the power of Spain at a time when Spain was the greatest power in the world. Intermix with them a strain of those inflexible French Huguenots who gave up home and fortune and left their country for ever at the time of the revocation of the Edict of Nantes. The product must obviously be one of the most rugged, virile, unconquerable races ever seen upon earth. Take this formidable people and train them for seven generations in constant warfare against savage men and ferocious beasts, in circumstances under which no weakling could survive, place them so that they acquire exceptional skill with weapons and in horsemanship, give them a country which is eminently suited to the tactics of the huntsman, the marksman, and the rider. Then, finally, put a finer temper upon their military qualities by a dour fatalistic Old Testament religion and an ardent and consuming patriotism. Combine all these qualities and all

these impulses in one individual, and you have the modern Boer—the most formidable antagonist who ever crossed the path of Imperial Britain. (BW, 1–2)

The Boers were trained by fighting with the most savage of beasts; their bloodlines, their "strains," linked them to historically famed warriors, much like Dracula's martial lineage; and they were hardened to their tropical climate, forging themselves a defense against endemic tropical illness.[72] It is significant that although Doyle describes the Boers in somewhat brutish terms, they nevertheless "evolve," a trait that no doubt emerges from the fact that they come from European stock, in contrast to a population like the Zulus. Thus, they are a kind of perfect storm of primitivism and evolution, not unlike Dracula. The Boers' military prowess can be read through the logic of immunity in light of the previous section's readings, insofar as the Boers developed their strength through exposure. The British, by contrast, lack the same inoculation through consistent exposure to hazardous, physically trying warfare.[73]

One often-cited example of military failure that has been linked to Doyle's fascination with invisible threats such as bacteria is the Boer guerrilla tactic of digging trenches and hiding in vantage points to slaughter British soldiers with trained snipers.[74] Doyle was critical of the reluctance of British commanders to adapt to modern warfare, citing the threat of "hidden guns" in both of his treatments of the war (BW, 95, 190, 331).[75] It is telling that even after the war, Doyle worked with the British on prophylactic techniques against invisible enemies, such as stealth attacks by submarines.[76] This shows how his medical and military interests coincided to make him a prominent figure in recirculating the martial metaphor within military discourse.

As Doyle suggests, the British army had not been hardened by warfare over the previous century in contrast to the Boers. This implication belies the social construction of the English body. Although Doyle doesn't address the nature of the English constitution in his text, we can take into consideration the consistent themes of corruptibility and degeneration in his earlier Holmes stories and the fact that even as the war was commencing, England had to come to terms with the vitality of its population. Although Doyle was rejected for his age, the fact that nearly two-thirds of recruits were simply not healthy enough for enlistment suggested endemic ill-health in the population. By 1901, the military had lowered its health standards, for instance by decreasing the height requirement, as height functioned as a proxy for robustness. This necessity contradicted the notion that the male middle-class body could be the index of national health—which by this time was equally susceptible to degeneration—as military vitality was not as contingent on him as it was on "the great unwashed." The country's labor and military body could no longer be viewed as immanently healthy enough. Moreover, even the upper classes proved defenseless against degeneration as his later fiction reveals.

The second way the Boer War taxed the British was in terms of military medicine and infectious disease. As in Crimea, the British fought disease alongside robust human foes, and the former produced significantly more casualties. The enemy here was not unlike cholera. In this case, it was typhoid, also a waterborne pathogen and frequently spread by poor sanitation around waterworks. The Boers carried out a form of biological warfare,[77] seizing the waterworks and giving the British no choice but to drink from a contaminated water supply in Bloemfontein during their long entrenchment.[78] Doyle knew that typhoid was waterborne and caused by bacteria, but the military culture was less concerned despite its experiences earlier in the century, and hygienic measures were not enforced. Doyle wrote, "If bad water can cost us more than all the bullets of the enemy then surely it is worth our while to make the drinking of unboiled water a military offense" (BW, 371). In the end, poor hygienic measures combined with a contaminated water supply led to a massive outbreak. In the end, Doyle was able to fight the disease only after it seized a soldier's body. Hygienic measures aside, an antityphoid vaccine existed that showed a promising success rate before the war broke out. Sir Almroth Wright developed it in 1896 while working as a professor at the Royal Army College at Netley. The vaccine itself, the same one that would be made available to civilian populations, was developed from military research, like so many other medical technologies and practices. Doyle campaigned unsuccessfully to have the army inoculate soldiers with it before the war. He wrote, "All through the campaign, while the machinery for curing disease was excellent, that for preventing it was elementary or absent.... With precautions and with inoculation all those lives might have been saved" (BW, 371). These critiques would draw medicine into a closer relationship with war, showing that in logistical terms, it was an essential part of the maintenance of an army, and by extension a nation.[79]

Reflecting on this time, Doyle invoked the rhetorically coupling of medicine and war to suggest this failure was not inevitable: "We lost more from enteric than from the bullet in South Africa, and it is sad to think that nearly all could have been saved had Almroth Wright's discovery been properly appreciated. . . . If the army had all been inoculated, this would, I think, have been absolutely the healthiest war on record."[80] The irony of a healthy war was perhaps lost on Doyle, as it was congruent with the social Darwinism of the period and his penchant for enjoining the medical and the military.[81] This use nonetheless shows the recursive nature of the martial metaphor as it reentered military discourse in a very literal way. Of course, even if they had adopted Wright's vaccine, that healthiest group of military men would not have been a representative sample of English health, according to the infamous recruiting statistics cited above. The anxieties surrounding degeneration and the lack of healthy recruits still contradicted Doyle's speculation. Doyle's autobiography, *Memories and Adventures* (1924), was followed three years later by "The Adventure of the Blanched Soldier," his only work of fiction to deal with disease and the Boer War.

In his 1900 letter to the *British Medical Journal*, "The War in South Africa," Doyle makes a case for the common orderly as a soldier, citing the dire conditions at Bloemfontein and the medical efforts to combat them. He contends that the outbreak of enteric fever involved a "calamity and magnitude" unrivaled in modern warfare.[82] In contrast to his earlier espousal of physicians and scientific researchers—and even the wonders of Sherlock Holmes—in this letter Doyle's primary focus is the work of medical men and orderlies in battling the disease.

Doyle makes a point of explicitly contrasting actual war with medical work. However, as in the case of Kingsley's sanitary lectures, the rhetorical move of making disease look worse than war only affirms the martial metaphor. The orderly "is not a picturesque figure," Doyle writes. He is instead, a humble, working-class man, one who enjoys not officially commendable martial heroics but the real work of saving lives.

> We have not the trim, well-nourished army man, but we have recruited from the St. John Ambulance men, who are drawn, in this particular instance, from the mill hands of a northern town. They were not very strong to start with, and the poor fellows are ghastly now. There is none of the dash and glory of war about the sallow, tired men in the dingy khaki suits— which, for the sake of the public health, we will hope may never see England again. And yet they are patriots, these men;

for many of them have accepted a smaller wage in order to take on these arduous duties, and they are facing danger for twelve hours of the twenty-four, just as real and much more repulsive than the scout who rides up to the strange kopje or the gunner who stands to his gun with pom-pom quaking at him from the hill.[83]

On the surface, this does not seem to romanticize fighting typhoid in the field hospital. But in refusing to romanticize the medico-military battle, Doyle indicates that the "grunt work" of medical men and orderlies not only has value and requires bravery but also sustains the army and the empire at large.

This construction of heroism does invoke a kind of romantic military hero. The orderlies working on the front line against enteric fever encounter disease up close and personally—"face-to-face"; it is just as real as, and more repulsive than, the gunner firing from a distance or the scout taking a hill. This comparison situates the orderly as a frontline infantryman and contrasts his work with the guerrilla tactics of the Boers, as in the case of the distant rifleman who is targeted by distant artillery. Doyle's espousal of intimate combat with disease, analogized to war, is remarkably consonant with early-twentieth-century fetishization of the bayonet by British military thinkers in the face of increasingly mechanical warfare and increasing distance between combatants.[84] The image of the working-class man that would face the bacterium in the closest of quarters makes fighting disease a matter of English pride for people from all walks of life, even at the lowest socioeconomic level. Their work is not only gruesome but, because of the contagious nature of typhoid, dangerous. By characterizing medical heroes this way, Doyle conveys hope in the power of the English laboring body to defend the nation against pathology and degeneration—a position that is ultimately contradicted in much of his fiction. Doyle's letter does suggest that medical warfare against declining inherent health and foreign infections is a matter of national pride. But with respect to the medical campaign of the Boer War, as with the charge of the Light Brigade during the Crimean War, "someone had blundered." These working-class heroes were there because of poor decisions by the officials in charge of the Royal Army Medical Corps. The rate of infection among vaccinated soldiers was 2 percent, in contrast to 14 percent among the unvaccinated.[85] The vaccine that Doyle espoused so strongly emerged from military medicine, but it never made it to the men on the ground.

Doyle's campaign to make the antityphoid vaccine compulsory was part of a larger, drawn-out debate that began with the Boer War and continued into the beginnings of the Great War. By the end of the first year of World War One, citing the number of deaths to typhoid in the Boer War and convinced by the most recent research, the Royal Army Medical Corps ensured that 90 percent of the troops were vaccinated, resulting in a typhoid incidence in World War One of 2.5 per 1,000, compared to 105 per 1,000 during the Boer War.[86] While the debate between the vaccinationists and antivaccinationists was a contentious one,[87] closely mirroring twenty-first century debates, the Boer War ultimately showed the British that the best offense was in fact a good immune defense aided by inoculation. As Anne Hardy has contended, what drove the debate over compulsory vaccination for soldiers during the Edwardian era was the tension between individual freedom, under the aegis of liberalism, and the increasingly political jurisdiction over public health in disease prevention,[88] which as we have seen was the central tension in the nexus of medicine and politics in the nineteenth century. This debate over compulsory vaccination reflected the larger stakes of the acceptance of modern epidemiological measures, post-bacteriology, in the public imaginary. Hardy writes, "In the autumn of 1914, therefore, battle was joined between the medical proponents of antityphoid inoculation and the anti-vaccinationists over the hearts and minds of Britain's fighting men—who, representatives of the common man, of the general public will, were required either to demonstrate their faith in the new immunology, or to reject it outright."[89]

By 1915, the organizational efforts of the Royal Army Medical Corps and its massive propaganda campaign to influence the opinions of soldiers with pressure from officers and fellow enlisted men, compelled those individuals who still held out. Sir William Osler, one of the most renowned physicians of the late nineteenth century, who had battled the antivivisectionists alongside Doyle, made the case that medicine was a crucial weapon in war. An influential Oxford penny pamphlet, widely circulated during the war and taken from his address at Camp Churn on the Berkshire Downs, was aptly titled *Bullets and Bacilli*. In it, he made the case for vaccination by appealing to the military ethos: "It can be prevented," wrote Osler; "it *must be prevented*; but meanwhile the decision is in your hands, and I know it will be in favor of King and Country."[90] In this case, Osler's choice of words helped internalize the medical war in the enlisted men, to disciplinarily shape their own conduct and choose vaccination.

Although the debate continued after the war, historical cases of military medical dealings with vaccination and infectious disease influenced the development, testing, and deployment of the vaccine in civilian public health. The vaccine was never made compulsory during the Great War, however; rather, the majority individual soldiers accepted it voluntarily.[91] What is critical here is the resistance to overt, juridical imposition of public health on the individual; in the case of the soldiers, we see Foucault's docile bodies. Although Doyle advocated for compulsory vaccination, the mobilization of medicine as war was part of the larger movement to get enlisted soldiers, and the working class that they came from, to accept this intervention into personal liberty and into the body. Beyond vaccination, the Boer War proved to be another occasion for Doyle to reflect on how populations were medically governed.

The Biopolitical Labs of Modernity in South Africa

The British management of civilian populations during the Boer War proved to be a significant moment in biopolitical history, demonstrating a nexus of medicine, the military, and colonial politics, an ideal breeding ground for the martial metaphor to thrive in. It was during the South African conflict that the British developed concentration camps to manage the women, children, and other noncombatants of the territory they seized. I have previously mentioned Agamben's contention that the camp emblematizes the state of exception, citing the most obvious case of the Nazis.[92] Agamben does connect the camps to colonization historically, but in a more philological capacity. But with the Boer War camps, the connection was quite material. They were precursors to the later colloquially associated point of reference, the Holocaust, in accordance with Mbembe's suggestion that biopolitical techniques and experiments were exercised in the colonies before the homeland. Aidan Forth extensively documents the history of Britain's "barbed wire imperialism," manifesting most visibly in the form of concentration camp during the Boer War, but having earlier legacies in famine control and measures like the Poor Law. The camps more proximately develop from responses to "states of emergency," the exercise of sovereignty, which was justified as an exception to the increasingly endemic crises of famine, war, and disease. Responses to epidemics of plague and cholera, population management in India, and, not surprisingly, the exemplar of the CD Acts played an important role in shaping the idea and practice of encampment, responding to "metaphors of social danger and contagion."⁹³ The concentration camps can be viewed as one of the many instances in which a colony serves as a "lab of modernity,"⁹⁴ in their iterations of welfare and social control between Britain and its "colonial periphery."⁹⁵ Thus, their construction drew from governmentalities in Britain while also serving as a place for testing biopolitical techniques before deploying them in Europe, the martial metaphor being a medium and justification for such practices.

Death and disease were rampant in the British camps during the Boer War. Furthermore, the British exercised a scorched-earth policy, making farmland unusable for the foreseeable future. The practice here was an explicit letting-die by controlling the material conditions of existence: food, water, sanitation, and the circulation of bodies. This tactic also disrupted communication between soldiers and civilians. We can understand this biopolitical exercise as a form of offensive medical warfare pursued in response to the Boer's guerilla tactics and their "biological warfare." By controlling social determinants of health, the camps acted as a countersiege that attacked the very thing the Boers were at war to protect: their land and population. In attacking the Boer's civilians, the British laid siege to the biopolitical foundation of their army and population. This marked a turning point in the nature of war: by targeting the Boer guerrillas' base of support through a military intervention on civilians, the British exercised counterinsurgency.

With respect to the campaign against disease and sickness, Doyle didn't just participate in the war, he actively advocated for it and defended it after its conclusion. He offered defenses against the charges of British atrocities in the camps in *The Great Boer War* and, even more assertively, in *The War in South Africa: Its Causes and Conduct*. For this defense of empire in addition to his medical service, Doyle was knighted in 1902. Because of his celebrity, Doyle had enough influence to justify Britain's actions. His work has been credited by some with changing much of the world's opinion on Britain's conduct during the war.⁹⁶ This imprimatur of Doyle's defense of the empire, both as a doctor and as an author, signals the significance of his position to propagate the martial metaphor in the service of national and imperial interests. By following the logic that the British were protecting the Boer civilians and insisting that their deaths were due to their failure to adopt hygienic standards and refusal of medical care in favor of more native practices, Doyle announced that the violence of the camp—its state of exception—was justified in the service of civilization. He claimed that most of the deaths were due to the measles, but he actually acknowledges that the measles outbreaks were a result of the creation of the camps.

> We cannot deny that the cause of the outbreak of measles was the collection of the women and children by us into the camps. But why were they collected into camps? Because they could not be left on the veldt. And why could they not be left on the veldt? Because we had destroyed the means of subsistence. And why had we destroyed the means of subsistence? To limit the operations of the mobile bands of guerillas. At the end of every tragedy we are forced back to the common origin of all of them, and made to understand that the nation which obstinately perseveres in a useless guerilla war prepares much trouble for its enemy, but absolute ruin for itself. (WS, 85)

This biopolitical exercise was, in Mbembe's terms, warfare in "service of civilization."[97] Under the guise of humanitarianism to protect the Boers and ensure a rapid peace, this inversion of public health was strategic and psychological warfare. In Doyle's eyes, the ultimate cause was the Boers themselves, as the British, he claimed, were merely responding defensively by forestalling the conditions required for guerrilla groups to exist; the Boers, then, were ultimately responsible for their own civilian deaths. By intervening destructively in their means of subsistence and public health, the British military used medicine, in its larger biopolitical context, as a weapon against the Boers. One consequence of the martial metaphor, then, is the recruitment of medical epistemologies and technologies as weapons of war. The example of the camps shows how the logic of the martial metaphor leads to the conflation of medicine and war and to material, biopolitical effects that oppose the values espoused by medical practice.

Beyond the invention of the concentration camp, what the military medical concerns of the Boer War did on a larger scale was link disease on foreign soil to medical anxieties back home, much as Kingsley did with Crimea. The failures of enlisted men's health during the Boer War fostered reinvestment in the fight against disease in all orders of life, from governmental intervention to personal hygiene and self-care. In this way, the martial metaphor was a useful tool for mobilizing mass social treatments, both in public health and, less overtly, in medical biopolitical management. Unsurprisingly, given the history of biopolitics and sexuality as articulated by Foucault, the target of this vital investment was the children, the future of the race. For instance, after the Committee on Physical Deterioration reported in 1904 on the health of the working class, prompted by the recruitment problems, free school lunches and other benefits were introduced for the urban poor to improve salubrity.[98] The medical aspects of the war contributed to new biopolitical techniques for fostering security by raising health standards. It was ultimately because of the need to revitalize a biologically and militarily enfeebled nation, aided by Doyle's firsthand experience with military medicine, that disease appears in two Holmes stories after the war as a central plot device in a military tenor.

Biological Warfare and Military Fitness

Of the countless letters Doyle received with respect to Holmes, one was written by his friend and mentor Dr. Joseph Bell on May 4, 1892. Bell wrote to Doyle early in his success with the Holmes stories to suggest a plot revolving around a "bacteriological criminal." Doyle replied, "I think a fine thing might be done regarding a bacteriological criminal, but the only fear is that lest you get beyond the average man, whose interest must be held from the first and who won't be interested unless he thoroughly understands."[99] By the time the Boer War had come and gone, bacteriology was much more widely circulated and popularly understood. Moreover, the medical problems surrounding the war—both the bacteriological and the racially constitutional—gave Doyle a reason to change his mind about featuring infectious disease as a plot device.

Bell couldn't resist positing the idea himself in his introduction to the 1893 edition of *A Study in Scarlet*, drawing on connections among detection, national borders, and bacteria. Recalling his contention regarding bacteriological research being the greatest medical advance in recent history, and comparing the work of detection to the microscopic gaze, he speaks of disease as a matter of Occidental security: "Poison a well at Mecca with the cholera bacillus, and the holy water which the pilgrims carry off in their bottles will infect a continent, and the rags of the victims of the plague will terrify every seaport in Christendom."[100] This incursion narrative by a biological enemy, which now reads like contemporary bioterrorism, invokes the alien elements that previously took the form of foreigners or lumpenproletariat and shrinks them down to microscopic bacteria. Here, the side effects of the martial metaphor appear much more visibly: if the British military can weaponize medicine, then medical knowledge can be weaponized and used against England. This possibility compounds Kingsley's preoccupation with the nature itself being inimical and ramifies Stoker's representation of individuals and other races being a diseased infiltration, because what is naturally pathological could now be harnessed intentionally.

In "The Adventure of the Dying Detective," the martial metaphor operates in these terms of biological weaponry. What makes the plot different from either the use of alkaloid poisons or the Boers' seizure of the waterworks is that in "The Dying Detective," bacteria themselves are used as a murder weapon.[101] Holmes, apparently dying of the mysterious Sumatran disease "Tapanuli fever," asks Watson to seek out one Culverton Smith, "a well-known resident of Sumatra now visiting London. An outbreak of the disease upon his plantation, which was distant from medical aid, caused him to study [the disease] himself with some rather far-reaching consequences."[102] Holmes's illness is an illusion, however. He previously suspected Smith of murdering his own brother with a culture of the disease brought from Sumatra. As revenge, Smith sent Holmes a booby-trapped package and Holmes only pretends to have been a victim of the ploy: "I would not touch that box. You can just see if you look at it sideways where the sharp spring like a viper's tooth emerges as you open it. I dare say it was by some such device that [Smith's brother], who stood between this monster and a reversion, was done to death" (*DD*, 444). The puncturing device, echoing the other penetrating mechanisms in *Dracula*, expresses angst about the permeability of the individual's supposedly hermetic boundaries.[103] By comparing a technological device—the spring-loaded lancet—to a biological one—the viper's tooth—Doyle highlights the way foreign, inimical nature, such as the poisonous snake or the bacterium, can be shaped by medical knowledge for malevolent ends. After having Watson bring Smith for "help," Holmes tells Smith that he received a box in the mail that drew blood by way of a spring mechanism when he opened it, whereupon Smith reveals his murder plot: "You have the truth now, Holmes, and you can die with the knowledge that I killed you" (*DD*, 442). Holmes plays along to get Smith to further implicate himself.

The characterization of Culverton Smith speaks to the broader but recurring discourse of medical anxieties over colonial-borne degeneration. He embodies the sickness he brings back to the metropole. As Watson observes, "I saw a great yellow face, coarse-grained and greasy, with heavy, double-chin, and two sullen, menacing gray eyes which glared at me from under tufted and sandy brows" (*DD*, 436). Watson continues, "The skull was of enormous capacity, and yet as I looked down I saw to my amazement that the figure of the man was small and frail, twisted in the shoulders and back like one who has suffered from rickets in his childhood" (*DD*, 437). Smith, however, is not a lumpenproletariat: he lives in a respectable area of London and is associated with wealthy British farmers in Sumatra. This ties him to a history of colonial greed and disrepute in which British farmers and government representatives failed to aid the local Aceh people against a blockade by the Dutch despite their protests to the British government. Smith's connection to this scandal undermines a central myth of British imperialism: "its palliative and moral motives for global development."[104] Like many of Doyle's corrupted Englishmen, Smith bespeaks colonial guilt. Disease, both infectious and degenerative, reveals Britain's failure to live up to its own mythology, which is contingent on its exerting political and military pressure. The repeated emphasis on twistedness, the mention of childhood disease, and the oversized skull allude to contemporaneous views of degeneration and criminal anthropometrics, except that Smith represents a higher class (in contrast to someone like Jonathan Small) being infected with the vices of empire. Thus, the contagion of empire spreads beyond class boundaries, infecting not just the masses but also the privileged.

The second concern the story raises is the fact that Culverton Smith is "not a medical man," signaling the dangers of the circulation of biomedical knowledge. In fact, Smith's use of a biological weapon suggests an inverted internalization of the martial metaphor, as he uses medicine to fight his own personal battles by spreading disease rather than eliminating it. Like a pathologically inverted Holmes, he is a self-trained professional. And when Watson calls on him, Smith compares his own talents to Holmes's: " 'I am sorry to hear this,' said he. 'I only know Mr. Holmes through some business dealings which we have had, but I have every respect for his talents and his character. He is an amateur of crime, as I am of disease. For him the villain, for me the microbe. There are my prisons' " (*DD*, 437). Pointing to jars on a table, he continues, "Among those gelatine cultivations some of the very worst offenders in the world are now doing time" (*DD*, 437). Smith deploys medical knowledge for his own ends, following through on the sort of threat depicted in H. G. Wells's "The Stolen Bacillus" (1895), in which a foreign anarchist feigns interest in a London bacteriologist's work in order to steal a sample of cholera and poison the city's water supply, a fulfillment of Joseph Bell's premonition. The misuse of bacteriology, like that of toxicology, rematerializes the military in the medical through the very literal weaponization of medicine.

Finally, of particular note in Culverton Smith's confession is his experimentation with the disease on colonial subjects. As Holmes malingers and groans in morbid pain, Smith gloats: "Painful, is it? Yes, the coolies used to do some squealing towards the end" (*DD*, 441). The knowledge Smith obtained this way not only helped his plantation deal with the disease but gave him personal knowledge of how to handle, transport, and weaponize the disease without risking self-infection. This work is a more concentrated realization of the martial metaphor than the biopolitical experimentation in South Africa with respect to colonial bodies. The bodies of the "coolies" perform the clinical labor required to produce bacteriological knowledge; these clinical "trials" foreshadow the Nazis' medical experiments,[105] which alongside later biological warfare research stand out as the most extreme cases in which redeploying the martial metaphor into military operations enables rather than forestalls death and human suffering.

Holmes's malingering itself signals another weak point in the British social body both at the level of the narrative and in contemporaneous medical history. At the narrative level, Holmes never really infected himself and is able to neutralize the threat; this plot betrays the confidence that Britain projects in its ability to protect against foreign, weaponized contagion. Holmes cures the disease through simple investigation and deception: by providing "alternative etiologies" and "controllable causes" for the symptoms of a diseased empire, he constructs a misreading that saves the empire from self-induced toxicity.[106] This narrative technique raises a specter of doubt in the face of the very real possibility of biological attack. Outside the scope of Holmes's and Doyle's narrative control, however, the historical tale resists such facile allayment. The idea of using bacteria as weapons came to fruition in both homicide and war. The Culverton Smith scenario actually occurred in 1933 in Calcutta, where one Amar Penday was murdered by his step-brother with the help of a physician, who infected Penday with septicemic plague using a hypodermic needle.[107] This was just the beginning of the biological weaponization that followed during and after the Second World War.

Holmes's malingering also calls into question his method of eliciting a confession. When "The Dying Detective" was published in 1913, the socioeconomic consequences of the decaying social body that were being discussed went back at least as far as the Boer War. That year, John Collie, a respected medical expert in actuarial matters, published *Malingering and Feigned Sickness*, detailing his experience detecting false compensation claims by workers for sickness and injury. Drawing on a military metaphor for industry, Collie writes, "The stricken soldier in the industrial warfare is, because of distrust, too often over-anxious, at all hazards, to guard himself against the possibility of future incapacity arising out of his disability."[108] Collie attributes the sickness of "the soldier in industrial warfare" not to a moral failing but to a psychological disorder caused by class warfare. What made England prosperous also produced the sickness of its laboring class, those on whom the continued prosperity of the nation depended.[109] Collie invokes the Holmesian gaze to diagnose the condition when he suggests, "Never was the old instruction of 'eyes first, ears second, hands third' . . . more necessary than in dealing with these cases. The patient should be carefully watched as he undresses . . . and the light should be the best possible."[110] Here, Collie demonstrates the influence of detective fiction on medicine itself. Although Holmes himself is acting, his British body's performance of the kind of diseased condition of colonial and British laborers links the two by way of a weaponized bacterial contagion. Read in the context of Collie's medico-detective work, this nexus shows the extension of the martial metaphor from the nation and the imperial defense more literally to industrialization. Thus, Holmes's malingering, though adopted for the purpose of catching a criminal, excites rather than allays concerns about the English race. The story, in effect, highlights both an external and internal medical war being waged in England: one by disease, and one by the system of medical discourse that pathologizes socioeconomic concerns through the language of war.[111]

On the subject of sick soldiers and class relations, in "The Adventure of the Blanched Soldier," Doyle deploys an instance of military medicine in the service of the martial metaphor. Written well into the twentieth century but taking place in 1903, just three years after the South African War, the story has Holmes face the medico-socio implications of the Boer War. James Dodd, an exemplary specimen of physical, military fitness, visits Holmes to learn the fate of his comrade-in-arms from that war, Godfrey Emsworth. After Holmes investigates, despite Emsworth's recalcitrant father, he reveals that Godfrey has been hiding in his family home because of what he believes to be a case of leprosy acquired in the war.

Recalling Holmes's ability to read Watson as a military man in *Scarlet*, Doyle has Holmes quickly ascertain that Dodd too is a military man and served in South Africa, before Dodd can even recount his case: "When a gentleman of virile appearance enters my room with such tan upon his face as an English sun could never give, and with his handkerchief in his sleeve instead of in his pocket, it is not difficult to place him."[112] In this characterization, Holmes supplants the image of the diseased, debilitated army, weak from typhoid and decaying constitutional health, with one of vitality and fitness: he reads Dodd's military background in his virile appearance. Holmes thus rejects the central anxieties of the Boer War and the worry that empire was physically degrading the English race.[113] In this way, Dodd's constitution disavows Britain's troubled medical history with respect to the war.

The other central character, however, challenges this embodiment. Dodd's fitness puts him in stark contrast to Godfrey, who reveals that after being wounded in battle he took shelter in a Boer leper hospital and was infected with the disease. In the nineteenth century, leprosy was associated with the tropics and the colonies, with the savage and the premodern. It was a disease that physically marked degeneration, through discoloration and disfigurement of the face and extremities, in addition to harkening back to the quarantine measures of Biblical times. When Dodd first glimpses Godfrey's blanched face, he sees "something slinking, something furtive, something guilty, something very unlike the frank, manly lad that I had known" (BB, 545–46). The "slinking" and "furtive" appearance connotes the Boer's stealthy tactics, those that changed the old narrative of gentlemanly warfare.[114] And this reference to the Boer influence in conjunction with the demasculinization suggests that a feminine, foreign presence has infected a prominent English family,[115] one with an upstanding genealogy of military service, no less, as Godfrey's father is a well-respected officer from the Crimean War. Read in this light, Godfrey's illness signifies the corruption of a bloodline that seemingly stood for the masculine, commanding defense of the nation.

The link between Godfrey's disappearance and the Boer War takes the form of disease, drawing a connection between British imperial war and the subsequent infection of the metropole and the British upper class. Once Holmes tells Godfrey's father that he is aware of Godfrey's "leprosy," the colonel grants Holmes and Dodd access to the missing soldier. Godfrey recounts his experiences in the leper hospital through a Gothic lens: "The African sun flooded through the big, curtainless windows, and every detail of the great, bare, whitewashed dormitory stood out hard and clear. In front of me was standing a small, dwarflike man with a huge, bulbous head, who was jabbering excitedly in Dutch, waving two horrible hands which looked to me like brown sponges" (BB, 554). Continuing the trope of deformation and degeneration—the large bulbous head recalls Culverton Smith's oversized skull—Godfrey comments on the other patients: "Not one of them was a normal human being. Every one was twisted or swollen or disfigured in some strange way" (BB, 554). The connection between the degenerate humanoids in the hospital and Godfrey's own corrupted body implicate war in the biological segregation of someone who had previously been a model specimen of a military man, like Dodd. It is important to recognize, however, that leprosy was not caused by the British military. It existed already in South Africa, and the circumstances of the war merely exposed Godfrey to it. Deploying the familiar trope of medicine as the ur-war, the only other English patient says to Godfrey, "Man alive! You are in far greater danger here than ever you were on the battlefield. You are in the Leper Hospital, and you have slept in a leper's bed" (BB, 555).

As in *Dracula*, this interaction brings the sexual ordering of society into a military context, drawing attention to the martial metaphor's, as a medical deployment of sexuality for racial purity, military genealogy. There are two possible agents of infection in this scene. One is the "dwarflike man" who assaults Godfrey with his "deformed hands," making contact with an open wound out of which fresh blood flows: "He had laid his deformed hands upon me and was dragging me out of bed, regardless of the fresh flow of blood from my wound" (BB, 554–55). The other is the bed that the English speaker identified as contaminated by leper patients. In both cases, military discourse frames the infection: in the first, through the physical altercation between a foreigner and a soldier, the former making contact with the latter's combat wound; in the second, through Godfrey's catching the disease "in bed," which binds his corruption to venereal disease,[116] a significant problem for the British military, leading to the CD acts, a policy Doyle which strongly subscribed to.[117] The venereal component, moreover, contributes to the idea that Godfrey's corruption in the war also polluted a great military and socially ranked bloodline. This connotation returns to Dodd's initial hypothesis about Godfrey's disappearance, that it involved guilt and shame over his conduct in the war. Godfrey's unmanly appearance, his "guilty" and "slinking" demeanor, seem to allude to the fact that British conduct during the Boer War was not altogether "manly."[118] In both cases, microbial infection is caused by war, which, on the one hand, destabilizes the martial metaphor but, on the other, reinforces the need to defend the British social body against infections of this nature, which reinforce the biopolitical techniques birthed from military medicine and utilized to shape the health of the British race through sexuality and reproduction.

The assemblage of Dodd, Holmes, and Holmes's medical expert reinforces the need for the martial metaphor to reveal and fight against what ails England—biologically, socially, and now, psychologically. Dodd frames his questions about Godfrey's disappearance in military language, approaching the house in a "frontal attack" but running into problems when he finds that it is "so large and rambling that a regiment might be hid away in it and no one the wiser" (*BB*, 546). Dodd's military-style inquiry leads him to find a physical and possibly criminal problem with Godfrey. Consequently, he seeks out Holmes, who with his medico-forensic detection makes his own initial diagnosis and discounts the criminal hypothesis. Holmes's hypothesis is finally confirmed by Saunders, the specialist in tropical medicine. This convergence of medicine, the military, and detection illustrates the ways these discourses become intertwined in surveillance, diagnosis, and treatment by way of the martial metaphor.

Doyle's foray into Boer War medical military fiction conveys an ambivalent position on the effects of equating medicine with war. The narrative at once espouses the martial metaphor as a narrative strategy for promoting British national interests and undercuts the viability of such a formulation. By offering an alternative etiology for Godfrey's "leprosy" and "controllable causes" for the side effects of imperialism, Holmes constructs a misreading that allows England to avoid self-toxicity; "The Blanched Soldier," however, suggests that as time passed it became more difficult for Holmes to exert this narrative control in a credible way.[119] This shows the contradictory nature of the martial metaphor with respect to British medicine in the early twentieth century: the fact that this representation has been narratively, fictionally constructed by national and military commitments rather than existing naturally in the British constitution. In this case, it is Doyle's documented commitment to sanitizing the British image in the light of the Boer War atrocities. Furthermore, while Godfrey's apparent leprosy seems to undercut Dodd's fitness, its psychological origin could assuage fears of biological ill health in the upper classes.

In his unique position as a writer, medical practitioner, and military doctor, Doyle wrote the martial metaphor into various developments of modernity both medical—bacteriology, immunology, toxicology, forensic medicine— and political—the Boer War, the Physical Committee on Degeneration, and Compulsory Vaccination. His work shows how the martial metaphor informed the medicalization of society, most prominently through linkages to detection, policing, and the ordering of the natural world. The underlying connections between the military underpinnings of the martial metaphor link Doyle's imperial and military imperatives with detection.

From Doyle's earliest Holmes fiction and medical writings to those written well into the twentieth century, it is clear that he conflated biological threats with military and cultural ones. Even though his early fiction doesn't invoke the martial metaphor overtly, the underlying logic of that metaphor, by way of the advent of immunology, toxicology, and bacteriology, is what makes Doyle's medical writings consonant with his Holmes stories. If the Holmes stories gave him a way to reflect narratively on the anxieties over the colonial, the degenerate, and the microbial, the stories also became a mode to communicate developing understandings of medicine to the lay reader, especially given his fin de siècle popularity. Indeed, there are countless medical publications, from the early twentieth century to the present articulating the acuity and accuracy of medicine in Doyle's fiction. There was not only an impact on public knowledge, but also the medical profession as his mode of investigation became its own metaphor for diagnosis. And yet, it was not only the fictional Watson but Doyle himself who embodied the martial metaphor, through his stint in the Boer War. Moreover, his enthusiastic defense of the British Empire, read in the context of his medical military concerns about enteric fever and vaccination, provides a background for the appearance of bacteriological disease in "The Dying Detective" and "The Blanched Soldier." Ultimately, Doyle's medical writing invokes the martial metaphor in the defense of Britishness as an identity and an index of health; his fiction simultaneously upholds and undercuts this proposition in the service of British imperialism. In effect, while Doyle's corpus puts into question the structures that the martial metaphor was deployed to sustain, taken as a whole, his work solidified the metaphor's place in medical culture and writing, suturing together the figure of the doctor as detective with that of the soldier.

5

Modernist Refractions of Tropical Medicine in Joseph Conrad's *Heart of Darkness*

Introducing a historical account of malaria in ancient Greece and Rome, military surgeon and tropical medicine specialist Sir Ronald Ross writes that in the war against disease, "we must welcome every possible ally,"[1] referring in this case to the historian. As I have shown in the previous chapters, authors like Kingsley, Stoker, and Doyle took up the role of allies to the physicians who were fighting this war "on the ground." Joseph Conrad was not one of these authors.

If the contradictions in Doyle's relationship to the martial metaphor trouble its validity as a narrative of social and medical order, then Conrad's modernist treatment of it radically foregrounds its pathogenic and destructive character. Although the lines between health and sickness blur in Conrad's writings, his position on the martial metaphor, unlike Doyle's, is unequivocal in showing how Englishness is being corrupted and is weakening. He reveals how the martial metaphor contributes to the production of the deaths of colonial others.

There is no question that Conrad's *Heart of Darkness* (1899) is plagued by the idea of illness. With its images of dying natives and mad, feverish Europeans, the book tempts us to read it as a warning against crossing the imperial threshold, that dark jungle kingdom beleaguered by some primordial miasma waiting to pollute the white body of the colonizer. But this reading reinscribes Western projections of exoticism and primitivism while missing the nuances of how sickness and health function in the novella in the larger context of tropical medicine. This chapter develops an extended reading of the novella's construction of tropical disease and how that reflects the martial narratives of tropical medicine specialists in popular and professional publications. Most medical readings of *Heart of Darkness* tend to focus on Kurtz's psychological maladies, building on Patrick Brantlinger's reading of "the myth of the Dark continent," in which Europeans bring the light of civilization to primitives at great risk of degenerating into subhumans themselves—"going native" or being "maddened by the tropics."[2] Cheryl Hindrichs contends that the aesthetics of illness and lack of closure in the novel compels readers to do their own work of sympathetic connection, producing "an ethical vantage from which to interrogate gender, culture, and race expectations."[3] I address how embodied forms of tropical disease and health operate in the novella. Conrad does destabilize Victorian cultural constructions, using disease to signify the effects of European imperialism and the health that sustains it. As his text reveals, health can be quite sickening. Conrad shows how this kind of pathogenic health is a function of the martial metaphor.

Heart of Darkness challenges notions of European health and even its own textual constructions of naturalized African insalubrity by implicating European colonials as pathogenic agents of what I refer to as *coloniopathy*: the physical sickness in the Congolese caused by colonialism. In line with the text's oft-cited indeterminacy, illness in the Africans both demonstrates the pathogenic effects of colonialism and reflects Western notions of Africa as an unwholesome environment. Even while Conrad critiques the morbid effects of empire, he is unable to avoid using its tropes. European health, bolstered by advances in medical science, also carries a complication: on the one hand, it denotes positive resistance to lethal disease; on the other, it signifies the capacity to perform genocidal work in the colony and an immunity to the horrors of that work. It is in this tension that the novella troubles the deployment of tropical medicine, a subdiscipline that had begun to develop out of parasitological research in equatorial areas and which, especially among the British, was supported mainly by the military, as one of its primary functions was to protect military personnel. Not surprisingly, the practitioners of tropical medicine mythologized their work through the martial metaphor, evident in Ross's proclamation above.

By showing how the novella's ambiguous relationship between health and sickness bears on tropical medicine, I also contribute to the discussion of *Heart of Darkness*'s problematic representations of race. Questions of whether Conrad was racist and whether his work has any merit, given its construction of natives as primitives, have occupied a number of Conrad scholars and postcolonial scholars in recent decades, such as Ian Watt,

Patrick Brantlinger, Chinua Achebe, and Edward Said. My reading of coloniopathy in *Heart of Darkness* takes account of the ambiguous representation of disease as both European and African in origin, by drawing from Said's argument that even though Conrad critiques empire, he cannot escape it as a guiding ideology for his critique. In terms of the martial metaphor, this suggests that Conrad challenges the differential production of health wrought by tropical medicine and the military infrastructure that the field developed co-constitutively; in doing so, however, he replicates some of the very tropes of primitivism on which that system relied.

This coloniopathic reading of Conrad promises three insights. First, it lays out a nuanced account of how literary genre destabilized the history of tropical medicine and its militarized narratives in the late Victorian popular and medical press. Conrad's own experiences of illness shaped his use of impressionism and modernist indeterminacy to challenge the Victorian imperial, military narratives attached to the heroes of tropical medicine. He ascribed his lifelong invalidism to infections acquired in the Congo. It was his sickness, however, that made his writing possible: his correspondence makes it clear that had he not been struck by disease, he would more than likely have continued his maritime career instead. His ill-health, especially his crippling gout that he attributed to tropical disease, made writing difficult, but as one of his friends notes, his recovery in the hospital gave him time to "do nothing and reflect."[4] This was an opportunity for him to work through how health and sickness had been and were being parceled out in the Congo. Conrad's ironic structure and impressionistic techniques reveal how tropical medicine contributed to rather than alleviated the "Dark Continent's" becoming "dark" and, analogously, how Africa was constructed ideologically and materially by imperialism as an inherently diseased environment,[5] one that needed to be colonized by the civilized world with medical force. In this way, the novella shows how tropical medicine itself was pathogenic to the native populations.

Second, this chapter shows how imperialism and its military infrastructure were linked to the development of tropical medicine. Countries like Germany and Britain funded tropical medicine to gain cachet on the world stage as bearers of the light of science to the benighted Africans, and the race to publish findings fueled aggressive research. Alongside this competition, though, medical knowledge was shared through the academic and popular publications, and states cooperated in advancing the martial metaphor to portray this as an effort of the "human race" against disease, as seen in the development of Belgian tropical medicine with help from British practitioners and institutions. The problem with this figuration, however, was who would and who would not be counted as part of the "human race," a prominent tension in Conrad's text.

Although tropical medicine emerged as a transnational network of cooperation and competition among European states, as Deborah Neill has suggested,[6] Conrad unravels specific nodes in this network. His novella draws attention to connections between Belgium and England in terms of military medicine, showing the complicity of British tropical medicine in what was called "the Crime of the Congo," after Arthur Conan Doyle's work (1909) by the same name, in the form of a necropolitical technology. We often think of medicine in terms of Foucauldian biopolitics, as a technology of governance that targets populations to maximize utility. Although Foucault qualifies this as the power to "make live" while letting some die, the focus is on producing vital and resourceful populations. But a less obvious way to think of medicine is in terms of what Achille Mbembe has called "necropolitics," the subjection of life to the power of death, by a sovereign power in a colonial space: the "capacity to define who matters and who does not, who is disposable and who is not."[7] In necropolitics, power lies in the ability not only to kill but to maintain life in a state of injury as a tool of labor. I suggest that tropical medicine enabled the conferral of this "living dead" status on the Congolese natives.[8] Understanding how the novella speaks to this necropolitical relationship between the Belgians and the Congolese enables us to see both the possibilities and the limits in Conrad's critique of the way European health triumphed over Congolese bodies.

Third, the novella brings to the surface a particular moment in epidemiological and pharmacological history that radically changed the way medicine "fought disease." The interventions in the Congo by European tropical medicine helped bring about Huxley's "pharmacological torpedo" in the form of German chemist and physician Paul Ehrlich's "magic bullet." The epidemic of sleeping sickness (trypanosomiasis) was exacerbated by colonization and gave tropical medicine researchers a lab to develop and test the first synthetic agents for targeting disease while to a degree sparing healthy tissue. In this context, Conrad exposes a history of coloniopathic disease behind arguably the most significant medical development of the last 200 years: antimicrobial, chemotherapeutic pharmacology. This linkage calls into question the logics that shaped the heroic, martial narratives of antibiotics as a "weapon."

In this concluding chapter, I outline the connections between tropical medicine and the mythologized, if not romanticized, constructions of its military medical heroes, such as Ronald Ross, Patrick Manson, and Thomas Heazle Parke, and the explorers such as Henry Morton Stanley whom their work supported. The role these men played as imperial heroes exposes the historical connections between tropical medicine and the representations of health and sickness in the novella. This first section primarily addresses the history of tropical medicine in reference to Conrad's representations of the Congo. In the second section, I show how native illness and death are produced out of European health, which I understand through Achille Mbembe's theory of necropower. Conrad emblematizes European health in the figure of the General Manager, who is entangled with both the natives' and Kurtz's illnesses, specifically via an epidemiological event contemporary with the novella: Henry Morton Stanley's catalysis of one of the worst epidemics in African history. I conclude by linking this epidemic with the rise of modern-day drug therapies, showing how colonialism enabled the development of a militarized pharmacological discourse that frames the antibiotic relationship between humans and microbes.

The "Civilizing" Mission to Beat Down Africa's Natural Defenses

Both as a material practice and as an ideological edifice, tropical medicine was a significant factor in and result of the Scramble for Africa, an imperial drive that took Europe by storm between the 1880s and 1914, and is consequently both a cause and a result of the use of the martial metaphor. But, however civilizing tropical medicine was meant to be, like so many other epidemiological technologies its history lies in the military. Not only were the majority of its early practitioners military officers, its central purpose was to support colonization in environments that had earlier been deemed inhospitable to the European body—Africa and India most notably. The "golden age" of tropical medicine, which allowed Britain to capture scientific renown of the sort previously held by Koch and Pasteur, came mostly from military researchers. In addition to the work of Patrick Manson and Ronald Ross, there was David Bruce's discovery of the bacteria that cause brucellosis (1887) and trypanosomiasis (1905), and Charles Donovan's discovery of the cause of donovanosis (1905). Meanwhile, researchers and military physicians also developed the field by institutionalizing it, as in John Sinton's founding of the Royal Society of Tropical Medicine and Hygiene (1907).[9] This birth of the tropical clinic was nurtured by and aided the military apparatus.

While the field's technological developments and protocols did reduce the incidence of disease among colonizers, the idea of progress that it espoused also fueled the scramble. That is, bringing European medical science to Africa became the medical component of the civilizing mission, the "white man's burden." At the European conference where King Leopold II of Belgium lobbied countries to accept his absolute control over what he called the "Congo Free State," he declared that his mission was "to open to civilization the only part of our globe which it has not yet penetrated," adding that "to pierce the darkness which hangs over entire peoples is, I dare say, a crusade worthy of this century of progress."[10] In reality, Leopold ruled the Congo as his private domain of resource extraction and a state of exception with his private army, the *Force Publique*.[11]

A central part of the "darkness" Europeans saw as haunting the Congo, along with the rest of Africa, was the inherently diseased and medically "backward" condition they attributed to the natives. Tropical medicine was part of the civilizing remedy for this. Two of its primary focuses were sleeping sickness and malaria. While both were significant inhibitors of empire, malaria had a viable treatment in the nineteenth century, which became an attractive technology to European explorers and militaries.

Quinine greatly mitigated malaria's impact on colonizers. It actually treated the disease, but it also boosted confidence in the viability of the imperial project and its "civilizing mission."[12] Though its causal relationship with imperial expansion is debated by medical historians, I would characterize quinine as instrumental in expediting the Scramble for Africa and as one of tropical medicine's weapons of empire; its material and ideological functions helped give Europeans unrestrained access to the continent.[13] This use of ideology along with medico-scientific technologies follows Laura Otis's claims that Robert Koch's visit to East Africa to treat German malaria victims was not just to make them physically healthier but also to make German colonizers "confident" enough to maintain the colony.[14] This confidence boost had a kind of placebo effect, inspiring support for colonization across Europe—especially, in Britain and Belgium. Closely tied to quinine, the work of British researchers such as Ross and Manson garnered support for tropical medicine and its role in increasing the cultural capital of British science and expanding empire in India and Africa.[15]

Conrad had personal experience with quinine. He diagnosed and treated a number of sailors with it during his maritime work.[16] This history is present in both his *Congo Diary* and his novella *The Shadow Line* (1916), where it serves as a plot device: "I pinned my faith to it. It would save the men, the ship, break the spell by its medicinal virtue, make time of no account, the weather but a passing worry and, like a magic powder working against mysterious malefices, secure the first passage of my first command against the evil powers of calms and pestilence."[17] The protagonist of *The Shadow Line* takes command of a new ship and finds that the quinine supply had been sold by the previous captain and replaced with inert white powder. He is thus unable to treat the deranged first mate, who believes the ship is haunted. Conrad was well aware of the drug's power to shape the course of expeditionary endeavors outside Europe. The framing of colonization being enabled through the martial metaphor was a central narrative of tropical medicine: these specialists defused the Dark Continent's "natural defenses" against colonialism. Men like Manson and Ross were portrayed as soldiers defending the nation by developing measures against insect-borne parasites, thanks in large part to their deployment of the martial metaphor in public addresses and medical publications. Even in death, many tropical medicine specialists where framed as soldiers for their medico-scientific work. A Dr. Dutton, for instance, was eulogized this way in *The Truth on the Congo Free State*, a periodical put out by the "Federation for the Defence of Belgian Interests Abroad": "He was one of that admirable assembly of learned men, which several European monarchs, King Leopold among them, have called upon to try and victoriously fight against the terrible diseases which ravage and depopulate Africa; the members of this Association have already done much towards finding a remedy against sleeping-sickness and their work is carried on so cleverly and actively that we may hope soon to be able to successfully fight against that devastating scourge."[18]

With an identifiable literary flair,[19] Ross, a surgeon-major who was often described as a polymath for his literary endeavors, crafted prose, poetry, and public addresses in the language of the martial metaphor. A notable example is his address to the Northumberland and Durham Medical Society in 1904, "The Battle for the Health of the Tropics."

Drawing repeatedly on the martial metaphor, which turns medicine into the ur-war of the British and of human civilization by extension, Ross opened his address with, "Gentlemen, is there anything more supremely important to men than the investigation of those great diseases which destroy them by millions? What are politics, laws and philosophies to us, compared with disease and death? The principal battle of all is the battle against disease—physical, intellectual and moral."[20] He made a similar claim in a historical context, likening disease to the fall of nations, in an introduction to William H. Jones's *Malaria, a Neglected Factor in the History of Greece and Rome* (1907), cited in the opening of this chapter: "The student of biology is often struck with the feeling that historians, when dealing with the rise and fall of nations, do not generally view the phenomena from a sufficiently high biological standpoint. . . . [T]hey seem to attach too much importance to individual rulers and soldiers, and to particular wars, policies, religions, and customs; while at the same time they make little attempt to extract the fundamental causes of national success or failure."[21] Here, Ross makes a case for the martial metaphor in historiographical terms, suggesting that such an intervention would "help in the war which is now being conducted against the disease in many countries."[22]

Ross discovered the malarial vector's life cycle in 1897. Together with Manson's previous work on mosquitoes, and the discovery of the tsetse fly as the vector for sleeping sickness five years later, this led to great strides in the actual prevention of disease with mosquito nets and other hygienic protocols.[23] On discovering the parasite's life cycle in the anopheline mosquito, Ross wrote the following poem:

> This day relenting God
> Hath placed within my hand
> A wondrous thing; and God
> Be praised. At His command,
> Seeking His secret deeds
> With tears and toiling breath,
> I find thy cunning seeds,
> O million-murdering Death.
> I know this little thing
> A myriad men will save.
> O Death, where is thy sting?
> Thy victory, O Grave?[24]

Recalling the way Kingsley framed the martial metaphor as a way to understand God's natural laws, Ross writes of discovering the malaria *germ*—with the word meaning both "seed" and "microbe," a duality Conrad deploys too—in the form of the malarial plasmodium. Moreover, he challenges Death's weaponized "sting," alluding to the verse in Corinthians (1, 15:55) describing the futility of death in the face of the Christian afterlife. In addition to its material consequences, Ross's research had significant ideological impact. It changed people's perception of the relationship between the white European and the tropics and of the real and perceived effects of quinine. Explorers, military troops, and biomedical researchers advanced at great risk, and the massive edifice of tropical medicine was built to protect their work.[25]

This imperial militarism recurred in Ross's 1902 Nobel Prize reception for his discovery of the malarial parasite's life cycle, where he was described as "a hero from Africa who had been occupied in a war, not against his fellow men, but against a most insidious enemy to mankind."[26] In Ross's own words in the *Journal of the Royal Army Medical Corps*, malarial fever had "withheld an entire continent from humanity—the immense and fertile tracts of Africa."[27] This echoes the mythological valence of the metaphor that Manson deployed in describing malaria as "the Cerberus that guards the African continent,"[28] and Leopold II's justifications when seeking the world's blessing to colonize the Congo. Tropical medicine reclaimed that continent "for humanity." The unwitting irony in Ross's statement is that the ideology and material technology that this work contributed to facilitated a "war" on the Congolese that was justified precisely by their exclusion from the rubrics of "humanity" and "mankind."

The discovery of the malarial parasite and its life cycle in the mosquito was significant because it overturned the attribution of the disease to the climate and the land, as inhospitable to Europeans. Jessica Howell has recently complicated the spatiotemporal logics of malaria, showing that malaria narratives, fictional and nonfictional, grapple with the endemic and epidemic uncertainty of the disease.[29] While still retaining an element of miasmic uncertainty, Conrad partook in the military ethos of tropical medicine when he followed the trope of constructing Africa, specifically its coasts, in a defensive posturing that repels Europeans. The figuration of tropical disease as having "withheld" Africa is analogous to Marlow's characterization in the novella of the miasmic darkness that permeates the coastline as he approaches the Congo, "where the merry dance of trade goes in a still and earthly atmosphere as of an overheated catacomb; all along the formless coast bordered by dangerous surf, as if Nature herself tried to ward off intruders; in and out of rivers, streams of death, whose banks were rotting into mud, whose waters, thickened into slime, invaded the contorted mangroves that seemed to writhe at us in the extremity of an impotent despair."[30] The way Conrad constructs the land here follows the Victorian trope of "the white man's grave," where the land's material filth breeds diseased air. The mangroves, which appeared frequently in descriptions of tropical rivers, also bespeak disease, as they were treated as warnings of malaria in both anticontagionist and parasitological etiologies—in the former because of their rank and decaying odor, in the latter because of their linkage to insect vectors.[31]

In opposition to the coast's "warding off intruders," Conrad figures the entropic effects of the martial metaphor. Marlow comes across a French man-of-war anchored offshore and firing indiscriminately into the jungle.

> There wasn't even a shed there, and she was shelling the bush. It appears the French had one of their wars going on thereabouts. Her ensign dropped limp like a rag; the muzzles of the long six-inch guns stuck out all over the low hull; the greasy, slimy swell swung her up lazily and let her down, swaying her thin masts. In the empty immensity of earth, sky, and water, there she was, incomprehensible, firing into a continent. Pop, would go one of the six-inch guns; a small flame would dart and vanish, a little white smoke would disappear, a tiny projectile would give a feeble screech—and nothing happened. Nothing could happen. There was a touch of insanity in the proceeding, a sense of lugubrious drollery in the sight; and it was not dissipated by somebody on board assuring me earnestly there was a camp of natives—he called them enemies!—hidden out of sight somewhere. (HD, 14)

This scene is often read in terms of waste and inefficiency,[32] and the avaricious and destructive nature of French colonialism specifically, which compounds Conrad's critique of Belgium's violent colonization of the Congo. The line about firing into the coast, in a context in which crew members "were dying of fever at a rate of three per day" (HD, 14), presents a failure of military-backed colonization, where the land itself fights back with disease. This is not so much a failure of the martial metaphor, though, as a reinscription: The French are fighting back against the land's pathogenesis, blindly, with weapons of war. Rather than showing the metaphor's failure, Conrad exposes the material damage that results from it. The description of the French's attack, however, their "blind firing," suggests that their response was entirely military, and missing the medical component: the work of tropical medicine specialists who could make the land habitable for them. Rather than firing blindly, tropical medicine attacked diseases precisely, by targeting their insect vectors and later the parasites within the insects themselves—leading, as I argue in the final section, to the realization of pharmaceutical torpedoes.

However, even with the targeted approach of men like Ross and Manson, the Congolese suffered medically in turn. With the growing success of tropical medicine at the end of the century, the idea that white men were constitutionally unable to withstand the pestilent heart of darkness was no longer tenable.[33] Climate does figure prominently in Conrad's work as a source of disease, fever, and neurasthenia in Europeans, but Conrad was quite up to date with medical discourse and the discovery of germs and parasites. In *Heart of Darkness*, climate serves as a metonym for the place where disease-causing elements, such as parasite-bearing insect vectors, reside. With tropical medicine as their weapon, Europeans could conquer both the parasites and the continent. They could avoid the mosquito with nets and prevent infection with quinine. These material effects, coupled with the ideological reconstruction of Africa as safer for white men, did not eliminate death; instead, they shifted its target population. Moreover, the insights and technologies birthed from tropical medicine did not just help the British conquer parts of Africa and India; they also helped the Belgians conquer the Congo. Leopold took advantage of the transnational network of tropical medicine research to cultivate his private colony and his public image. The effect was that tropical medicine helped turn the "white man's grave" into the native Congolese's grave.

Germs of Empire

Modernism afforded Conrad a grammar to articulate the contradictory image of Europe as simultaneously healthy and diseased with respect to the Congo. *Heart of Darkness* is fraught with contradictions. Binaries such as light and darkness become unstable, as in the city where the Belgian

Company resides: a "whited sepulture" at once light and sanitary on the outside and dark and putrid on the inside (*HD*, 9). The play between the conventional positive valences of "light"—civilization, progress, science, health, and life—and the negative ones of "darkness"—primitivism, degeneration, vacuity, disease, and death—follows the complexity of the text's narrative and thematic temporality.

Conrad blurs the boundaries that subtend the martial metaphor. This blurring is evident in the way Marlow's experiences and "impressions" shape the narrative structure: moments from the past are interjected into the narrative present, while his own thoughts and feelings splice together fragments of dialogue in what Ian Watt has called "delayed decoding."[34] This technique is essential to Conrad's impressionism: a style that leaves the reader with impressions from the author or narrator and an atmosphere that is filtered through subjective sensory perceptions, and embraces ambiguity and indeterminacy.[35]

To this effect, Marlow qualifies his tale before he starts it in order to show how these impressions shape his narrative: "I don't want to bother you much with what happened to me personally, yet to understand the effect on me you ought to know how I got there, what I saw. . . . It was the farthest point of navigation and culminating point of my experience. It seemed to throw a kind of light on everything about me—and into my thoughts" (*HD*, 7). Marlow's experience at the core of the heart of darkness, his meeting with Kurtz, reveals the significance of all that came before it because it structures the way he tells the very story after the experience. Conrad's own story in the Congo operated analogously: it was cut short by illness, which gave him a "kind of light" to throw relief on what he saw there. The narrative that became the novella was filtered through Conrad's individual impressions, impressions that reflected his critique of empire, and of tropical medicine just when it was rising as an institution. On an allegorical and authorial level, drawing attention to death and disease as seemingly immanent to the African darkness also throws into sharp relief the conditions that produced it, namely those of European health or "light."

This impressionistic technique helps Conrad implicate colonial powers, especially the British, by way of tropical medicine, in the Belgian production of death in the Congo. Marlow's visual impressions of the Scramble for Africa reflect how Conrad assigned but also blurred the blame for colonial atrocities. On the surface, Marlow seems to hold the British Empire in higher esteem than the other European colonizers. In the Company's office in Belgium, he sees a multicolored map "marked with all the colours of a rainbow representing the different European interests in Africa" and remarks that "there was a vast amount of red—good to see at any time, because one knows that some real work is done in there" (HD, 10). Although Marlow travels to the Belgian Congo, "the yellow," his status as an Englishman bespeaks his reference to "the red," representing Britain's interest in Africa. Marlow clearly looked more favorably on British imperialism at this point in his past. But this is undercut by his general chastisement of the imperial impetus, delivered before he recounts his story. He claims that the great men of empire were "conquerors" and "for that you only want brute force—nothing to boast of, when you have it, since strength is an accident arising from the weakness of others. . . . The conquest of the earth . . . mostly means the taking away of it from those who have a different complexion" (HD, 7). Marlow's reference to "real work" in the context of this preface adds irony to his younger self's positive affirmation of British "work" in Africa. Furthermore, "strength," refers not just to military developments like the automatic Maxim gun, but also to the power arising from technologies of European health.[36] This tension between Britain's work, the Congo, and European imperialism addresses the ostensibly altruistic work of tropical medicine. Read as a network of such medicine, the map identifies the "real work" being done by the British medical enterprise, suggesting that it is a civilizing mission or some testament to progress; yet, it does so ambivalently. Britain's strength arises from the disease the empire projects onto the colonized. But, Conrad resists the notion that these values are absolute and tied to their respective positive and negative connotations; he suggests that they are, instead, differential. This difference is evident in the way in which tropical medicine produced health for the colonizer, and not only in a way that was different to medical evaluation of the colonized but in some cases to their detriment.

The historical linkage between British tropical medicine and the Belgian Congo reveals how the enterprise functioned as a tool of necropower, as a weapon that enabled death rather than forestalling it. Before the British advancements, the continent's own power over European life hindered the potential of colonialism. King Leopold wanted to take part in the Scramble for Africa but needed the knowledge and experience of British explorers and medical specialists. It is thus no coincidence that the two greatest producers of tropical medicine specialists and knowledge arose alongside Leopold: The London and Liverpool Schools of Tropical

Medicine. The Liverpool school, founded in 1899, was supported primarily by Sir Alfred Jones, a British shipping magnate. Jones had clear economic and political motives for funding the institution: he held a monopoly on commercial traffic between the Congo and Antwerp, and he was King Leopold's consul for Belgium in Liverpool.[37] Leopold relied on London and Liverpool for information and training for some Belgian doctors, whose primary directive was not in fact humanitarian because it focused only on treating Europeans.[38] They really turned to native health only when the sleeping sickness epidemic became a threat to production and came to be discussed around the world.

In 1901 and 1903, Leopold invited members of the London School of Tropical Medicine to inspect the Congo Free State, help deal with the epidemic, and eventually to conduct drug trials for the organoarsenical atoxyl, a chemotherapeutic agent I will discuss at length with respect to pharmacological medical-war. After Ross won the 1902 Nobel Prize, Leopold invited him and other military physicians and scientists to Belgium to celebrate, awarding him *L'Ordre de Leopold* and donating funds to the school in addition. Letters in Ross's archive at the London School of Tropical Medicine suggest that some of Ross's friends were less than thrilled at his accepting this distinction. His close friend John Holt writes, "I'm sorry to see you accept 'honors' from King Leopold. 'He' does you 'no' honor by anything he can bestow. Your work has been to save human suffering and human life. What his has been you know."[39] Leopold strove to profit from his relationship with the British institution. To deploy the knowledge and technologies he had received from them, he founded the Antwerp School of Tropical Medicine, designed on the British model, in 1906, two years before he was forced to abdicate his control of the Congo.

Apart from Alfred Jones, the explorer Henry Morton Stanley served as a nexus between British medicine and the Belgian colonial project. Stanley set up routes, infrastructure, and trading stations in the Congo Basin for Leopold in the late 1870s and the 1880s—*Heart of Darkness*'s "inner station" is the fictional correlative of Stanley Falls Station, Conrad's uppermost destination during his own expedition. In his relationship with the development of British pharmaceuticals, Stanley promoted the idea of British health as it was tied to the country's development of quinine and tropical medicine more generally. Admired by both the British and the Belgians, he was knighted for his colonial work in 1899, the year Conrad published *Heart of Darkness* and the year the London School of

Tropical Medicine was founded. Explorers like Stanley held significant interest for the public; for instance, his book *In Darkest Africa* (1890) sold more than 150 thousand copies.[40] And before his expedition for Leopold, Stanley led his famed search for Dr. David Livingstone, whose own mid-century use of quinine had demonstrated the medicine's efficacy, especially when used prophylactically.

Later in the century, Leopold and Stanley both benefited from the specifically British hype surrounding quinine, the validation of its effectiveness, and the increase in supplies of it by the British military in the 1880s.[41] The pharmaceutical company Burroughs Wellcome and Co. even marketed a "Livingstone Medicine Chest" stocked abundantly with quinine. Stanley vigorously endorsed the British brand, urging in *The Founding of the Congo Free State* (1885), "Obtain your medicine pure and well prepared. Messrs. Burroughs and Welcome [sic] will equip you with tropic medicine in chest and cases. . . . They have sought the best medical advice."[42] When Stanley went on the Emin Pasha relief expedition (1886–1889) his doctor, Thomas Heazle Parke, an army surgeon with experience in tropical medicine, gave a similar testimonial, citing his treatments of Stanley, his men, and himself with the drug.[43] Parke was hailed as a hero in the medical press after his death and the publication of his journal and his *Guide to Health in Africa* (1893). One reviewer wrote that he "furnishes the standard for the career of a medical hero."[44] While Parke's journal does describe some of the drug's failures, he writes of the importance of its prophylactic use and the impression it gave of British health in the Congo: "The Belgian officers, stationed at Stanley Pool, told us that our exception from fever was most extraordinary and unusual."[45] The health of Stanley's unit stood in stark contrast to that of the Belgians, and Parke writes that it "impressed us all so strongly with the prophylactic treatment, that, so far as our stock of quinine permitted, we pursued it all through our entire expedition."[46] In addition to its antiparasitic effects, the drug inspired a kind of confidence that imbued British tropical medicine with the image of triumphant health, which became an ideological catalyst for seizing charge of African land and bodies. I suggest that it is this kind of health—a material effect of the martial metaphor—that Conrad embodies in the figure of the General Manager.

Conrad's experiences in the Congo and his writing and publication of *Heart of Darkness* were thus part of a significant cultural moment when tropical medicine and imperial expansion existed in a mutually constitutive relationship for Britain and Belgium. Stanley was a significant actor in this moment. As he had become a kind of celebrity adventurer, his and Parke's espousal of the Burroughs-Wellcome pharmacopeia gave British tropical medicine significant cultural purchase as a technology of civilization, one that was certainly appealing to Leopold. If the Maxim gun gave Stanley and his men tactical advantage and ideological support against the native populations, British pharmaceuticals gave them both the confidence and the protection from disease they needed to develop the Congo. The analogy between weaponry and medicine highlights tropical medicine's efficacy as a tool for subjugating Congolese life to the colonizer's ability to maim, kill, and instrumentalize it. Brantlinger suggests that Stanley's work for Leopold was essentially the same as that of the Company's mercenary army, the Eldorado Exploring Expedition, in *Heart of Darkness*: "To tear treasure out of the bowels of the land was their desire, with no more moral purpose at the back of it than there is in burglars breaking into a safe" (*HD*, 30). This work was supported by both the material efficacy and the idea of quinine, and by its intimate ties to the British Empire and its supporting industries. Conrad was in the midst of the imperial work of British pharmacology, alongside the work of tropical practitioners like Parke and researchers like Ross and Manson, during his time in the Congo and his time writing about it.

Heart of Darkness links this imperial zeitgeist with the perception of microbial pathogenicity. Early expanders of empire like Stanley, and their supporting medical specialists like Ross, Mason, and Parke, were seen as heroes, forgers of empire. This explains why Dr. J. L. Todd, a member of the London School of Tropical Medicine who went on the 1903 expedition sent by Leopold to inspect the Congo, wrote that "the future of imperialism lay with the microscope."[47] But Conrad's novella challenged these constructions, linking the military rhetoric of tropical medicine with its imperial imperatives and pejorative effects.

In the opening of *Heart of Darkness*, the narrator evokes the sentiments of imperial soldiers, signaling the martial rhetoric surrounding tropical medicine's part in colonial expansion. He frames the heroes of empire as knights-errant who resonate in the "great spirit of the past in the lower Thames": "The tidal current runs to and fro in its unceasing service, crowded with memories of men and ships it had borne to the rest of home or to the battles of the sea. It had known and served all the men of whom the nation is proud, from Sir Francis Drake to Sir John Franklin, knights all, titled and untitled—the great knights-errant of the sea" (*HD*, 4–5). Emilie Taylor-Brown has noted how fin-de-siècle parasitologists constructed themselves in a similar image and were viewed by the public as mythic heroes of empire,[48] an ethos similar to the one *Dracula*'s Crew of Light drew on when battling Dracula. Ross and Manson, and certainly Stanley and Parke, fit the model of the "knights" the narrator so admires in Marlow's opening. These were men who opened once-unconquerable lands to the sacred fire of civilization, the light of medical science. The narrator closes his apology for the knights of empire who embarked from the Thames: "Captains, Admirals, the dark interlopers of the eastern trade, and the commissioned 'Generals' of the East India fleets. Hunters for gold and pursuers of fame they all had gone out on that stream, bearing the sword, and often the torch, messengers of might within the land, bearers of a spark from the sacred fire. What greatness had not floated on the ebb of that river into the mystery of an unknown earth! . . . The dreams of men, the seed of commonwealths, the germs of empires" (*HD*, 5). Conrad explicitly names the military component of colonialism, linking the "sword" with the "spark" of civilization and noting the military aspect of Britain's control of India through the privatized East India Company.[49] Furthermore, he associates these military roles with microbial pathogens. In terms of germ theory, we see the knights of empire who emanate from the Thames being linked with cholera during the mid-century. Both *germ* and *seed* denote an origin, but these knights too are germs insofar as they are pathogens of empire.

These seeds are simultaneously points of origin and microbial parasites: they grow and create, but they do so only by draining life from the native host. Martin Bock argues that Conrad's diary, letters, and fiction show his knowledge of the germ theory of disease. He cites a number of instances of Conrad using the word *seedy* to denote sickness, and links this terminology to the contemporaneous spread of germ theory in medical and popular discourse.[50] With Bock's assertion in mind, we can see how a germ functions as an origin, one that will grow into a disease for native populations, and we can see how these knight-germs of empire, like so many agents of tropical disease, are parasites.[51] In this way, the passages lead us to ask who or what exactly becomes the "cunning seed" in Ross's poem. These knights-as-parasites come to represent both material and metaphorical disease in the novel, reflecting the health and sickness that tropical medicine brought to the Congo. Disease was naturalized as part of the land and the natives, because of their assigned primitive, unhygienic ways and the environment's hospitality to parasites. In this opening, Conrad begins to demythologize this naturalization which validated tropical medicine's intervention as part of the civilizing mission but ironically led to a recursive propagation of disease and a necropolitical death-world for the Congolese.

Coloniopathic Work and Necropower

In *Heart of Darkness*, as the parasitic agents consume more ivory and "eviscerate the land [and tear] treasure out of its bowels," the native population withers from privation and tropical disease (*HD*, 30). This process shows the health of the colonizer becoming a necropolitical weapon. Consider one of the most memorable scenes in the novella, the "grove of death."

> Black shapes crouched, lay, sat between the trees, leaning against the trunks, clinging to the earth. . . . They were dying slowly—it was very clear. They were not enemies, they were not criminals, they were nothing earthly now,—nothing but black shadows of disease and starvation lying confusedly in the greenish gloom. Brought from all the recesses of the coast in all the legality of time contracts, lost in uncongenial surroundings, fed on unfamiliar food, they sickened, became inefficient, and were then allowed to crawl away and rest. . . . I began to distinguish the gleam of eyes under the trees. Then, glancing down, I saw a face near my hand. The black bones reclined at full length with one shoulder against the tree, and slowly the eyelids rose and the sunken eyes looked up at me, enormous and vacant. . . . Near the same tree two more bundles of acute angles sat with their legs drawn up. . . . [A]ll about others were scattered in every pose of contorted collapse, as in some picture of a massacre or a pestilence. (*HD*, 17)

The natives live and die as "black shadows of disease." They exist as "bare life," biology stripped of political significance and protection. The banality of this scene documents the way death and diseased life are business as usual in the colonial space.[52] The native bodies become part of the background, even of the earth—yet remain an ethereal part of the darkness that imbues the Congo. The men Marlow sees are nearly indistinguishable from the tree that their bones or "bundles of angles" recline against. The synecdoche here is both a result of necropower and an indication of Conrad's critique.

The fragmentation into parts, a result of "pestilence" caused by the labor conditions, also reflects the colonial project's necropolitics, which Achille Mbembe defines as the "instrumentalization of human existence and the material destruction of human bodies," based on a racial divide that characterizes not only the life but even the death of the natives as not human.[53] Kiel Hume, in his necropolitical reading of Conrad, describes this scene as one of modernism's most "sustained representations of bare life."[54] For Mbembe, necropolitical spaces are those, such as the colony or the slave plantation, where people are not necessarily killed outright—although they can be at any time—but are "subjected to the conditions of life which confer upon [populations] the status of *living dead*." What makes this scene—a representative picture of the labor conditions in Leopold's Congo—readable as necropolitics is the way the natives are at once killable and "kept alive but in a state of injury."[55] In the European view of Africa, natives were a kind of inexhaustible natural resource. They could always get more laborers from other regions, from other slave traders. The idea was that human capital, much like rubber and ivory, seemed to exist in infinite supply in this region; Stanley himself had reported on the rich supply of natural and human resources.[56] Conrad's construction of the natives as a bodily mass that merges with the jungle, together with his denial of agency to the natives for most of the text, contributes to this imperial ideology.

The way Conrad thinks through sickness here shows his understanding that the representation of the body was not only a way to make necropower visible in his critique; it was also a tool the colonial system used to impose necropower. The depiction of the Congolese as inhuman is a proposition in the kind of logic that facilitates genocide. Even though Marlow rejects this cruel treatment of the natives, the presentation of his critique reflects the larger problem of racial representation and its relation to death in the Congo. The Congolese die like animals, part of the "natural" environment. But this primitivization is not a regression in time to "the very beginnings of the world," as Marlow suggests (*HD*, 33); rather, the natives' naturalized death is "a product of modern political design . . . an entirely cultural process."[57] Even as Marlow denounces their treatment, his representation of the Africans in this scene and elsewhere as animals undergoing cruel treatment employs the very logic that facilitates colonial atrocities. Conrad may be denouncing the Belgians, but he is still writing his critique under the aegis of an imperialistic civilizing mission based on racial difference. As Edward Said suggests, the "non-European darkness" Conrad writes of "cannot see the non-European world *resisting* imperialism."[58]

This problem speaks to why Conrad's text does not present us with the full scope of necropower. Though Mbembe's necropolitics is mainly concerned with the death-producing work of colonization and war, an often-overlooked valance of the theory is the way necropower functions as a tool of both the colonizer and the colonized. An example of the latter is the martyr or suicide bomber. By assuming agency over one's own death, one takes up a form of political agency and resistance.[59] The fact that native resistance through suicide is missing from Conrad's novella is telling; it supports Said's contention that Conrad can't see the Congolese resisting imperialism.[60] Yet there were in fact historical accounts of natives committing suicide as a result of Belgian rule. For instance, Conan Doyle writes in *The Crime of the Congo* (1909), "Suicide is not natural with [sic] African, as it is with some Oriental races. But it has come in with the other blessings of King Leopold's rule," citing the example of a native who hanged himself but was resuscitated.[61] A counterpoint that contributes to the construction of naturalized insalubrity in Africa is the only mention of a suicide in *Heart of Darkness*: a reference to a "Swede" who hanged himself, perhaps because "the sun" or "the country" was "too much for him" (*HD*, 15). Even Doyle's reference to a native trying to seize necropower "from below" is fraught with racist and primitivist rhetoric. Moreover, this attempt to gain agency through death was forestalled by medical intervention. The lack of agency in death mirrors the lack of agency in native life in *Heart of Darkness*. Conrad's racially problematic constructions reveal themselves through his narrative and modernist techniques; Marlow's many references to going back in time contribute to the assumptions underwriting this necropolitical exercise. Part of the reason the natives appear as bare life is that they are constructed as existing before modern time, and thus before politics.[62] Thus, they lack *bios*, or political life—"human rights," as we might, however problematically, say today.

One consequence of using primitivism to represent bare life was that it allowed Europeans to colonize under the imprimatur of evolutionary science and humanitarian aid. In the case of tropical medicine, even after the discovery of insect vectors, disease was understood as contiguous with the land and people, justifying European intervention. Conrad shows us how this made tropical medicine into a necropolitical weapon. Medicine in the Congo was directed at the few Europeans who were there to "civilize," per Leopold's lip service to progress. In giving Europeans a means—defense against disease—as well as a reason to penetrate the Congo, tropical medicine helped them confer a living-dead status on the natives, one that kept them barely alive for labor power that was inefficient but could easily be replaced when they died.

Heart of Darkness discloses the practical, logistical problems of what came to be known as the "Leopoldian" system. In contrast to the biopolitical calculus of birth rates and death rates in liberal European states, where the imperative was to make some live while letting others die, in the Belgian Congo it was the profligate expenditure of life and death that fueled "the tendency of imperial capitalism . . . toward monumental forms of waste and inefficiency; the entire operation of managers and accountants, waystations, steamboats, agents, rifles and rivets, [was] dedicated to keeping a 'trickle of ivory' out of the Congo."[63] But ultimately, there would be no bodies to extract labor from, no hosts to parasitize, without a shift in the economies of health. This turn finally came in the early twentieth century, when Leopold abdicated control of the Congo. Thus, while it might seem contradictory for the Leopold's Congo to have allowed such an entropic use of labor power as appears in the grove of death, the way Africa and the natives were figured as a natural resource made this a marginal concern, one of the differential productions of health that was made thinkable and feasible by the martial metaphor.

The labor problems caused by population loss in Leopold's necropolitical state—eight to ten million by some estimates—were connected to a shift in the imperatives occupying tropical medicine between its inception in the nineteenth century and its later developments in the mid-twentieth. The reaction to the Leopoldian system did eventually lead to a more African-centered public health system after his abdication. Part of this was public relations, but it did result in some "real advances in health policy and practice."[64] The involvement of biomedicine in empire passed through two phases in this period, as Margaret Lock and Vinh-Kim Nguyen have argued.[65] In the "imperial" phase (before 1920), biomedicine and its associated technologies were deployed to protect settlers and soldiers and focused on fevers like malaria and sleeping sickness—the kind of imperative we see in Conrad. It wasn't until after 1920, when the native people were recognized as an indispensable resource to colonial economics, that the focus shifted to managing the health of the local people by shaping them into viable, self-sustaining, and hygienic populations.[66] I would characterize this as a shift in emphasis from necropolitical to biopolitical regimes.

It is not just forced labor and overexertion that induce sickness; the "grove of death" passage suggests that Europeans actually caused disease among the native populations by displacing them: they were "brought from all the recess of the coast" and were "lost in uncongenial surroundings, fed on unfamiliar food" (HD, 17). This displacement might seem less savage than forced labor and starvation, but it was just as devastating. Neill suggests that even during the sleeping sickness epidemic, most people recognized a relationship between colonial projects, military conquest, and the spread of the disease.[67] Epidemiology is largely determined by ecological setting. Africans who had historically lived around the foci of disease outbreaks existed in a "tolerant relationship" with the sleeping sickness parasite.[68] Westerners disturbed this balance when they displaced populations, introduced new carriers, and violently changed the environment through colonial development. This suggests that the movement of people was a significant factor in the necropower-induced material pathology of the grove of death—what Marlow describes as "the work that was going on. The work!" (HD, 17). His word choice and repetition are significant, as they recall not only his earlier use of the word with respect to the "real work" done by the British in Africa, but also mirror Stanley's memoir of his work for Leopold, the subtitle of which was: "A Story of Work and Exploration."

Stanley's expedition is the historical correlative of the colonial work that facilitates disease in Conrad's novella. Stanley was a pathogenic agent in the Congo in a material sense: medical historians generally agree that he contributed significantly to the dispersal of sleeping sickness. When setting up Leopold's routes in the continent and in his search for the Emin Pasha, Stanley at least exacerbated the sleeping sickness that was endemic to the western part of the continent, spreading it into the central and eastern Congo when he established trading stations, disrupting populations and ecologies.[69] Moreover, as *Heart of Darkness* so vividly illustrates, forced labor and privation produced in Leopold's Congo the ideal conditions for sleeping sickness and other tropical diseases to move across Africa and thrive.[70]

In stark contrast to the inhabitants of the grove of death is the General Manager, who represents the inverse relationship between health in Europeans and sickness in Africans. His most striking characteristic is his health. Marlow does not ascribe any efficacious qualities to him, "no genius for organising, for initiative or for order even. . . . He had no learning and no intelligence" (*HD*, 22). He seems to have no particular aptitude for administration, either: "His position had come to him—why? Perhaps because he was never ill. . . . He had served three terms of three years out there. . . . Because triumphant health in the general rout of constitutions is a kind of power in itself" (*HD*, 23). The Manager simply has the stamina to do his job—in effect, managing the forced labor of the natives and sending other colonial agents to seize ivory. His health recalls the impression that Parke describes Stanley's outfit making on the Belgian officers, how their exemption from sickness was "extraordinary and unusual."[71] Reading Parke's journal as a historical context for the Manager exposes how his health is linked to the perception of British health in the Congo. The Manager, like Stanley and his staff, has the triumphant health to do the work.

Conrad's careful word choice, "triumphant health," is telling in terms of necropolitics. The history of British tropical medicine and its complex entanglement with King Leopold and his Congo Free State demonstrate how the production of white health promoted necropower in the Congo. Medicine advanced European health to allow for further conquest and for the state of exception in the colony. In this context, tropical medicine specialists functioned as parasites because they enabled the parasitic relationship between the empire and the colonies. When the Manager and his uncle discuss their competitor, the rogue ivory agent Kurtz, the uncle assures him that "anything can be done in this country, I say; nobody here, you understand me *here*, can endanger your position. And why? You stand the climate—you outlast them all" (*HD*, 32, emphasis in the original). The Manager's ability to operate outside the law is linked with his vitality—his salubrity in a pathogenic environment. His savagery and his constitution are both functions of what is inside him. And perhaps, we are told, "there was nothing within him. . . . Once when tropical diseases had laid low almost every agent in the station he was heard to say, 'Men who come out here should have no entrails'" (*HD*, 22). This image of there being nothing inside the Manager but dark vacuity subverts the projection of darkness onto the "savage" tropical environment by reflecting it back inside the healthy European body. As darkness is made to carry the connotation of disease, we can read the Manager's inner darkness as a kind of contagion, the living contagion of imperialism's pathogenic effects—a coloniopathic infection. This is the "uneasiness he inspires," the *dis-ease*.

The Manager's anatomical vacuity serves two functions: first, it lets him resist falling prey to tropical disease, as he has no organs to infect; second, it gives him immunity to the "natural" human response to abject stimuli—the death and disease around him, the necropolitics he practices. He has no digestive organs to produce the normal human response of nausea to the noxious and objectionable—he can "stomach" the savagery he commits because he has no stomach. This metaphorical lack of entrails is figured as a kind of degeneration gained through science, a trope we start to see in late nineteenth-century Gothic, horror, and science fiction. On the one hand, it makes him fit for survival in the Congo; on the other, it associates him with criminal and, ironically, atavistic savagery. By fitting it into the medical history of the time period, the cultural moment of tropical medicine, we can view the Manager's health as a kind of evolution gained through medico-scientific progress, one which is also, in effect, an ethical degeneration—in other words, a truly savage product of civilization. The contradiction of the Manager's body—its unnatural, inhuman, and pathogenic health—helps us see how health and medicine do not fall into familiar binaries in Conrad's novella. His physical health is a moral sickness, the disease of colonial parasites; medicine, the enabling technology.

Kurtz is diametrically opposed to the Manager's vitality. Conrad does not say what he is dying of, and I will not attempt a forensic diagnosis of a literary text. I would like to draw attention to how medicine operates in the text as a tool for controlling both life and death and as a contingency for colonial atrocity. Kurtz, like the other Belgians, would have been given medical supplies consistent with Parke's prescription, including quinine to prevent and treat malaria. His devotee and nurse, the Russian, has also done his best to "keep [Kurtz] alive" despite the fact that "there hasn't been a drop of food or medicine or a mouthful of invalid food for months. [Kurtz] was shamefully abandoned" (*HD*, 58). The implication here is that medicine was being supplied, but when or before Kurtz took ill, the vital provisions—the medical weaponry keeping tropical disease at bay—were withheld.

The way the Manager facilitates Kurtz's death speaks to how "triumphant health" works "as a kind of power." Marlow repeatedly mentions the Manager's jealousy and hatred of Kurtz, whom the Manager claims "wants to be Manager" (*HD*, 32). According to the Manager, Kurtz threatened the colonial order by resorting to native savagery. His "unsound methods" and "lack of restraint," exemplified by the display of severed heads outside his camp (*HD*, 57), recall the Belgian *Force Publique*'s methods in the Congo, as a number of contemporaneous accounts document.[72] Their procedures for making natives meet production quotas included taking hostages, burning down villages, and hanging, rape, and mutilation; perhaps most notoriously, they required "soldiers" to return with severed hands to account for bullets used.[73] This horror is not without irony; as a mark of efficiency, it stands in direct contrast to Belgium's entropic use of native populations with respect to health and hygiene. While Kurtz's literal disease is a result of the withdrawal of medical supplies, his metaphorically diseased state, his "savagery," is caused by imperialism itself. He turned the disease of European tropical health against itself when he created competition for official colonial agents and started operating under his own imperative—which detachments of the *Force Publique* also did in remote regions, for private gain. If Kurtz is "diseased," psychologically or devolutionarily, we might think of him as a kind of autoimmune response to the larger system of empire, along the lines of Roberto Esposito's understanding of immunity and biopolitics.[74] The figuration of Kurtz as a disease that is the result of a system attacking itself speaks to what Esposito views as the problematic conceptualization of immunity, in both the political and biological sense—the one marked by distinguishing the self from the other in an exclusionary relationship, one of the martial metaphor's problematic effects.

In response to the Company's allergic reaction to Kurtz's extreme methods, the Manager withdraws from Kurtz the health that enabled him to operate without restraint. Marlow overhears the Manager and his uncle discussing "the affair": "The climate may do away with this difficulty for you. Is he alone there?" (*HD*, 31). Indeed, ironically, the climate fosters conditions for colonial parasites to thrive. The exchange suggests that without colonial—medical—support, Kurtz will die. Marlow listens more closely: "The 'scoundrel' had reported that the 'man' had been very ill—had recovered imperfectly . . . I heard: 'Military post—doctor—two hundred miles—quite alone now—unavoidable delays—nine months—no news—strange rumors'" (*HD*, 32). The Manager's logistical control over Kurtz's health is supplemented by his calculation that disease will do his dirty work for him. If in the eyes of the Company, synecdochally the Manager, Kurtz is metaphorically corrupting the health of their empire, it is because "he plays the game all too well."[75] The "rescue" the Manager organizes for him is merely a show, like many of Leopold's initiatives, such as supporting British tropical medicine and inviting its specialists to "save" the Congolese from their "naturally" dark and diseased country.

For Conrad, the imperial imperatives of tropical medicine, the excess of life and health of the European body, and its confluence with microbial life produce this darkness, the subjugation of colonized life to death. Imperial health produces the vacuous carapaces of modernity: hollow men, savage germs of empire. A coloniopathic reading of *Heart of Darkness* reveals that Conrad himself was challenging the civilizing mission of tropical medicine during the very period when it was emerging as a tenet of empire; this extends our reading of Conrad's critique of civilization beyond madness, degeneration, and resource extraction. However, the critique itself is framed within an imperial ideology that constructs Africa as inherently insalubrious to the nonmedically fortified European and represents the natives' death and disease through tropes of primitivism.

Just as medicine facilitated colonial atrocity, disease enabled the very revelation of that fact: in Conrad himself, through his sickness and its influence on the denunciation of Leopold; in the novella's treatment of the Manager's health vis-à-vis the natives' sickness; and in the case of British tropical medicine and empire. Beyond simply giving it literary representation, Conrad calls into question the very work of tropical medicine, revealing that even while militarized imperial medicine and British nationalism led the charge in the civilizing efforts of empire, through a romantic narrative of conquest by "knights" like Manson and Ross or Stanley and Parke, it was not, in fact, producing "triumphant health" for all. Instead, it was abetting the same colonial atrocities that British nationals were charging Leopold's Congo Free State with. This brings the connections between death and politics to bear on the history of tropical medicine beyond the conventional biopolitical understanding, suggesting that the effects of tropical medicine at the fin de siècle enabled the regulation not only of life but of death—a form of necropower. Conrad's novella, like that indeterminate emblem of pathogenic health the General Manager, inspires profound unease. Like Marlow, we too are meant to "have a little fever" when we read his tale and form our own impressions (*HD*, 41). As Conrad suggested in a letter to publisher David Meldrum, "Perhaps true literature (when you 'get it') is something like a disease one feels in one's bones, sinews, and joints."[76]

The Legacy of War and the Congo in Ehrlich's Magic Bullets

Heart of Darkness sheds light on how the deployment of the martial metaphor in its tropical capacities affected medicine as a discourse more broadly. If the concentration camps in the Boer War functioned as biopolitical laboratories of modernity, the Congo became a research laboratory much more literally. At this moment, the metaphor became enmeshed with the development of the pharmacological "weapons" against disease that would become the foundations of treatments that are still used today for illnesses against which medicine was once defenseless.

Huxley's dream of a pharmacological "torpedo"—a medicine that would "find its way to some particular group of living elements, and cause an explosion among them, leaving the rest untouched"[77]—was realized early in the twentieth century when Paul Ehrlich, a German physician and chemist and a colleague of Metchnikoff, did research on trypanosomiasis. This, in conjunction with his work on industrial dyes and staining techniques in the late 1880s and his immunological work on drug chain theory, led to the burgeoning field of antimicrobial chemotherapy: specific chemical compositions that would precisely target microbial pathogens; in Ehrlich's words, "the use of drugs to injure an invading organism without injury to the host."[78]

The significance of this development is the thinking that lay behind this kind of treatment, and how it conceptually differed from earlier therapeutics. The pharmacological torpedo materialized as a specific compound designed to attack a specific pathogenic entity. Earlier pharmacologic treatments, like quinine, had been researched and tested for efficacy, and even the failure of Koch's tuberculin prompted discussion of validity, research transparency, and replicability. But in the case of quinine, the mechanism of action was not fully understood, and the drug had originated in what we might call botanical therapeutics—the use of drugs from "natural," usually alkaloid, sources that entered the Victorian pharmacopeia through anecdotal use and folk-medicine traditions. Vaccines and antitoxins, likewise, were derived from cultures and serum. Although pharmacological developments continued to be drawn from botanical and other related sources, Ehrlich's chemotherapy was focused on those that could be developed synthetically, could be built with a target in mind, and were flexible enough to be modified. It was not just a matter of what worked, but of how and why: Ehrlich wanted to develop a biochemical foundation for pharmacology.[79] However, his method, like Bernard's, was based on "experiments of destruction," and he advocated firmly for experimental pharmacologists to replicate or evince pathologies in live animals rather than testing drugs in healthy animal or human tissue.[80]

The logic of planning and targeting and the language of injury and weaponry framed the birth of modern therapeutic pharmacology. This birth marked a significant period for the martial metaphor in terms of a discursive parallel with the industrial militarism of the twentieth century. Although Ehrlich did envision drugs like quinine, naturally derived but not fully understood, as suitable for other kinds of infections, what he imagined was building precise weapons with precise targets from a blueprint drawn with an understanding of chemistry, physiology, and microbiology. Huxley's "torpedo" became Ehrlich's "magic bullet." Ehrlich's contribution was to the creation of compounds that aimed at, or had an "affinity" for, pathogens: *Corpora non agunt nisi fixata*; or, "agents work only when bound." Together with his side-chain theory of immunology, this way of thinking about drugs and disease influenced drug-receptor theory, which is now a foundational premise of pharmacology. This marks the martial metaphor's central place in the origins of modern pharmacology.

At this nexus lies an arsenical compound and the Belgian Congo. In 1905, Ehrlich was doing research into chemotherapeutic dyes and read a paper by Henry Wolfesteran Thomas, a Canadian who had tested an arsenic-based compound known as atoxyl in live animals for the Liverpool School of Tropical Medicine. When the drug began to show success, it became the center of a medico-military program to control the sleeping sickness epidemic and test the drug's efficacy. Manson and Ross believed that atoxyl could be for sleeping sickness what quinine was for malaria. Ross suggested that it was "the biggest thing [their] school had ever done."[81] The epidemic and the experimental deployment of atoxyl thus began this transition. The testing followed strict military protocols of the cordon, using what were known as *lazarets*, prison-camp-like quarantines where natives were forcibly held if thought to have sleeping sickness, and many were forcibly tested with atoxyl. As Lyons has suggested, the inspiration for Belgium's military policy in the Congo was the work of the Liverpool School.[82] Thomas's medical trials of the drug were conducted in 1905 in Uganda and the Congo. While there was some debate among Belgian officials and tropical medicine specialists over whether they should impose the experimental atoxyl on the colonized Congolese, ultimately any native who showed the symptoms was forced to give blood and lymph samples, cordoned off in an isolation camp, and given the drug. Doctors in the Congo Free State were required to research subjects, under penalty of disciplinary action. The drug frequently caused violent reactions or death, and in up to 30 percent of cases blindness. The focus of the trials was, indeed, more on research than treatment.[83]

This drug testing was emblematic of the network of tropical medicine, particularly the points of contact between British tropical medicine and Leopold's Congo Free State. The development of the trials constituted spatial and social relationships that were typical of the colonial system, but it was also "the beginning of a new configuration of science, industry and medicine unfolding between metropole and colony, and across imperial borders."[84] Leopold benefited from the research insofar as it promised to ensure a future labor source and countered the campaigns against his rule that the Casement Report had incited in the world press.[85]

Although Ehrlich had tested atoxyl in the late nineteenth century, he had done so in a culture of trypanosomes in vitro. Thomas demonstrated that it worked in live animals, either by stimulating an internal immune response or by metabolizing into another agent active against the parasite.[86] Ehrlich began working with a manufacturing chemist to determine the relation of the compound's structure to its effect, and more importantly, how they could be modified. Bertheim writes of this foundational moment of modern pharmacology when "probably for the first time . . . a biologically effective substance existed whose structure was not only known precisely but also—unlike the alkaloids—was of a simple composition and extraordinary reactivity, which permitted a wide variety of modifications."[87] The drug's very name, derived from that of the mythically toxic element arsenic, suggests a mitigation of the compound's toxicity—its damage to healthy human tissues—implying the drug was "atoxic" or "nontoxic." Atoxyl was in fact quite toxic. Ehrlich and Bertheim, however, discovered they could modify the compound's toxicity,[88] which led them to synthesize hundreds of variants in an effort to find the best magic bullet. What had amounted to antimicrobial pharmacology before the magic bullet theory had in some capacity resembled Conrad's inefficacious French man-of-war, firing aimlessly into darkness. Huxley himself evokes this connection in his essay through a frequently cited parable in nineteenth-century medical periodicals regarding the state of pre-pharmacological medicine: "A scorner of physic once said that nature and disease may be compared to two men fighting, the doctor to a blind man with a club, who strikes into the melee, sometimes hitting the disease, and sometimes hitting nature . . . He had better not meddle at all, until his eyes are opened, until he can see the exact position of the antagonists."[89] Dating back to French scientist and philosopher Jean le Rond d'Alembert in 1749, this parable frames the metaphorical battle of medicine not so much between human technological intervention and disease, but rather between the body's natural capacity for health (*vis medicatrix naturae*) and disease processes.[90] This, as discussed previously in terms of humoralism, reflects more the restorative, balancing quality of medicine and less the militarized elimination of disease for purity and defense. Medical science, personified as the blind man, intervenes indiscriminately, sometimes arresting the disease, other times damaging the inherent bodily functions that work to return the body to homeostatic balance after a pathological discord. By the 1880s when Huxley gave his speech, and certainly by the turn of the century when Conrad reflected on tropical medicine and figures like Ehrlich, Bertheim, and Thomas, doctors and scientists' "eyes were open" and they began to know "the exact position of the antagonists." The epistemological construction of this microscopic and biochemical vision, however, was understood as reconfigured battle; the new parable resulting in the medicine and disease fighting. This tunnel vision came at a price, one that became evident when the martial order of the microscopic world is scaled up again to the individual body and, more so, to the epidemiological level of populations. That cost is materialized in the lives that either threaten the nationalistically defined social body, or those that are expendable, as collateral damage in the process.

In the case of the Congo, the battle that was waged by tropical medicine took its main enemy to be the microbe, ignoring the natural and social environments in which the epidemic emerged.[91] A central issue with this military quarantine protocol was its surveillance and forcible containment. Tropical medicine researchers transformed the infected

Congolese into pure "receptacles of the disease"—recalling Foucault's idiom of the medical gaze—simple transporters of trypanosomiasis. By contrast, any European who showed signs was treated as a patient.[92] Indeed, the battle between tropical medicine specialists and the trypanosomiasis parasite took place in the Congolese bodies, leaving plenty of collateral damage in the form of blind and dead natives, without accounting for the cultural, environmental, and psychological trauma the medico-military imperative caused.

The deployment of atoxyl in the Belgian Congo was a definitive point of inflection in the European imperial project's management of life and death in the colonies. While Conrad's novella, as I have shown, speaks to the necropolitical function of tropical medicine, the use of atoxyl begins to signal the investment in colonial life by means of tropical medicine. This is not to absolve European colonizers; it simply marks the turn to a biopolitical regime. It might seem curious, given the history of tropical medicine in the Congo, that there were documented debates about the ethics of imposing this kind of experimental care on local populations. I suggest, following Margaret Lock and Vinh-Kim Nguyen, that this is an example of a shift that began in the twentieth century in the goals of medical care in the colonies. Around 1920, the involvement of biomedicine in empire passed from its necropolitical "imperial" phase, with medical technologies deployed mainly to protect Europeans from local fevers, to its biopolitical phase (in a Foucauldian sense), focused on managing the health of local populations now seen as economically indispensable. The new model aimed to produce rather than negate life. In response to the scandal surrounding Leopold and the entropic, unsustainable production methods in the Congo, the colonizer began to make the colonized live.

The chemotherapeutic research into trypanosomiasis had effects beyond the colony. Ehrlich's work birthed new classes of drugs that significantly altered the course of medical and military history. In 1909, he began working with arsenic derivatives to find a synthetic compound that could target the *Treponema pallidum* of syphilis, a disease that had been devastating armies for some time, as evidenced in chapter 3. After hundreds of analogues were tested, "Preparation no. 606" proved to be an effective antisyphilitic agent. The drug was first synthesized by Bertheim in Ehrlich's lab in 1910, tested in the Congo in 1912, and eventually marketed under the trade name Salvarsan (arsphenamine), "the arsenic that saves lives."[93] In 1932, sulfa drugs derived from industrial azo dyes joined the developing antibiotic pharmacopeia. Recall from the previous chapter that Ehrlich's earliest research and MD thesis (1878) had been on histological staining, and these dyes increased the visibility of microbes under the microscope during the booming decades of germ theory. The line of reasoning was that if a dye could have an affinity for, or "target," a particular type of cell while avoiding others, then a synthetic magic bullet compound for that type of cell could be derived from the dye. Ehrlich had theorized as early as 1905 that dyes could kill bacteria but—foreshadowing our own post-antibiotic era—found that protozoa quickly developed resistance. He turned his interest to atoxyl, which also eventually turned out to produce resistance.[94] Salvarsan, however, became the standard treatment for syphilis and was the most widely utilized antimicrobial until 1940.[95] By World War Two it was being mass produced, and at the end of the war penicillin and, a few years later streptomycin, started to displace sulpha drugs.

Ehrlich's work was well known, and as a result chemotherapeutics and pharmacology became new points through which the public came to know the martial metaphor. That is, it came to be known not just in angst, fear, and defense, but in the medico-scientific weaponization of biochemistry. This was in large part due to Paul de Kruif, a Dutch-borne microbiologist and journalist who served in the US military during World War One. De Kruif redoubled the martial metaphor as the operative grammar and vocabulary of modern medicine in the minds of early-twentieth-century readers of popular science. In his best-selling *Microbe Hunters* (1926), he described the heroics of men like Koch, Ross, and Ehrlich in heavily militarized and dramatic language: "No serum or vaccine of the modern microbe hunters could come near to the beneficent slaughtering of the magic bullet, compound six hundred and six."[96] The book is widely considered one of the most influential texts in bringing microbiological science to the public, and it is both highly romantic and unsurprisingly martial in its language,[97] so it is tempting to credit it with the public circulation of the martial metaphor, especially as supplemented by his *Men against Death* (1932), which draws from his frequent framing of microbiologists as "fighters of death." However, a number of other medical histories focused on antimicrobial therapies, such as Boris Sokoloff's *The Miracle Drug* (1943).[98] While there is no doubt de Kruif and others of his time were influential and did propagate the metaphor during the antibiotic golden era, we have seen that mid-twentieth-century authors who espoused the martial metaphor were riding the crest of a much larger and older wave, one that was just as literary as it was journalistic and even medical in its textual expression.

By the mid-twentieth century, the work Victorian authors did to circulate the martial metaphor had been appropriated by the film industry. Salvarsan was the first widely known antimicrobial and led the martial metaphor's pharmacological iteration to make its way into the film through the adaptation of de Kruif's *Microbe Hunters* in *Dr. Ehrlich's Magic Bullet*, released in 1940 by Warner Bros. This film and its magic bullet metaphor were linked to the sex-hygiene films of the early twentieth century, such as the 1918 *Fit to Fight*, which was developed through a cooperative effort by the US military and public health officials.[99] In this capacity, Ehrlich's use of the metaphor was deployed by the regulatory apparatus to control female sexuality, reinscribing the kind of battle that was fought on the female body in Stoker's *Dracula*. The magic bullet and its scaffolding of modern-day antibiotic therapy carried with it the legacy of Victorian authors' engagement with the martial metaphor.

꽃

The martial metaphor gained a new level of traction in the twentieth century. What Conrad exposes is that although Victorian authors, through their influence and wide circulation, transfigured material military medical imperatives and histories into metaphor in their writings—showing that literature was in large part responsible for inscribing the metaphor in the public imaginary—that very mode could be turned against itself. We saw early on in Shelley's apocalyptic Romanticism, writing during the beginnings of the martial metaphor's extension from military medicine to civilian life, her use of the sublime and frame narration to denaturalize the martial metaphor. The Condition-of-England novel gave Kingsley a pulpit to politicize and espouse the martial metaphor during the mid-century sanitary movement. By the time germ theory changed the etiological landscape, late Victorian Gothic and detective fiction aligned themselves with the medico-military logics and anxieties surrounding the British social body when faced with colonial threats, while beginning to show evidence of the martial metaphor's contradictions and failures. Modernism afforded Conrad a venue for unraveling the muddled connections between imperialism, the military, tropical medicine, and modern pharmacology. It provided a means to shatter the imperial and nationalist narratives that had been building from the mid- to the late nineteenth century. Like his "germs of empire" and his pathogenic figure of preternatural health, the General Manager, Conrad's *Heart of Darkness* draws attention to the complex encounters between medicine, empire, and the military at the moment when the West began its campaign against microbes through modern pharmacology. Indeed, tropical medicine and Elhrich's magic bullet, as civilizing and modernizing lights of medical science wrought horror for some as instruments of militarism. The novel refracts the martial metaphor just enough to shed light on its consequences in tropical medicine: the material effects of making the colonizer fit for conquest at the expense of the colonized's health; the imperial ideology it fostered and justified; and the very way the metaphor occludes its social and fictional construction.

If *Heart of Darkness* disrupted the assumed humanitarian and simplistic logic of the martial metaphor, it would not remain a heap of broken images for long. The grander narratives of triumphant health, microbe hunters, and miracle drugs would prevail in the twentieth century. This was the moment when the martial metaphor's expansion out from under the researcher's microscope and into patients' bodies via pharmacological compounds—and the language used to describe them. This became a moment of total war, which certainly signaled the beginning of a period of increased health and longevity for many; yet, it continued the use of medical discourse to justify xenophobia and produce differential social determinants of health by the West, and, in time, our current global crises with antibiotic resistance. If anything, then, the literary and cultural history of the martial metaphor reveals it as an instrument of antibiosis, one that often worked as much against life as it did for it.

Collateral Damage

An Afterword

In these chapters, I have indicated the value of examining the genealogy of the martial metaphor for changing how we think about medical history and literature in Victorian studies. *Medicine Is War* shows how literature not only reflected the process of the martial metaphor's development and cultural work but also helped forge its naturalization. Its representation in literature obscured the metaphor's military origins and the biopolitical work it performed in moving between fiction, the popular press, and medical discourse; however, by considering its narrative, figurative, and ideological work in conversation with medical and military history, we can unravel these discursive threads and trace their present entanglements and continuities. This work, then, provides a resource for literary scholars, medical historians, and scholars in the health humanities to examine the martial metaphor critically. To close my treatment, I would like to touch on some of the current implications of the martial metaphor. In doing so, we can see how investigating its cultural history lets us not only fill a scholarly gap in Victorian studies but rethink certain aspects of medical ethics, politics, and communication. I will briefly consider these points with respect to a select few instances of the metaphor relative to contemporary medical concerns: specifically, antibiotic resistance, the catachresis of immigration and infectious disease, and the oft-cited "war against cancer."

While tropical medicine wrought triumphant health in the colonial space, the failures of British health at home, of such concern to Conan Doyle, would continue to be entangled with militarism in the twentieth century. The connection between "warfare and welfare" was a major factor in the development of the National Health Service. The most recent historiography traces the national insurance welfare state's political foundations to World War One, not only the implantation of health services that occurred after World War Two.[1] It was of course during this time that antibiotics were mass-produced out of the military industrial complex in the United States, drawing from scientific research in Britain, both very much in need of penicillin for wartime infections, including syphilis, echoing the military impetus of the CD Acts. The antibiotic era that emerged from the 1950s became part of the so-called golden age of medicine, when several new antibiotics were discovered or created in rapid succession. This was a short period, approximately two to three decades, before increased longevity—in large part due to the reduction of mortality from infectious diseases—would draw into sharp relief the emergence of terminal and chronic diseases that medicine could treat but not cure; the time before HIV; before renewed attention to zoonosis and "emerging disease"; the time before the post-antibiotic apocalypse.

I have alluded to the way the martial metaphor, through its centuries-long deployment, has played a significant role in the development of antibiotic resistance. It has been estimated, not without contention, that by 2050 deaths related to antibiotic resistance will eclipse cancer.[2] There have been no new classes of antibiotic drugs since 1987. Indeed, if the martial metaphor structured the war on germs from the early twentieth century until the end of the golden age of medicine in the 1980s, then it has evolved into an apocalypse; or, at least that is how the popular press and scientific publications have been articulating, for the past decade or so, the failure of the total war on bacterial infections.[3] Some strands of posthumanist scholarship, microbiological ecology, and clinical medicine have turned their attention to the symbiotic evolutionary relationship between humans and the microbial life that lives on and inside the body, conceptualized as the microbiome.[4] This work has called into question the militarized theories of immunity and the ideologies contingent on bounded, autonomous liberal subjectivity, especially given the discoveries after this microbiomial turn, such as the "mind-altering effects" of the brain-gut axis.[5] As I suggested in the introduction regarding the National Academy of Science's Forum on Microbial Threats (2005), it seems bacterial evolution has perhaps given us no choice but to change metaphors, an opportunity to respond responsibly to the already extant postantibiotic apocalypse—perhaps returning to a model of balance, a form of humoral logic or *vis medicatrix naturae*. Chapter 1's historization of humoral theory vis-à-vis the martial metaphor helps us appreciate and account for the cultural logics embedded in what and who is balanced, so as not to reinscribe some of the racial discourses of the early nineteenth-century cholera epidemics. But as of 2020, inequality, xenophobia, and racism under medical aegis and in the idiom of nationalism, to be sure, remain much too with us.

The nationalist and liberal politics associated with the Victorian investment in the martial metaphor have continued into the next two centuries. From the mid-1800s to the first decade of the twentieth century, in response to the cholera epidemic and high rates of syphilis, Kingsley, Stoker, and Doyle blurred the lines between disease, the foreign, the biological and the social body through the martial metaphor. Likewise, as the problem of antibiotic resistant infections grew from the 1980s into the twenty-first century, British politicians conflated it with economic and immigration agendas. In 2004, for instance, Conservative opposition leaders planned to impose compulsory MRSA screening of immigrants prior to their departure. They associated the rise in MRSA infection with immigrants and the inefficacy of socialized medicine. In 2005, Conservative leader Michael Howard would use the number of cases of MRSA as "pathologically symptomatic of national malaise within caring institutions and Britain as a whole,"[6] playing on loose associations deployed to foster fear and anger in partisan salvos such as, "[T]axes are up, crime up, immigration up, waiting time up, MRSA up. . . . Take home pay down. Pensions down. Productivity growth down. Manufacturing employment down. Detection rates down."[7] At the same time, during the first decade of the twenty-first century, Britain invested in research, education, and outreach toward addressing antibiotic resistance; in fact, much like in Victorian era, this complex problem was circulated through cultural productions. The Wellcome Trust and National Endowment for Science Technology and the Arts (NESTA) funded a number of creative projects to address the problem: *Infectious Futures* (2015), a short story anthology; *Surgeon X* (2017), a graphic novel; and, *Superbugs* (2016), a mobile video game. In 2017, the BBC commissioned science fiction author Val McDermid to write a radio drama *Resistance* that would later be remediated as an audiobook. Ironically, despite all this investment in education and humanistic inquiry, the consequences of the Brexit vote will have a dramatic impact on the future possibility of mitigating this postantibiotic apocalypse. A number of medical practitioners, researchers, and policy makers have expressed concern over the consequences of Brexit vis-à-vis global health, and specifically antibiotic resistance.

The NHS and consequently the health of British citizens will suffer due to the economic consequences and shortage of medical personnel.[8] This will certainly be compounded by the cruel irony of headlines like "'Dickensian Diseases' Are Making a Comeback in the UK," appearing in 2019.[9] Kingsley's idealized vision of English history as an emblem of resilience and futurity seems, unfortunately, to have become relevant again, stoked by "Brexit's toxic nostalgia."[10] The clash of the modern and the antiquated so aptly embodied in the contest between the foreign Dracula and the Crew of Light might materialize into an all too real nightmarish form when the failure of antibiotics, the infrastructure of so much contemporary health and health care, will bring medicine back "to the dark ages."[11] Beyond Britain, Brexit will disrupt funding and collaborative scientific research, especially in the field of global health, effecting negative consequences to the health of hundreds of millions, if not billions of people both within and outside of Britain's borders. While *Medicine Is War* does not consider the genre of science and postapocalyptic fiction in terms of the late-Victorian and early-twentieth-century inflection, as I have discussed elsewhere,[12] it is worth considering the fact that all of the extant reflections of antibiotic resistance look to these genres to educate and reflect on this very present reality.

Yet, as with the case of tropical medicine refracted through *Heart of Darkness*, while the phenomenon of antibiotic resistance has implications for humankind, like so many other health issues, it also operates differentially. Antibiotic resistance has a major socioeconomic component. Poverty is a driving factor: sharing medications, using left-over antibiotics, and buying foreign antibiotics without a prescription have been cited as contributing to resistance in the US. This problem is magnified in the context of global health, especially in countries such as India, Mexico, and the Philippines.[13] Antibiotic resistance is commonly understood as an emblematic tragedy of the commons; however, limiting the problem to national scopes is not only unethical, but harmful, as the "costs of antibiotic resistance are both local and global."[14] Given the martial metaphor's contribution to the overuse of antibiotics and the fact that social determinants such as poverty limit access to adequate care and education, the metaphor's material effects only magnify these inequalities and injustices.

Of course, the problem has as much to do with individualism and anthropocentrism as it does with nationalism and imperialism, if we could even think of these rubrics discreetly. Some recent work on infectious disease, microbiology, and pharmacology of antibiotic alternatives has moved away from solely considering etiologies that are attributed to a singular pathogen, looking not toward antibiosis but rather dysbiosis. Microbiota dysbiosis is defined as the imbalance between species of bacteria living in or on the human body that results in a pathology.[15] Infections certainly still occur from the introduction of a new pathogen that affects the body in negative ways, such as *vibrio cholera*, which introduces the cholera toxin (CT), producing the signs and symptoms associated with the disease. However, the dysbiosis paradigm accounts for all factors that alter the fine balance of organismal ecology in the body; in dysbiosis, when the internal microbiomial relations among organisms is disrupted, an underrepresented or normally controlled growth of particular pathogens amplifies and can become pathogenic. Perhaps the most resonant example, considering the martial metaphor's history, is *Clostridium Difficile*, infections which often occur after the use of broad-spectrum antibiotics that level the gut microbiome. Out of such scorched earth therapies, opportunistic bacteria, like *C. difficile*, become dominant and fill the territorial void. Many readers will be aware that we must be careful about antibiotic overprescription and pressuring medical practitioners to give us something to fight that infection that probably is not bacterial. It is important, however, to keep in mind this book's unpacking of the historical tensions between the individual and the social and to remember to look beyond our own individual guts.

One of the obstacles to effectively tackling antibiotic resistance is that we tend to think about it too individualistically, misunderstanding its evolutionary mechanisms and scale. Focus group and metanalyses have shown that many people understand antibiotic resistance in terms that are not unlike the pharmacology of dependence or receptor downregulation, in other words, that an individual's body stops responding to the drugs due to overexposure.[16] This insular, anthropocentric kind of thinking fails to account for resistance being a characteristic of bacteria rather than the human body. This kind of thinking is precisely a function of the martial metaphor's relationship to bounded, autonomous liberal subjectivity. This is not even to mention that the resistance phenomenon extends far beyond a singular pathogen. Resistance is a hyperobject, so massive in space and time that the scale of the bacterial resistome—the collection of vertically and horizontally transferred genes across pathogenic and commensal bacteria that makes them resistant to antibiotic drugs—is difficult to comprehend.[17] Through environmental reservoirs, livestock, oceans, and soil, the resistome becomes a posthuman linkage of species, environments, technologies, and humans. *Medicine Is War* has focused on allopathic medicine, but it is crucial to recognize that one of the leading causes in the most recent surge in resistance is its use by the agriculture industry as a growth-promoting agent in livestock. This deployment of antibiotics is a significant determinant in the spread of antibiotic resistance genes into the food chain and into the water supply via animal waste, allowing these genes to traverse across environments and economies. If anything, *The Last Man*'s representation of a global plague, fluid like an ocean, touching together distant lands and populations, should be illustrative and instructive for understanding the scale and reach of the resistome.

Moving from bacterial to viral discourse, the 2014 Ebola pandemic showed us tropical medicine's redeployment of nineteenth-century colonial narratives. It not only asserted the martial metaphor in the defense of the Western world and body, it also espoused the use of the cordon sanitaire in a continent that was seemingly still dark and dangerous in Western perceptions. The outbreak narrative that forms Richard Preston's *The Hot Zone*, which continues to inform media coverage and popular discourse surrounding Ebola two decades later, is intertextually structured by *Heart of Darkness*. Preston draws extensively on the tropes of the Dark Continent, the absent voices of native populations, and the metonymic amalgamation of a people, a geography, and a disease.[18] The script of conflating immigrants and foreigners with diseased invasion follows the same logic as treating cholera, parasitism, and vampires as invaders from the East: Asia's cultures are associated with (H5N1) avian flu, Africa's with Ebola. Yet, this conflation does not only occur on a longitudinal axis. In 2019, leading up to Donald Trump's declaration of a national emergency in response to the approaching "caravan" of migrants from Central America, one right-wing publication ran an article titled "Will the Migrant Caravan Kill Your Child—With Disease?" not long after which a former immigration agent went on Fox News to declare that these migrants were "Coming in with diseases such as smallpox and leprosy and TB [tuberculosis] that are going to infect *our people* in the United States."[19] The attribution of diseases like leprosy and tuberculosis to immigrants follows the same Victorian script of ascribing disease to primitivism that becomes a biological threat to the civilized world. Cultural histories and ideological discussion aside, there are plenty of reasons such a claim is fallacious: it is worth noting that 95 percent of the population has immunity to leprosy, and, not discounting its severity, it is also easy to treat; the CDC screens inbound migrants for TB; and that smallpox, to use Budd and Simpson's language, has been completely "stamped out," eradicated from the human population since 1977. These persisting conflations of immigration and infectious disease in bellicose idioms don't even account for the heightened fears about bioterrorism post-9/11, which have been used to evoke similar nationalistic and militaristic thinking.[20]

The martial metaphor still drives social iniquity and inequality in global public health, an effect that is often supported by the xenophobic association of foreigners with disease using tropes of primitivism and degeneration. And as in *Dracula*, the martial metaphor continues to draw from popular culture. To cite one example, in 2014, a small number of West African immigrants prompted a zombie-narrative response when their boat approached a nudist beach in the Canary Islands. Because of fears of Ebola, they were quarantined in the hot sun until they had tested negative, after which they were transported in the back of a dump truck.[21] Another news story prompted fears that an Ebola victim had risen from the dead in Africa; this hoax was based on a doctored image from the film *World War Z* (2013).[22] Like *Dracula*'s vampire, the zombie today connotes infectious disease, racialized bodies, and degeneration, and almost always does so in the context of a military-like response. In *Bioinsecurities*, Neel Ahuja notes that the figures of the zombie and vampire among others "persistently racialize representation of disease and environments" to generate "political crises that intensify feelings of public of hope and fear," along with "specific forms of govermentality."[23] Notably, the xenophobic and cordoned response to the 2014 Ebola outbreak from the Western public, especially in the United States, shows the continued construction of the developing world as pathogenic and a threat to the salubrity and safety of the West. Militarized "top-down quarantine" responses can foster disease as much as they delimit it, a concern that was regularly raised in the debates between contagionism and anticontagionism, as we saw in chapter 2. Research into the deployment of the cordon during the 2014 Ebola epidemic in Liberia indicates that this militarization is not only ethically unjustified but often counterproductive; misinformation and fear that prompt dangerous behaviors and noncompliance, in both quarantined and nonquarantined populations, are just a few of its problematic effects which include stigmatization, such as attaching labels of "Ebola people" to many who are not even infected; and the occurrence of secret burials—borne of the desire to avoid cremation and believed by medical personal to create greater risk of infection.[24]

Like infectious disease, cancer too has biopolitical dimensions that are socially determined. The debates surrounding health care and insurance in the United States provides a striking example. In *Notes toward a Performative Theory of Assembly*, Judith Butler cites the case of Ron Paul, a former practicing physician, who in a 2011 GOP Tea Party debate was posed the hypothetical question: who would pay for an individual who opted not to purchase health care and then became suddenly gravely ill and slipped into a coma? Would "[Paul] let him die?" While the specific illness was not identified, it was read by some as, and certainly does fit, the model of cancer.[25] Paul rhetorically maneuvered his way without giving a definitive answer—defending freedom of choice. He contended that "The individual, private charity, families, and faith based groups should take care of people not the government." Paul's response aside, what Butler notices, and what I would suggest is most disturbing, is the interjection by the crowd before Paul answered: "A shout of joy rippled through the crowd, according to published reports [and evident in the video recording]. It was, I conjecture, the kind of joyous shout that usually accompanies going to war or forms of nationalist fervor . . . The implications clearly that those who are not able to achieve jobs with health care belong to a population that deserves to die and that is finally responsible for their own death."[26] Nowhere in the exchange are there any explicit references to anything military, metaphorical, or literal. Whether the enthusiasm of the audience's interjection "Yeah!" in response to Wolf Blitzer's direct follow-up question to Paul, "Are you saying society should just let him die?" rises to the degree of a war cry may be arguable. However, Butler's analogy is entirely felicitous. It makes sense because it is supported by the innumerable examples of politicians rallying around wars against x, y, and z: cancer, drugs, and terrorism, some targets less metaphorical than others. Furthermore, her analogy is subtended by the fact that such wars bring certain groups of people together in direct opposition to, or at the expense of Others. In the case of the Tea Party, those political targets and expendable lives are those who cannot responsibly acquire health care, those who, it is assumed by some, "rightly contract disease, suffer accidents, and will rightly die as a consequence."[27]

Given the associations between military medicine and the metaphorical militarization in medicine documented in the previous chapters, it is perhaps not surprising that cancer has not only analogical connections to war, as Butler's example demonstrates, but also historical, material ones. The same era that birthed antibiotics saw the development of chemotherapy, as the term is most commonly used today to encompass pharmacological agents that destroy cancer cells. In this history, we see how the exchange between medicine and the military was bidirectional: if medical culture received the metaphor from military applications and imperatives, then the effects of the martial metaphor on medical culture—such as the magic bullet—returned to the military in a very material way. In a fitting irony for practicing medicine as war, one of the compounds produced in the development of arsenical derivatives from atoxyl was Lewisite, a lethal respiratory, vesicant chemical weapon developed in 1918 by the US Army Chemical Weapons Division and stockpiled aggressively after the First World War. Military medicine in the form of chemical weapons led to the first effective agents for "fighting cancer," arguably the most frequent target of the martial metaphor in modern times. The first chemotherapeutic agent was developed from Mustargen, derived from mustard gas. Physicians from both the US and Britain noticed a correlation between mustard gas exposure and a drop in white blood cell count, and speculated that the agent might be of use for leukemia patients, who suffer from rapid overproduction of white blood cells. This led researchers to isolate nitrogen mustard and experiment with lethal and therapeutic dosages. This discovery was not a silver lining to the vesicant cloud of cytotoxic gas. The research produced collateral damage. The movement from observation of chemical weapon to medical research entailed medical experimentation of American and Canadian soldiers after World War One and well into World War Two.[28]

The governmental scale of funding that drove this nexus between military science and medicine to oncology was birthed from the transformational event of World War Two. Government attention to experimentation that would serve the interests of the state allowed for the explosion in support for medical science from the 1930s to the 1960s. As a result, federally funded teams replaced isolated research.[29] The unsettlingly entangled history of chemotherapy and chemical warfare is of course just the tip of the iceberg, as the cross-pollination between the military and medicine notably created other weapons of mass destruction, as it created effective therapeutics through research into nuclear and germ warfare. While the development of chemotherapy did not cure cancer, this weapon offered more hope than anything before, especially in the case of radiation resistant cancers. Consequently, the American Cancer Society began a major funding effort in 1958. The research effort began crossing economic, political, and discursive boundaries. Against the backdrop of the Cold War and President Nixon's declaration of the War on Cancer (heralded by the signing of the National Cancer Act in 1971), the business executives of the ACS followed the engineering logic of the space and arms races/wars. Eventual cures to cancer, then, were understood under this paradigm as solely a function of time and money.[30] One epidemiologist would later recall a day when managers from NASA came to coach the CDC on tactics and strategy: "They had the entire war on cancer mapped out on one huge drawing. All the known technologies about cancer and viruses were on the bottom left, and all the things we needed to fill in, so to speak, were at the top right. To get from one to the other, it was all just supposed to be a matter of filling in the blanks to comply with their engineering requirements."[31] In the decades that followed, it became clear that cancer's complexity made materializing Huxley's pharmacological torpedo qua chemotherapy much more elusive than getting a man to the moon or building the atom bomb.[32] As with the case of antibiotics—and the new field of antibiotic alternatives and antivirulence agents—the pharmacological paradigm of oncology has now looked toward immunotherapies, aiding the body's internal mechanisms to mitigate abnormal growth rather than killing disease head on.

While mustard gas, the ACS, and Richard Nixon reveal some problematic, constellatory links to the medico-military-industrial complex of the twentieth century, it is hard to argue against the very personal encounters with cancer that seem to lend themselves so easily and reasonably to the language of war. Having addressed the larger, aggregate implications of the martial metaphor, we must consider individual bodies, their immune systems, and medical narratives. Fighting cancer has become a convention in the contemporary genre of pathography. In its use with terminal diseases like cancer, the martial metaphor makes meaning in a way that imbues agency in the face of what is out of the individual's control and so often stochastic: the results of genetics (in the case of cancer),[33] or the chance encounter with a pathogen one doesn't have resistance to (in the extreme case of Ebola, or, more prosaically, a freshly mutated rhinovirus causing an upper-respiratory infection acquired by touching the wrong door handle). I don't wish to oppose or disparage the use of the martial metaphor per se; I certainly empathize and espouse the right of individuals to make their own meanings out of their experiences with illness. And there are, indeed, positive effects of the use of this and other metaphors by patients and doctors in medical narratives. For instance, some studies have shown both increased medical compliance and knowledge acquisition from the use of a video game—"Re-Mission 2"—in which patients "blast" enemy cancer cells. The history I have discussed in terms of biopower, especially in the case of Kingsley's fiction and prose, shows how a martial-medical video game could serve a disciplinary yet clearly affirmative function. I don't want to deny the beneficial effects of the martial metaphor, whether in behavioral or medication-related compliance or even placebo-like improved immune response.[34] What I do want to insist on, however, is a critical awareness of the implications its use carries: subjecting patients into failures when they succumb to disease, conceptual opposition to palliative care, and continued deployment of what some might still call heroic medicine qua chemotherapy with drugs of last resort and radiation in extremis. Recent editorials, going along with a trend in medical humanist inquiry, have made the case that the war metaphor is not universal. Many cancer patients find it an imposition to follow the cultural script of bravely fighting disease. Mary Elizabeth Williams, author of A Series of Catastrophes and Miracles (2016), describes her experience this way in a recent interview: "Whenever I hear someone say 'I beat cancer,' it just feels so disrespectful to others. . . . It divides us into winners and losers."[35] As we have seen, literature can show us how we got to this zero-sum narrative, and affords a unique perspective to examine and contest the martial metaphor's expansive set of cultural complicities and implications.

While Medicine Is War is a cultural study of literature and history rather than a practical or theoretical text on narrative medicine, its readings and conclusions can bring Victorian studies to bear on the narratological humanistic inquiry into medical communication.[36] I have made the case that it is important, given the naturalization of the martial metaphor, to acknowledge its history, even though it works as a valuable rhetorical shorthand for understanding how medicine developed or for understanding how the immune system and medication work. In the same way, medical professionals training in narrative medicine and humanistic inquiry might be better served by not just thinking about alternative metaphors, or necessarily discouraging patients from thinking about medicine as war, but by considering the conditions that fostered this and other metaphors' emergence. This can help parse the social, cultural, political, and ethical tensions that fold into our now default way of approaching human morbidity and mortality. This line of inquiry opens a space for doctors and patients to ask what war allows for and delimits in terms of treatment. But beyond single patients and their health care providers, I follow Olivia Banner's recent call to consider the medical humanities in terms of structural competency in addition to the empathic imperative—to look at the larger context in which medical interactions take place and replicate cultural norms and social inequalities.[37] In this capacity, tracing the martial metaphor's history and literary representation helps us think about what structures not just doctor-patient interactions, but medicine as a larger system that is bound up in social and political relations—as much as malignant histological and pathogenic microbial ones.

Addendum

A Surge of Epilogics in the Midst of the War against COVID-19

It is August 5, 2020. I have been told over the course of the past few months—the "first wave" of COVID-19—that my book is especially timely. This addendum is an expression of the complicated feelings, events, and entanglements that, for whatever it is worth, might validate that statement. What follows is a record gleaned from diary entries, social-media posts, e-mails, and text messages during the period between the publisher's approval of my manuscript for production and the final moments of copyediting. How these fragments have been placed in sequence will be made manifest in the reading of them.

December 31: The starting gun: "There is some important and disturbing information coming out of China right now re severe pneumonia with similarities to SARS, and etiology currently not yet confirmed. See the following @ProMED_mail post: http://promedmail.org/post/6864153."[1]

January 4: The World Health Organization (WHO) reports that there is a cluster of pneumonia in Wuhan, China, with no fatalities.[2]

January 12: The manuscript of *Medicine Is War*, with all the revisions done and the formatting changed, is submitted. Chinese authorities have shared the sequence of a novel coronavirus to be named severe acute respiratory syndrome coronavirus 2 (initially nCoV; later SARS-CoV-2), which was isolated from some clustered cases.[3]

January 18: I have a case of the flu (strain B, they think). Unremarkable case, they say. It has been hard to finish plans to schedule copyediting for the book in the midst of personal illness and emerging reports of the emergent disease.

January 25: There is a novel zoonotic disease, and I still feel sick. Fatigue, depression, cognitive impairment. "You look very pale." For most of January, like many, I felt confident that biosecurity protocols and international collaboration would contain the virus. Many experts do not share this optimism.

January 29: I have been diagnosed with iron-deficiency anemia, unknown etiology. Declined a blood transfusion and proceeded to see a hematologist. Yes, this all feels a bit *Dracula*. Explains severe fatigue, memory problems, depression. The irony that this is "oh so very Victorian" is not lost on my friends and colleagues. I begin biweekly iron infusions for the foreseeable future. I admit feeling discomfort being around other immunocompromised patients at the infusions center (most of the others are there for chemotherapy). I worry about their safety and my own.

January 31: The WHO declared a global health emergency yesterday. Today, Donald Trump restricts travel from China.[4]

February 7: My friend and colleague Dr. Travis Chi Wing Lau, an Asian American health humanist, "goes viral" with the following tweet: "Cleared my throat and coughed in an elevator today and got my first ugly look from someone who clearly was afraid I had coronavirus. Because I'm petty, I decided to cough some more, and as they were leaving, I yelled 'racism is more contagious.'"[5]

February 17: Conspiracy theories multiply, suggesting that SARS-CoV-2 is a bioweapon. Virologist Dr. Angela Rasmussen and other scientists have taken up arms, given their time, and risked their personal safety in the face of violent threats via direct messages to become the scientific communicators we need during the so-called infodemic.[6] Our family decides to exercise caution; we begin to socially distance and, later, quarantine. I have stopped keeping track of how often the martial metaphor appears in social and news media.

February 18: My production editor at SUNY Press reaches out regarding the process of reviewing my manuscript. I have been working for weeks to try to fill in citational gaps and make lists of necessary changes, given the relevant scholarship that has been published recently or that I have found in the past month. But then came 2020, bringing an entirely new set of data that was all too intimately entangled with my book's very specific line of historical inquiry—in very present lineaments. I draft an e-mail asking if I can add a short addendum to the afterword, one that addresses the current militarized state of the medical world as it appears in social and news media.

February 27: Dr. Monica Green, renowned historian of medicine and health, on Twitter: "#twitterstorians A lot has happened since I first posted this list of sources to follow for regular information on #COVID19. These remain voices to trust. As historians, we have the ability to help our communities understand change—over—time, esp. important now as this unfolds."[7]

March 5: Surgery scheduled for April 1 to fix the apparent cause of my anemia.

March 11: Lehigh University, my home institution, announces, "As of Monday, March 16, classes will be taught remotely and students are expected to return home or remain home to continue their coursework for the next two weeks."[8] This arrangement will become permanent a few weeks later. My students are concerned, as am I. One who is currently in Spain asks me for advice about what she should do—it is not very bad there, yet. I'm unsure how to advise her.

March 14: President Trump bans all incoming flights from Europe. There are increasing reports of a vast shortage of personal protective equipment for health workers; most notably, the N95 masks.[9]

March 17: I write this around thirty days into voluntary quarantine. I feel an affective charge from as well as an inescapable entanglement with the 100,000 words preceding this addendum, feelings that elude poetics, figuratives—and academic discourse, generally. Five years of writing about a metaphor's history and fiction, extrapolating and theorizing its relation to the present fields of Victorian studies and health humanities, means the martial metaphor is at the forefront of my mind, my body, and—on a larger scale but still a local one—the political machines and actors who have mangled nearly all opportunities to address our encounter with this novel virus successfully. Cases of COVID-19 increased 40 percent in twenty-four hours in the United States. There are 220,000 deaths worldwide but no new cases in China.[10] People have been citing the film *Contagion* for what feels like an eternity. Hydroxychloroquine and the term *magic bullet* have been shot back and forth. Like many, I underestimated the danger of SARS-CoV-2. When I wrote the sections of this afterword that precede these closing remarks, while doing what I thought would be the final revisions of the manuscript in December 2019, never did I expect to live through a pandemic of this severity, despite knowing it was a possibility that biosecurity experts had warned us about. This pandemic has fulfilled the nightmare prophecies of *The Coming Plague*, *Spillover*, and the like. It also, admittedly, has shifted my attention from antibiotic resistance (a matter that remains of the utmost exigency, which I have given voice to above). I now begin to entertain the necessity of the rhetoric of war for the sake of solidarity and urgency—perhaps drawing on metonymic connection, military logistics could stop this. I recall Christos Lynteris's prescient point about animal vectors in his collection *Framing Animals as Epidemic Villains* (2019): the "practical and political limitations" of multispecies intimacies, microbiome studies, entanglement frameworks in medical anthropology, and the like "are revealed each time there is an actual epidemic crisis. . . . Then all talk of One Health, multispecies relationships and partnerships melt into air, and what is swiftly replaced is an apparatus of culling, stamping out, disinfection. . . . What remains is the maintenance of this militarized apparatus."[11]

March 18: That new turn of mind on my part did not last. We cannot resign to the martial metaphor's dangerous misuse. Today, President Trump tweeted, "I only signed the Defense Production Act to combat the Chinese Virus should we need to invoke it in a worst-case scenario in the future. Hopefully, there will be no need, but we are all in this TOGETHER!" The martial metaphor's history is all condensed here: the facile use of war as a call to arms to unify nationalist ideology against a racialized other. We are clearly not all in this together. Without question, underserved populations suffer differentially under this pandemic. Black people, people of color more broadly, and the economically disadvantaged are already becoming acceptable losses; their suffering is even being attributed to their cultures and "lifestyles."[12] The compounding factor of police violence against Black people, among other social determinants of health, has yet to reach national public consciousness, although public health and critical race scholars have drawn attention to this for some time.[13] The visibility of this will change in the wake of the murder of George Floyd on May 25, and the Black Lives Matter protests that follow.

March 30: Between March 16 and today, Trump has publicly, emphatically, and repeatedly referred to SARS-CoV-2 as "the Chinese virus." Most states have issued stay-at-home directives.[14] My surgery has been canceled, "indefinitely." Because of the work I've done for this book, news media and others have contacted me for comments about the pandemic, but I have thus far been at a loss, unable to provide much of substance.

March 31: I am not alone in thinking that going to the grocery store feels like an episode of *The Walking Dead*.[15] I begin to look for Lysol, water, toilet paper, and paper towels on gray markets.

April 10: I give a virtual lecture and then have a long discussion with twenty-two second-year medical students at the University of Southern California, for their elective course War, Wounds, and Words: Narrative Medicine for the Pandemic, led by Dr. Pamela Schaff and Dr. Erika Wright. I am overwhelmed by their engagement with my work, their thoughtfulness, and their rigorous questions: "Do you think the medical community has a responsibility to explicitly disavow this connection and do you have any ideas on how that could be effectively done?" or "NPR reported that thirty-three percent of hospitalized patients were African American, even though only thirteen percent of the population was considered African American. In light of this news, I have seen many headlines naming COVID-19 as a 'racist' virus. My question is What are your thoughts on these headlines?"[16] So many, but I try to reply cogently and succinctly.

April 21: It has been nearly a month, it seems, since things have gotten really bad, although, admittedly, I cannot account for time in the same way as I could during what we now think of as pre-COVID times. But while COVID-19 has changed much of my thinking, it has not taken long for me to see that the martial metaphor's problematics, which history and literature document, are materializing again in this pandemic.

May 6: My surgery is rescheduled for today, with a week's notice. I arrive at the hospital exercising biosafety protocols that rival those of a BSL-4 laboratory. The doctors and nurses laugh, which is kind of reassuring. I will have three coronavirus PCR tests during this process, which will fortunately be negative. In the Oval Office, Trump decries China for not containing the virus: "There's never been an *attack* like this."[17] I am in tremendous pain, and my iron has a long way to go before it reaches normal limits.

May 26: George Floyd is murdered by three police officers under the pretext of resisting arrest. I cannot do justice to the dynamic this introduces to the pandemic in the United States, its systems of policing, and public health—let alone the history of racism in the United States, as evidenced by the months that follow. I refer readers to T. J. Tallie's incisive reading of Black people's specific "death potential" in the United States—what she terms "asymptomatic lethality."[18]

May 27: Worldwide, the coronavirus has now caused 353,000 deaths that we know of—there are likely many more. One hundred thousand of those deaths are in the United States alone.[19]

June 24: I received news that my application to Dartmouth's Master's in Public Health program has been accepted. I am less excited about this than I envisioned when I started the application in November 2019.

June 25: It is striking to me how the droplet/aerosol (as it has developed between researchers in different disciplines and lay people alike on social media) debate mirrors the miasma/contagion debate in many ways. The way that the political impinges on the medical, so that political and ideological impulses shape evidence and narrative, is especially striking. Readers may recall from chapter 2 that Kingsley gave a lecture on May 31, 1861, during the public fight against miasma. In it, he advocates for cleanliness, ventilation, and the purity of individual health subtended by breathing: "The breath which you give out is an impure air, to which has been added, among other matters which will not support life, an excess of carbonic acid. . . . I beseech you to remember at least these two—oxygen gas and carbonic acid gas; and to remember that, as surely as oxygen feeds the fire of life, so surely does carbonic acid put it out."[20]

In Palm Beach, Florida, on June 24, 2020, members of the public testified before the Palm Beach County Board of Commissioners, which was voting on whether masks should be required in public places. One citizen proselytizes: "And they want to throw God's wonderful breathing system out the door. You're all turning your backs on it. Can you prove that it's good for people to breathe carbon dioxide over and over and over again? God made it so that we would breathe in fresh oxygen, to go to our body, to every cell in the body. It has to have that to make energy."[21] This skeptical citizen echoes Kingsley, who talks about hygiene and the dangers of carbon dioxide (carbonic acid for him) but, as I argue in chapter 2, does so through the logic of sin and liberalism. Kingsley is more rhetorically sophisticated and accurate, even in terms of biochemistry and respiratory physiology, and he drives the point home that individuals have the right and the moral duty to be clean and healthy for the imperative of national health. The individual has a duty to the social to be healthy. This is not what is happening in the meeting in Palm Beach; however, there is a converging logic, one that follows the history of the individual, their health, and right against government control in the most adversarial of terms.

Here in Florida 2020, the focus is merely on "God-given" choice—and at that, a choice not to be healthy and instead be potentially a threat to an incalculable number of others, a choice clothed in a thin covering of religiosity and pseudoscience that has clearly divided the population in our current moment. The "war" against COVID-19 has produced a kind of parallel civil war—not without its material referents: militarized police and national guard exercising states of exception during protest; armed white-nationalist protesters demanding that lockdowns be ended. And lynchings.[22] This syndemic (a situation in which two epidemics interact in devastating synergy) of COVID-19 and racism, particularly against Black bodies in the United States, has been devastating. In the space of two months, we have seen massive, rapid resistance to police brutality as well as to racist legacies in the form of statues and other symbols. We can hope that resistance produces lasting change. Similarly, we can only hope that COVID-19 effects a complete rethinking of what it means to live with disease and with other people in a precarious future. Like Tsing's matsutake mushroom, this enmeshed history in the present cultural work of the martial metaphor might help us imagine what it will be like to live—in the human-microbiological-ecological sense specifically—without the "handrails" of mythologized "dreams of modernization and progress that offered a vision of stability."[23]

※

It has never been clearer that the martial metaphor is profoundly entrenched in our cultural imagination as a response to diseases. George Eliot's narrator in *Middlemarch* (1872) provides further insight here: "We all of us, grave or light, get our thoughts entangled in metaphors, and act fatally on the strength of them."[24] While we have never been so fatally attached to the martial metaphor—fatal in terms of both continuing to allow the causes of mass death and seemingly having no alternative—we are at the same time in a unique moment for change. At the same rate and speed at which the infodemic produced emerging, conflicting, erroneous, and also correct information about the disease, we have seen, in the popular press, in the social sciences, and in the humanities, a rapid and massive mobilization to examine the language, history, and politics at work in the COVID-19 pandemic. Examples of such work have appeared in publications such as *Vox*, the *Atlantic*, the *Washington Post*, and *Somatosphere* and *Nursing Clio*.[25] And that is not even counting the massive number of tweets by humanists and social scientists, along with work by epidemiologists and others in the vast expanse of fields needed to address problems with the language that shapes the infodemic, that socially and culturally determines the pandemic. Just three days ago, communication scholar Benjamin Bates published "The (In)Appropriateness of the WAR Metaphor in Response to SARS-CoV-2: A Rapid Analysis of Donald J. Trump's Rhetoric."[26]

What story will we tell about all of this in 100 years? What story will we continue to tell ourselves in the next 5? I can't say. What I can say is that there are plenty of alternatives, and as of this writing, the critical visibility of the metaphor is at an apex I would have never imagined it would have reached. Charlotte Brives has recently proposed the helpful frame of amphibiosis: "We can think about [the relationships between humans and microbes] through the idea of 'amphibiosis,' a term developed in the 1960s by microbiologist Theodor Rosebury to illustrate the changeable and dynamic nature of the relations maintained by different biological entities, depending on the place and time."[27] This is not unlike the rethinking of the host-pathogen relationship as one of relationality versus ontological essentiality that we see in the current development of antivirulence drugs.[28] There is plenty of research that complicates the inimical framing of viruses and looks to the beneficial roles they might be playing in the holobiont. Iona Walker, who researches alternatives to thinking of medicine as war and interdisciplinary approaches to mitigating antimicrobial resistance, recently pointed me to the #ReframeCovid initiative and its open-source document, which contains, in multiple languages, hundreds of cited alternatives to war metaphors. Walker and her research group suggest drawing on coevolution and ecological language in line with Haraway, specifically with respect to AMR.[29] Brian Resnick and Umair Irfan, in addition, elegantly characterize the complexities, sequences, and concerns of the immune system as an "orchestra."[30] In short, there are many alternatives to the martial metaphor and many people who are actively thinking about and communicating them.

I would like to cite, engage, and entangle this book's arguments with at least a dozen more texts and scholars. But I will limit myself to saying that the time is ripe to reframe the scalar language of humans, microbial life, morbidity, and mortality. This is no longer just a scholarly conversation among the medical and health humanists or a topic for Victorian studies; it has become very public. The linguistic moment, we can only hope, has reached the moment of its crisis.

If social distancing, voluntary quarantine, and wearing masks demonstrate anything, it is that "the effect of [our] being on those around [us can be] incalculably diffusive: for the growing good of the world is partly dependent on unhistoric acts." Those closing lines from Eliot's *Middlemarch* so effectively express the "incalculably diffusive"[31] good that we all—whether we are scholars, teachers, readers, or simply human beings—can do, flattening the amplitude of that ominous curve and changing the pathological cultures that are catalyzed by the martial metaphor and that produce health, morbidity, and mortality differentially.

We need not be the scientists who sacrifice themselves to secretly test an experimental therapy in some dramatic movie. If we think critically about how our language and metaphors can *make* health and life *with* rather than make morbidity and war *against*, we can be—collectively—part of the growing good of the world that remains in the ruins of this moment.

Notes

Introduction

1. While *infectious* is generally used to mean a microbial pathogen that can produce a pathological response in the body, in the early nineteenth century, the term specifically referred to disease transmission via air as *infectious*. Christopher Hamlin, *Cholera: The Biography* (Oxford: Oxford University Press, 2009), 74.

2. Military medicine encompasses a number of specialties, including combat traumatology, but here I refer to its primary directive of supporting combat operations and military deployments in terms of hygiene, epidemiology, and preventive medicine. Morbidity and mortality rates before World War II were due mostly to infectious disease. The primary determinant for military causalities, however, started changing with the development of the mechanistic and chemical weapons of World War I and the development of antibiotics, most notably penicillin, during and after World War II, when combat-related fatalities trumped infectious disease as the primary manner of death.

3. Mark Harrison notes that Park's text was the standard for military medical men at home and in the British colonies, between the 1860s and 1880s. *Public Health and British India: Anglo-Indian Preventive Medicine, 1859–1914* (Cambridge, UK: Cambridge University Press, 1994), 52. See also Pamela K. Gilbert, *The Citizen's Body: Desire, Health, and the Social in Victorian England* (Columbus: Ohio State University Press, 2007), 54. Other examples of military medical manuals following this pattern include John Martin, *Contributions to Military and State Medicine: First Volume* (London: J & A Churchill, 1881); James Irving, *A Concise View of the Progress of Military Medical Literature* (Edinburgh: Stark & Co., 1846).

4. See for instance, R. A. Pearlman and Tyler P. Tate, "Military Metaphors in Health Care: Who Are We Actually Trying to Help?" *American Journal of Bioethics* 16, no. 10 (2016): 17; Arthur Frank, *At the Will of the Body: Reflections on Illness* (New York: Houghton Mifflin, 2002), 83.

5. The September 2016 issue of the *American Journal of Bioethics* begins with an editorial, article, and series of responses as to the implications of using metaphorically militarized medicine. See this issue's introduction, Kayhan Parsi, "War Metaphors in Health Care: What Are They Good For?" *American Journal of Bioethics* 16, no. 10 (2016), 1–2.

6. George Eliot, *The Mill on the Floss* (New York: W. W. Norton, 1994), 117.

7. George Lakoff and Mark Johnson, *Metaphors We Live By* (Chicago: University of Chicago Press, 2003), 1, 5. For previous readings of this and other conceptual medical metaphors see Giovanni De Grandis, "On the Analogy between Infectious Diseases and War: How to Use It and Not to Use It." *Public Health Ethics* 4, no. 1 (2011); April D. Marshall, "Metaphors We Die By," *Semiotica: Journal of the International Association for Semiotic Studies* 161 (2006); V. L. Warren, "The 'Medicine Is War' Metaphor," *HEC Forum* 3, no. 1 (1991).

8. Many of the balance, journey, and dance metaphors follow language from Eastern medicine. Paul Hodgkin, "Medicine Is War: And Other Medical Metaphors," *British Medical Journal* 291, no. 6511 (1985): 1821. More contemporary Western symbiotic models follow current research into the microbiome. See M. P. Francino, "Antibiotics and the Human Gut Microbiome Dysbiosis and Accumulation of Resistances," *Frontiers in Microbiology* 6 (2015); Benjamin P. Willing, Shannon L. Russell, and B. Brett Finlay, "Shifting the Balance: Host–Microbiota Mutualism," *National Review Microbiology* 9, no. 4 (2011).

9. Institute of Medicine Forum on Microbial Threats, *Ending the War Metaphor: The Changing Agenda for Unraveling the Host-Microbe Relationship: Workshop Summary* (Washington, DC: The National Academies Press, 2006), 2.

10. Roger Cooter, "Of War and Epidemics: Unnatural Couplings, Problematic Conceptions," *Journal for the Society of the Social History of Medicine* 16, no. 2 (2003): 301; Abdulsalam Al-Zahrani, "Darwin's Metaphors Revisited: Conceptual Metaphors, Conceptual Blends, and Idealized Cognitive Models in the Theory of Evolution," *Metaphor & Symbol* 23, no. 1 (2008): 52. Gillian Beer speaks to some of the problems and benefits of analogy and, more specifically, metaphor in *Darwin's Plots: Evolutionary Narrative in Darwin, George Eliot and Nineteenth-Century Fiction*, 3rd ed. (Cambridge, UK: Cambridge University Press, 2009), 50.

11. Charles E. Rosenberg, "Disease in History: Frames and Framers," *Milbank Quarterly* 67, no. 1 (1989): 1.

12. Nikolas Rose, "Medicine, History and the Present," in *Reassessing Foucault: Power, Medicine, and the Body*, eds. Colin Jones and Roy Porter (London: Routledge, 1998), 50.

13. Priscilla Wald, *Contagious: Cultures, Carriers, and the Outbreak Narrative* (Durham, NC: Duke University Press, 2008), 58.

14. Richard Evans, "Ebola: From Public Health Crisis to National Security Threat." In *Biological Threats in the 21st Century: The Politics, People, Science and Historical Roots*, ed. Filippa Lentzos (London: Imperial Press, 2016). Representative

and recent examples include the following: Alan Bleakley, *Thinking with Metaphors in Medicine: The State of Art* (New York: Routledge, 2017); De Grandis, "On the Analogy"; Marshall, "Metaphors We Die By"; Warren, "The 'Medicine Is War' Metaphor"; Abraham Fuks, "The Military Metaphors of Modern Medicine," in *The Meaning Management Challenge: Making Sense of Health, Illness and Disease*, eds. Zhenyi Li and Thomas Lawrence Long (Oxford: Inter-Disciplinary Press, 2010); Institute of Medicine Forum on Microbial Threats, *Ending the War Metaphor*; Ann Mongoven, "The War on Disease and the War on Terror: A Dangerous Metaphorical Nexus?" *Cambridge Quarterly of Healthcare Ethics* 15, no. 4 (2006).

15. Susan Sontag, *Illness as Metaphor* (New York: Vintage Books, 1979); Tauber, *Immunity: The Evolution of an Idea* (Oxford: Oxford University Press, 2017), 1. Before Sontag, the earliest recognition of this metaphor and its relation to medical epistemology I found is Ludwik Fleck's 1935 *Genesis and Development of Scientific Fact* (Chicago: University of Chicago Press, 2008), first translated into English in 1975.

16. Mooney, *Intrusive Interventions: Public Health, Domestic Space, and Infectious Disease Surveillance in England, 1840–1914* (Rochester: University of Rochester, 2015), 6. Mooney uses this wording to challenge the idea that germ theory alone solidified the acceptance of public health to the general public.

17. Cooter, "Of War and Epidemics," 290.

18. Ed Cohen, *A Body Worth Defending: Immunity, Biopolitics, and the Apotheosis of the Modern Body* (Durham, NC: Duke University Press, 2009), 8–9.

19. Pamela K. Gilbert, *Cholera and Nation: Doctoring the Social Body in Victorian England* (Albany: State University of New York Press, 2008); Gilbert, *The Citizen's Body*.

20. Laura Otis, *Membranes: Metaphors of Invasion in Nineteenth-Century Literature, Science, and Politics* (Baltimore: Johns Hopkins University Press, 1999), 3–5.

21. Erin O'Conner, *Raw Material: Producing Pathology in Victorian Culture* (Durham, NC: Duke University Press, 2000), 53–59.

22. Tina Young Choi, *Anonymous Connections: The Body and Narratives of the Social in Victorian Britain* (Ann Arbor: University of Michigan Press, 2015), 134. Other scholars in Victorian studies have mentioned the metaphor in passing, such as Kristine Swenson, *Medical Women and Victorian Fiction* (Columbia: University of Missouri, 2007); Mary Wilson Carpenter, *Health, Medicine, and Society in Victorian England* (Santa Barbara, CA: Praeger, 2010).

23. Here, I draw from Rose's understanding that we cannot solely focus on medical discourse as representation and explanation, but must also consider the material, conceptual, and institutional means through which illness is made thinkable. "Medicine, History, and the Present," 62.

24. For more references to earlier instances, see Fuks, "The Military Metaphors of Medicine."

25. John Donne, *Devotions upon Emergent Expressions and Death's Duel* (New York, Cosimo: 2010), 124.

26. Thomas Sydenham, *The Works of Thomas Sydenham, M.D: Volume I*, ed. William A. Greenhill, trans. R. G. Latham (London: Sydenham Society, 1848), 267. On Fludd, see Laura Kassell, "Magic, Alchemy and the Medical Economy in Early Modern England: The Case of Robert Fludd's Magnetical Medicine," in *Medicine and the Market in England and Its Colonies, c. 1450–c. 1850*, ed. Mark Jackson (London: Palgrave, 2007), 96–98. See also Maurizio Meloni, *Impressionable Biologies: From the Archaeology of Plasticity to the Sociology of Epigenetics* (New York: Routledge, 2019), 49. This image of the body as castle will resonate with those readers familiar with Emily Martin's anthropology of immunology, which include a two-page illustration from a 1975 publication *How Your Body Works*, representing immune response as a medieval defense of a citadel. *Flexible Bodies: Tracking Immunity in American Culture from the Days of Polio to the Age of AIDS* (Boston: Beacon Press, 1994), 34–35.

27. I am indebted to Michael Brown for his helpful clarification of this idea as a heuristic device before the nineteenth century versus a means to shape who practitioners were and what disease meant in political, cultural, and ideological terms.

28. There are, of course, innumerable influences to consider, as detailed by the expansive scholarship on the medical profession and medical press. See Michael Brown, *Performing Medicine: Medical Culture and Identity in Provincial England, C.1760–1850* (Manchester: Manchester University Press, 2011); Ian Burney, "Medicine in the Age of Reform," in *Rethinking the Age of Reform Britain 1780–1850*, ed. Arthur Burns and Joanna Innes (Cambridge, UK: Cambridge University Press, 2009), 167–68; Christopher Lawrence, *Medicine in the Making of Modern Britain 1700–1920* (New York: Routledge, 1994); Kim Price, *Medical Negligence in Victorian Britain: The Crisis of Care under English Poor Law, c. 1834–1900* (London: Bloomsbury, 2016); On medical periodicals, William F. Bynum, Stephen Lock, Roy Porter, ed., *Medical Journals and Medical Knowledge* (London: Routledge, 1992); Megan Coyer, *Literature and Medicine in the Nineteenth Century Periodical Press: Blackwood's Edinburgh Magazine, 1817–1858* (Edinburgh: Edinburgh University Press, 2017).

29. Michael Brown, "Medicine, Reform and the 'End' of Charity in Early Nineteenth-Century England," *English Historical Review* 124, no. 511 (2009), 1353–38, 1360.

30. Brown, "Medicine, Reform and the 'End' of Charity," 1358, 1380–81, 1387.

31. Michael Brown, "Like a Devoted Army," *Journal of British Studies* 49, no. 3 (2010): 595.

32. There are numerous different intersecting and discrete theories of the body, disease, and therapeutics, along with their respective figurative language,

from antiquity to the late 1700s: vitalism, solidism, humoralism, iatromechanism, iatrochemistry, among others. For a more detailed survey, see W. F. Bynum and Roy Porter, eds, *The Companion Encyclopedia of the History of Medicine* (London: Routledge, 1993), in particular the sections on "Body Systems"; "Theories of Life, Health, and Disease"; and "Understanding Disease." It is important, however, to remember that the terminology we use to describe medical theories and schools of thought are rhetorical shorthands and were always less than fully systematic. Mary Lindemann, *Medicine and Society in Early Modern* Europe (Cambridge, UK: Cambridge University Press, 1999), 109.

33. The mechanist model also moved toward a form of vitalism (the physiological explanation of life premised on a "vital principle" that animated organisms) at the end of the eighteenth century that centered on nerves, force, and tone. William Cullen, for instance, believed that temperature, dampness, and effluvia, alone and in union could produce disease. His pathophysiology was concerned with vessels, pulse, structures, and evacuations as they were related to the nervous system. Emphasis on the primacy of the nervous system in medicine was mutually constitutive with the growing cult of sensibility in the late eighteenth and early nineteenth centuries. W. F. Bynum, "Nosology" in *The Companion Encyclopedia of the History of Medicine*, ed. W. F. Bynum and Roy Porter (London: Routledge, 1993), 364. Hisao Ishizuka, *Fiber, Medicine, and Culture in the British Enlightenment* (New York: Palgrave, 2016), 126–33.

34. Cooter, "Of War and Epidemics," 289.

35. Medical cosmologies are intellectual gestalts: "metaphysical attempts to circumscribe and define systematically the essential nature of the universe of medical discourse as a whole. They are conceptual structures which constitute the frames of reference within which all questions are posed and all answers are offered." N. D. Jewson, "The Disappearance of the Sick-Man from Medical Cosmology, 1770–1870," *Sociology* 10, no. 2 (May 1976): 225–44.

36. This ontological thinking had earlier roots in physiological models, such as those of Sydenham and Paracelsus that understood disease as things independent from the human body. Bynum, "Nosology," 351–52.

37. Michel Foucault, *The Birth of the Clinic: An Archaeology of Medical Perception*, trans. A. M. Sheridan Smith (New York: Vintage, 1994), xvii, 186, 221. As Ian Burney characterizes it, "Disease was not a specific entity (in either its causes, its course, or its physical signs), but was instead a disequilibrium of generalized elements, either solid, fluid, or both, which implicated the whole person." "Medicine in the Age of Reform," 167.

38. Xavier Bichat, *Physiological Researches upon Life and Death*, trans. Tobias Watkins (Philadelphia: Smith & Maxwell, 1809), 1.

39. Martin Willis uses the term "disease objects" when characterizing how germs became studied as objects of investigation leading to their consideration

as anthropomorphized agents that cause disease. *Vision, Science, and Literature, 1870–1920: Ocular Horizons* (London: Pickering & Chatto, 2011), 23.

40. Hamlin, *Cholera*, 45.

41. Pamela K. Gilbert, *Mapping the Victorian Social Body* (Albany: State University of New York Press, 2004), 208–9n15.

42. Erika Wright has also noted the way authors, such as Charles Dickens, posited an epistemological ambiguity between disease theories, although her reading focuses more on the narratological implications of such positions. *Reading for Health: Medical Narratives and the Nineteenth-Century Novel* (Athens: Ohio University Press, 2016), 80–82.

43. The East Asian medical tradition had forms of inoculation before Western Europe. Vivienne Lo and Michael Stanly-Baker, "Chinese Medicine," in *The Oxford Handbook of the History of Medicine*, ed. Mark Jackson (Oxford: Oxford University Press, 2011), 162. See also Travis Chi Wing Lau, "Inventing Edward Jenner: Historicizing Anti-vaccination" in *The Routledge Companion to Health Humanities*, eds. Paul Crawford, Brian Brown, and Andrea Charise (London: Routledge, 2020): 120–133.

44. Tim Fulford and Debbie Lee, "The Jenneration of Disease: Vaccination, Romanticism, and Revolution," *Studies in Romanticism* 39, no. 1 (2000): 140.

45. On Chadwick, see Christopher Hamlin, *Public Health and Social Justice in the Age of Chadwick* (Cambridge, UK: Cambridge University Press, 1998), 47. See also Florence Nightingale, *Florence Nightingale on Public Health Care: The Collected Works of Florence Nightingale* vol. 6, ed. Lynn McDonald (Ontario: Wilfrid Laurier University Press, 2004), 568. See Michael Brown, "From Foetid Air to Filth: The Cultural Transformation of British Epidemiological Thought, ca. 1780–1848," *Bulletin of the History of Medicine* 82, no. 3 (2008): 515–44, for a nuanced historization of the development of miasma as evidenced by figures like Smith.

46. Hamlin makes the case that Edwin Chadwick specifically authored a conservative and narrow version of public health, focusing more on filth as a cause of disease *and* poverty, putting less emphasis on poverty and deprivation. Hamlin, *Public Health and Social Justice*, 13. On the expansion and idea of public health surveillance, in a complex contestation with liberal subjectivity and articulation through the domestic, see Mooney, *Intrusive Interventions*, 12–17.

47. Erwin H Ackerknecht, "Anticontagionism between 1821 and 1867," *International Journal of Epidemiology* 38, no. 1 (2009): 9.

48. Joseph W. Childers, *Novel Possibilities: Fiction and the Formation of Early Victorian Culture* (Philadelphia: University of Pennsylvania Press, 1995), 14, 92.

49. Gilbert, *The Citizen's Body*, 38; Henry Mayhew's *London Labour and the London Poor* (New York: Dove, 1968), serialized in the 1840s and published as a collection in 1851, was emblematic of the racialization of the poor vis-à-vis sanitary discourse.

50. Proto-germ theories, such as *contagium vivum* had been hypothesized by those building off of the work of Anton van Leeuwenhoek and Robert Hooke, such as British physician Nicolas Andry (1700) who posited that diseases like smallpox were caused by living worms, or Richard Bradley who suggested poisonous insects were responsible for miasmic pestilence. Margaret DeLacy, *The Germ of an Idea: Contagionism, Religion, and Society in Britain, 1660–1730* (Basingstoke: Palgrave Macmillan, 2016), 75–101.

51. Arthur Conan Doyle, "The Adventure of the Copper Beeches," in *Sherlock Holmes: The Complete Novels and Stories: Volume I* (New York: Bantam Dell, 2003), 500.

52. Sontag, *Illness as Metaphor*, 65–66. Tauber, *Immunity*, 1.

53. I borrow the term here from Nancy Tomes, who provides an extensive account of the panic and promises of germ theory in American culture in the late nineteenth and early twentieth century. *The Gospel of Germs: Men, Women, and the Microbe in American Life* (Cambridge, UK: Harvard University Press, 1998).

54. Willis, *Vision, Science, and Literature*, 23.

55. See, for instance, Charles Darwin's discussion in *On the Origin of Species by Means of Natural Selection, or the Preservation of Favoured Races in the Struggle for Life* (New York: Signet, 2003), 84–85. While he uses the word *war*, he does so significantly less often than he uses *struggle* and *fight*. Gillian Beer and Devin Griffiths have noted the presence of that analogical form in Darwin's work. Beer, *Darwin's Plots*; Devin Griffiths, *The Age of Analogy: Science and Literature between the Darwins* (Baltimore: Johns Hopkins University Press, 2016).

56. Michael Brown, "Cold Steel, Weak Flesh: Mechanism, Masculinity and the Anxieties of Late Victorian Empire," *Cultural and Social History* 14, no. 2 (2017): 157.

57. Gilbert, *The Citizen's Body*, 8–9.

58. On the relation between biopolitics and statistics, see Ian Hacking, *The Taming of Chance* (New York: Cambridge University Press, 1990). For more recent work in Victorian studies in this vein, see Choi, *Anonymous Connections*; Emily Steinlight, *Populating the Novel* (Ithaca, NY: Cornell University Press, 2018).

59. Michel Foucault, *Society Must Be Defended: Lectures at the Collège de France, 1975–76*, trans. David Macey (New York: Picador, 2003), 243.

60. See Cooter's parsing of the problematic distinction between endemic and epidemic. "Of War and Epidemics," 287.

61. Foucault, *Society Must Be Defended*, 243. See also Michel Foucault *Security, Territory, Population: Lectures at the Collège De France, 1977–78*, trans. Graham Burchell (New York: Palgrave Macmillan, 2007), 104.

62. I follow Gilbert's broader, catholic, understanding of liberalism, which accounts for the economic theories of Smith and Mills which espoused social responsibility while retaining a Kantian understanding of the self as individual while specifically referring to the "overarching philosophy of government" in

the nineteenth century that developed from Enlightenment ideals. For example, government should be representative in some capacity and develop society; operate on consent rather than force; and be contingent on the free circulation of labor, capital, goods, and the "inviolability of property." At its core, liberalism was a "capitalist and possessive individualist vision." Gilbert, *The Citizen's Body*, 2n1.

63. Gilbert, *The Citizen's Body*, 8–9. "Britishness equals Englishness equals, by the end of the period, the healthy (clean, isolated), white masculine, middle-class body. Women became the privileged site of production of this body through their ability to construct an appropriately domestic sphere."

64. Erin O'Conner makes a similar case with respect to the pathological social determinants of industrialization and the its material effects on the body: "Victorian logics of embodiments sought certainty; they found a way out of the world by tautology, ordering culture by ordering the body by discovering in it in the germ of social structure." *Raw Material*, 14.

65. Julian Reid, *The Biopolitics of the War on Terror: Life Struggles, Liberal Modernity and the Defence of Logistical Societies* (Manchester: Manchester University Press, 2009), 13, 18.

66. Nathan K. Hensley, *Forms of Empire: The Poetics of Victorian Sovereignty* (Oxford: Oxford University Press, 2016), 11–13.

67. Hensley, 13–14.

68. Hensley, 12.

69. Cohen, *A Body Worth Defending*, 20. On the immune system as a defense system, see also Martin, *Flexible Bodies*; Donna Haraway, "The Biopolitics of Postmodern Bodies: Determinations of Self in Immune System Discourse," in *Biopolitics: A Reader*, ed. Timothy Campbell (Durham, NC: Duke University Press, 2013); Esposito, *Immunitas: The Protection and Negation of Life* (Cambridge, UK: Polity, 2011).

70. Jasbir Puar, "Introduction: Homonationalism and Biopolitics," in *Terrorist Assemblages*, ed. Jasbir Puar, *Terrorist Assemblages in Queer Time* (Durham, NC: Duke University Press, 2007), 9.

71. Wald, *Contagious*, 58.

72. On the role of the physician see Tabitha Sparks, *Doctor in the Victorian Novel: Family Practices* (Farnham, UK: Ashgate, 2010); see also Gilbert, *The Citizen's Body*, 53. The disciplinary function of the Victorian novel in the production of subjectivity has been well established. See D. A. Miller, *The Novel and the Police* (University of California Press, 1988); Nancy Armstrong, *Desire and Domestic Fiction: A Political History of the Novel* (Oxford: Oxford University Press, 1989).

73. Gilbert, *Cholera and Nation*, 4. See also, Hamlin, *Cholera*, 4; Brown, "Like a Devoted Army," 614.

74. Fuson Wang, "Romantic Disease Discourse: Disability, Immunity, and Literature," *Nineteenth-Century Contexts* 33, no. 5 (2011): 469.

75. Linda Colley makes this case in her cultural history of Great Britain from the Act of Union between England Wales and Scotland to the beginning of Queen Victoria's reign in 1837, contending that Britain's military campaigns over the course of the long eighteenth century forged an imagining of a communal national identity. *Britons: Forging the Nation 1707–1837* (New Haven: Yale University Press, 1992), 3–7.

76. Thomas H. Huxley, "The Connection of the Biological Sciences with Medicine," *Science* 2, no. 63 (1881): 426.

77. Josephine Butler, *The Constitution Violated: An Essay* (Edinburgh: Edmonston & Douglas, 1871), 91.

78. Foucault, *The Birth of the Clinic*, 196.

Chapter 1

1. Mary Shelley, *The Last Man*, ed. Pamela Bickley (Hertfordshire, UK: Wordsworth Classics, 2004), 196. Hereafter cited parenthetically in the text as *LM*.

2. This identity formation was of course not a complete political or cultural integration or homogenization; rather Britishness was superimposed "on an array of internal difference" through the rational, creative, and practical response to foreign invasion. Colley, *Britons*, 6.

3. Fulford and Lee document how Jenner became a military hero and his vaccination was metaphorized into a holy war in professional medical writing that was both "natural and political." They show how that reception emerged both from the connection of vaccination to the military and from smallpox's transformation from a disease caused within the body to one that came from the outside in. Fulford and Lee, "The Jenneration of Disease," 157.

4. Edward Jenner, *A Continuation of Facts and Observations Relative to the Variolae Vaccinae, or Cow Pox* (London: Sampson Low, 1800), 41. See Fulford and Lee, "The Jenneration of Disease," 160.

5. *Outbreaks* are defined by the sudden occurrence of an infectious disease in a community or area that has either never experienced it or experiences a significantly higher number of cases than in the past. *Epidemic* is generally interchangeable with outbreak but is usually used for larger geographic areas. *Pandemics* are epidemics that have spread to across an entire country, or more often, across multiple countries, and even more often, to multiple continents. *Endemic* refers to the ongoing or normal presence of a disease in a given area or population.

6. O'Conner, *Raw Material*, 44.

7. Anne McClintock, *Imperial Leather: Race, Gender, and Sexuality in the Colonial Conquest* (New York: Routledge, 1995), 5. See also O'Conner, *Raw Material*, 28–30.

8. Alan Bewell, *Romanticism and Colonial Disease* (Baltimore: Johns Hopkins University Press, 2003), 300. A number of other critics have discussed Shelley's

Last Man in terms of medical discourse. See Peter Melville, "The Problem of Immunity in The Last Man," *SEL Studies in English Literature 1500–1900* 47, no. 4 (2007); Fuson Wang, "We Must Live Elsewhere: The Social Construction of Natural Immunity in Mary Shelley's The Last Man," *European Romantic Review* 22, no. 2 (2011); Wang, "Romantic Disease Discourse."

9. The monolithic progressivism of the sanitary movement has indeed been demythologized, especially regarding the prominence of Edwin Chadwick. Chadwick's "techno fix," for instance, was one of many possible public health actions. He chose to focus on water and filth, rather than wages, working conditions, and food. Hamlin, *Public Health and Social Justice*, 11–14.

10. Bewell, *Romanticism and Colonial Disease*, 20–22.

11. Hamlin, *Cholera*, 33–35, 240.

12. Antonis A. Kousoulis, "Etymology of Cholera." *Emerging Infectious Diseases* 18, no. 3 (2012): 540; Hamlin, *Cholera*, 163.

13. "History of the Rise, Progress, Ravages, &c. of the Blue Cholera of India," *Lancet* 17, no. 429 (1831): 241. Gilbert notes the influence of the article. Gilbert, *Mapping the Victorian Social Body*, 143.

14. "History of the Rise," 241.

15. James Jameson, *Report on the Epidemick Cholera Morbus: As It Visited the Territories Subject to the Presidency of Bengal, in the Years 1817, 1818 and 1819* (Calcutta: Government Gazette Press, 1820), 16, 23, 45–67, 210–215. See also S. L. Kotar and J. E. Gessler, *Cholera: A Worldwide History* (Jefferson: McFarland, 2014), 8. The disease's "violence" can be understood in contrast to something like tuberculosis, which (not including the incubation period, but even from the point of showing symptoms) can take years to cause death. Erin O'Conner makes a persuasive case for the relationship to the rapidity of cholera's symptoms, empire, and industrialization. *Raw Material*, 22–25, 41–43. I am also grateful to Janis Caldwell for noting these qualities of cholera's symptoms in contrast to other diseases.

16. Ackerknecht, "Anticontagionism," 13. A notable exception is Jameson's *Report on the Epidemick Cholera Morbus*, chapter 6.

17. Gilbert, *Mapping the Victorian Social Body*, 142, 148; Ackerknecht, "Anticontagionism," 12.

18. Margaret Pelling, "The Meaning of Contagion," in *Contagion: Historical and Cultural Studies*, eds. Alison Bashford and Claire Hooker (London: Routledge, 2001), 21; see also Gilbert, *Cholera and Nation*, 71.

19. Gilbert, *Mapping the Victorian Social Body*, 209n15. Michael Brown has argued looking at the writings of Southwood Smith, contagionism also became aligned with despotism due to quarantines' effect of concentrating disease. "From Foetid Air to Filth," 525.

20. Anne McWhir, "Mary Shelley's Anti-Contagionism: The Last Man as 'Fatal Narrative.'" *Mosaic* 35, no. 2 (2002): 23.

21. David Arnold, *Colonizing the Body: State Medicine and Epidemic Disease in Nineteenth-Century India* (Berkeley: University of California Press, 1993), 64.

22. Bewell, *Romanticism and Colonial Disease*, 8–12.

23. Bewell, 246, 298–301. For a more extensive historical account of the military influences of cholera in India, see Arnold, *Colonizing the Body*; Mark Harrison, "Differences of Degree: Representations of India in British Medical Topography, 1820–c. 1870," *Medical History Supplement* 20 (2000); Hamlin, *Cholera*, 162.

24. "History of the Rise of Cholera," 214.

25. "History of the Rise of Cholera," 276.

26. Bewell, *Romanticism and Colonial Disease*, 246.

27. Hilary Strang, "Common Life, Animal Life, Equality: The Last Man," *ELH* 78, no. 2 (2011): 416.

28. Bewell, *Romanticism and Colonial Disease*, 300. The painting by Antoine-Jean Gros was commissioned by Napoleon and depicts the commander visiting his sick soldiers in what is now modern-day Israel. See Yvonne Hibbott, "'Bonaparte Visiting the Plague-Stricken at Jaffa' by Antoine Jean Gros (1771–1835)," *British Medical Journal* 1, no. 5642 (1969): 501.

29. Bewell, *Romanticism and Colonial Disease*, 301.

30. Byron joined the Greek War of Independence, fighting for the Ottoman Empire against the Greek Revolutionaries, but died of a fever in Missolonghi in 1824. Kari E. Lokke, "The Last Man," in *The Cambridge Companion to Mary Shelley*, ed. Esther Schor (Cambridge, UK: Cambridge University Press, 2003), 120.

31. Bewell, *Romanticism and Colonial Disease*, 313; Wang, "We Must Live Elsewhere," 242.

32. Peter Melville, *Romantic Hospitality and the Resistance to Accommodation* (Waterloo, ON: Wilfrid Laurier University Press, 2007), 156.

33. Melville, 162.

34. Bewell, *Romanticism and Colonial Disease*, 205–41.

35. Bewell, 302, 306.

36. See also Cohen, *A Body Worth Defending*, 212.

37. Mary Floyd-Wilson, *English Ethnicity and Race in Early Modern Drama* (Cambridge, UK: Cambridge University Press, 2006), 3.

38. Arnold, *Colonizing the Body*, 25. Harrison discusses how medical topography did not always make rigid racial distinctions and was in many ways ambivalent with respect to the British construction of Indian culture. The Indian and the British were still different (and the former still a threat to the latter) but often in terms of degrees and not kind. "Differences of Degree," 66.

39. Bewell, *Romanticism and Colonial Disease*, 18.

40. Emily Lyons, "'O Little Isle!': Landscape, Englishness, and Apocalypse in *The Last Man* and *The War of the Worlds*." *ISLE: Interdisciplinary Studies in Literature and Environment*, isz067 (2019), https://doi.org/10.1093/isle/isz067.

41. Lauren Cameron, "Mary Shelley's Malthusian Objections in *The Last Man*." *Nineteenth-Century Literature* 67, no. 2 (2012): 184.

42. This seasonal determinant is in line with the thought of the time, evidenced in the works of physicians of the period like Charles Maclean. Brown, "From Foetid Air to Filth," 522.

43. Bewell, *Romanticism and Colonial Disease*, 308.

44. Melville, *Romantic Hospitality*, 163.

45. This ambiguity was likewise the case with medical topographical understandings of India, from between the 1820s and 1870s: "Medical topography was a project born of crisis, demonstrating that feelings of vulnerability and superiority were two sides of the same imperial coin." Harrison, "Differences of Degree," 65.

46. Melville, "The Problem of Immunity," 838.

47. Melville, *Romantic Hospitality*, 167.

48. A number of scholars have previously established the sublime aesthetics of the novel. See, J. Jennifer Jones, "The Art of Redundancy: Sublime Fiction and Mary Shelley's *The Last Man*," Keats-Shelley Review 29, no. 1 (2015); Steven Vine, "Mary Shelley's Sublime Bodies: Frankenstein, Matilda, the Last Man," *English* 55, no. 212 (2006): 142.

49. Vanessa L. Ryan, "The Physiological Sublime: Burke's Critique of Reason," *Journal of the History of Ideas* 62, no. 2 (2001): 267.

50. Frank Kermode, *The Sense of an Ending: Studies in the Theory of Fiction* (Oxford, UK: Oxford University Press, 2000), 17.

51. Edmund Burke, *A Philosophical Inquiry into the Origin of Our Ideas of the Sublime and Beautiful* (London: N. Hailes, 1824), 34.

52. Ryan, "The Physiological Sublime," 266.

53. Burke, *A Philosophical Inquiry*, 31.

54. Burke, 33–34.

55. Timothy Morton makes a similar claim about miasma when he characterizes it as "the first hyperobject." Morton, *Dark Ecology: For a Logic of Future Coexistence* (New York: Columbia University Press, 2016), 50.

56. Quoted in O'Conner, *Raw Material*, 39.

57. Richard Nelson, *Asiatic Cholera, Its Origin and Spread in Asia, Africa, and Europe, Introduction into America through Canada* (New York: Townsend, 1866), 16. This quote is originally discussed by O'Conner, *Raw Material*, 24.

58. Hildebrand Jacob outlines a number of images, including war, that had been associated with the sublime by the first quarter of the nineteenth century. See "From *The Works* (1735)" in *The Sublime: A Reader in British Eighteenth-Century Aesthetic Theory*, eds. Andrew Ashfield and Peter de Bolla (Cambridge, UK: Cambridge University Press, 1996), 53.

59. See Pamela Bickley's note in Shelley, *The Last Man*, 383n72.

60. Morton D. Paley, *The Apocalyptic Sublime* (New Haven: Yale University Press, 1986), 1–4.

61. Avril Horner and Sue Zlosnik, "The Apocalyptic Sublime: Then and Now," in *Apocalyptic Discourse in Contemporary Culture: Post-Millennial Perspectives*, eds. Monica Germana and Aris Mousoutzanis (New York: Routledge, 2014), 59. On the sublimity of war and its relation to Kantian interpretations, see Michael Gelven, *War and Existence: A Philosophical Inquiry* (University Park, PA: Pennsylvania State University Press, 1994). See also François Debrix, "The Sublime Spectatorship of War: The Erasure of the Event in America's Politics of Terror and Aesthetics of Violence," *Millennium: Journal of International Studies* 34, no. 3 (2006).

62. Mary Shelley, *History of A Six Weeks' Tour through a Part of France, Switzerland, Germany and Holland: With Letters Descriptive of a Sail Round the Lake of Geneva, and of the Glaciers of Chamouni* (London: T. Hookham, 1817), 19.

63. Barbara Claire Freeman, *The Feminine Sublime: Gender and Excess in Women's Fiction* (Berkeley: University of California Press, 1997), 17.

64. Wang, "We Must Live Elsewhere," 26.

65. Steinlight, *Populating the Novel*, 70.

66. Ranita Chatterjee demonstrates the relationship between counting and biopolitics in "Our Bodies, Our Catastrophes: Biopolitics in Mary Shelley's The Last Man," *European Romantic Review* 25, no. 1 (2014): 46.

67. Steinlight, *Populating the Novel*, 71.

68. Chatterjee, "Our Bodies, Our Catastrophes," 4.

69. Cameron, "Mary Shelley's Malthusian Objections," 178.

70. Burke, *A Philosophical Inquiry*, 48.

71. Burke, 48.

72. Jones, "The Art of Redundancy," 30.

73. Ryan, "The Physiological Sublime," 277.

74. Jones, "The Art of Redundancy," 28.

75. Steven Vine also contends that Shelley writes against the Kantian sublime. "Mary Shelley's Sublime Bodies," 142.

76. Cited in Ryan, "The Physiological Sublime," 267. Emphasis in the original.

77. Percy Bysshe Shelley, *Queen Mab: A Philosophical Poem* (New York: Wright & Owen, 1831), 22; William Godwin, *An Enquiry Concerning Political Justice: And Its Influence on Virtue and Happiness*, vol. 2 (London: G.G.J. & J. Robinson, 1793), 86. See Bewell, *Romanticism and Colonial Disease*, 207.

78. Wang, "We Must Live Elsewhere," 240.

79. Wang, "Romantic Disease Discourse," 477.

80. Wang, "We Must Live Elsewhere," 244.

81. Steinlight, *Populating the Novel*, 70.

82. Mary Shelley to Claire Clairmont, 7 July 1845, "Letters (6) from Mary Shelley to Claire Clairmont," Ashley MS 5023, Ashley Manuscripts 19th Century–20th Century, British Library Archives, London, UK.

83. Cameron, "Mary Shelley's Malthusian Objections," 184.

Chapter 2

1. Gilbert, *Cholera and Nation*, 157; Carpenter, *Health, Medicine, and Society*, 33–34; Hamlin, *Cholera*, 87–95.

2. Gilbert, *Cholera and Nation*, 157.

3. On Kingsley's convergence of natural and national history see Jonathan Colin, "An Illiberal Descent: Natural and National History in the Work of Charles Kingsley," *History* 96, no. 322 (2011): 167–87.

4. By *governmentality*, I mean the simultaneous care for and technology of the self in terms of conduct, and that "ensemble formed by the institutions, procedures, analyses, reflections, calculations and tactics" that enable the exercise of biopower. Foucault, *Security, Territory, and Population*, 108. Lauren M. E. Goodlad details how governmentality operated differently in the British versus French context that Foucault articulates, focusing on the Victorian conceptualization of "character." *Victorian Literature and the Victorian State: Character and Governance in a Liberal Society* (Baltimore: Johns Hopkins University Press, 2003), 17–27. On the conduct of conducts, see Michel Foucault, *The Birth of Biopolitics: Lectures at the Collège De France, 1978–79* (New York: Palgrave Macmillan, 2008), 186.

5. Chris Otter, *The Victorian Eye: A Political History of Light and Vision in Britain, 1800–1910* (Chicago: University of Chicago Press, 2008), 11.

6. See Stefan Collini, "The Idea of 'Character' in Victorian Political Thought," *Transactions of the Royal Historical Society* 35 (1985): 26.

7. Gilbert, *Cholera and Nation*, 156.

8. Carpenter, *Health, Medicine, and Society*, 33–34; Hamlin, *Cholera*, chapters 2–3.

9. Choi, *Anonymous Connections*, 64–66.

10. Brown, "Like a Devoted Army," 610.

11. Choi, *Anonymous Connections*, 66.

12. Charles E. Rosenberg, *Explaining Epidemics and Other Studies in the History of Medicine* (Cambridge, UK: Cambridge University Press, 1992), 279.

13. David M. Goldfrank, *The Origins of the Crimean War* (London: Longman, 1994), 49.

14. E. Fee and M. E. Garofalo, "Florence Nightingale and the Crimean War," *American Journal of Public Health* 100, no. 9 (2010): 1591.

15. "The War: Naval and Military Intelligence," *Lancet* 63, no. 1599 (1854): 461.

16. Cooter, "Of War and Epidemics," 292.

17. Charles Kingsley, *Two Years Ago* (London: Collins Clear Type Press, 1903), 1. Hereafter cited in the text as *TY*.

18. Charles Kingsley, review of *A History England from the Fall of Wolsey to the Death of Elizabeth* by J. A. Froude, *North British Review* 25 (November 1856): 39, 41.

19. Kingsley, review of *A History*, 56.
20. Kingsley, 56.
21. Kingsley, 57.
22. Charles Kingsley, *True Words for Brave Men* (London: Keagan Paul, Trench & Co., 1888), 202.
23. Keith A. Francis, "Sermons: Themes and Developments," in *The Oxford Handbook of the British Sermon, 1689–1901*, eds. Keith A. Francis and William Gibson (Oxford: Oxford University Press, 2012), 39, 41.
24. Mary Wilson Carpenter, "Medical Cosmopolitanism: Middlemarch, Cholera, and the Pathologies of English Masculinity," *Victorian Literature and Culture* 38, no. 2 (2010): 513.
25. Catherine Hall bluntly suggests that "Kingsley scorned cosmopolitanism." Catherine Hall, "Men and Their Histories: Civilizing Subjects," *History Workshop Journal*, no. 52 (2001): 60.
26. Lyons draws heavily from and quotes Thomas Sydenham, who, as mentioned in the introduction, is one of the earliest users of the martial metaphor. Robert Dyer Lyons, *A Treatise on Fever or Selections from a Course of Lectures on Fever Being Part of a Course of Theory and Practice of Medicine* (London: Longman, Green, Longman, & Roberts, 1861), 2, 77.
27. Charles Kingsley, "The Study of Natural History for Soldiers," in *Scientific Lectures and Essays* (London: Macmillan, 1899), 196.
28. Lyons, *A Treatise on Fever*, 8.
29. Lyons, 8.
30. C. J. Wan-ling Wee, *Culture, Empire, and the Question of Being Modern* (Lanham, MD: Lexington Books, 2003), 8.
31. Stefanie Markovitz, *The Crimean War and the British Imagination* (Cambridge, UK: Cambridge University Press, 2009), 12–15.
32. Swenson, *Medical Women*, 44.
33. Carpenter, *Health, Medicine, and Society*, 17.
34. John Snow, *On the Mode of Communication of Cholera* (London: John Churchill, 1855), 26.
35. John Snow, "On the Chief Cause of the Recent Sickness and Mortality in the Crimea," *Medical Times and Gazette*, May 12, 1855, 457.
36. While Snow published the waterborne theory in 1854, it took several years for it to be fully appreciated and accepted. Without mentioning Snow, Kingsley does acknowledge the waterborne theory later in the century, as evidenced in his 1866 lecture on cholera. He lays blame not on the poor but on "those who supply poisoned water, and foul dwellings." Charles Kingsley, "Cholera, 1866," in *The Water of Life and Other Sermons* (London: Macmillan, 1879), 190.
37. Swenson, *Medical Women*, 36n39.
38. Elaine Hadley, "Nobody, Somebody, and Everybody," *Victorian Studies* 59, no. 1 (2016): 68.

39. Priti Joshi, "Edwin Chadwick's Self-Fashioning: Professionalism, Masculinity, and the Victorian Poor," *Victorian Literature and Culture* 32, no. 2 (2004): 358.

40. Charles Kingsley, "Physician's Calling," in *The Water of Life and Other Sermons* (London: Macmillan, 1879), 17. Hereafter cited in the text as *PC*.

41. The Medical Act of 1858 distinguished "qualified" and "non-qualified" professionals by creating a list of vetted practitioners and professional standards, although its precise influence has been debated. See M. J. D. Roberts, "The Politics of Professionalization: MPs, Medical Men, and the 1858 Medical Act," *Medical History* 53, no. 1 (2009).

42. Catherine Kelly, *War and the Militarization of British Army Medicine, 1793–1830* (London: Pickering & Chatto, 2011), 143.

43. Brown, "Like a Devoted Army," 595, 629.

44. Hamlin, *Cholera*, 106–8.

45. Charles Kingsley, "Lecture III: The Explosive Forces," in *Three Lectures: Delivered at the Royal Institution, on the Ancient Regime as It Existed on the Continent Before the French Revolution* (London: Macmillan: 1867), 88.

46. Gilbert, *Cholera and Nation*, 175–76.

47. "The War: Naval and Military Intelligence," 460.

48. Gilbert, *Cholera and Nation*, 163.

49. It is important to note the variety of heroic masculinities a work in *Two Years Ago*. Holly Furneaux reads Tom Thrurnall less as a "Christian Soldier" and more a "Christian Humanitarian" and finds her "military man of feeling" in the heartbroken Major Campbell. *Military Men of Feeling: Emotion, Touch, and Masculinity in the Crimean War* (Oxford: Oxford University Press, 2016), 80–81.

50. Mooney, *Intrusive Interventions*, 180.

51. Carol Helmstadter and Judith Godden have challenged the Nightingale paradigm, contending that the development of modern nursing was a more protracted process, beginning early in the century with the rise of scientific medicine. They also attribute many mid-nineteenth century nursing techniques to the Anglican sisterhood. *Nursing before Nightingale, 1815–1899* (Farnham, UK: Ashgate, 2011), 123.

52. Lynn McDonald, "Florence Nightingale, Statistics and the Crimean War," *Journal of the Royal Statistical Society: Series A (Statistics in Society)* 177, no. 3 (2014): 569–71.

53. Louise Penner, *Victorian Medicine and Social Reform: Florence Nightingale Among the Novelists* (New York: Palgrave Macmillan, 2010), 10.

54. Mooney, *Intrusive Interventions*, 180.

55. "Two Years Ago by C. Kingsley," *The British Quarterly Review* 25 (April 1857): 414.

56. See Mary Poovey, *Uneven Developments: The Ideological Work of Gender in Mid-Victorian England* (Chicago: University of Chicago Press, 1988); Swenson, *Medical Women*; Penner, *Victorian Medicine and Social Reform*.

57. Poovey, *Uneven Developments*, 169. Furneaux qualifies the mythologized figuration of Nightingale (in concert with Queen Victoria) as they provided reparations for the shame of military failures and the sanitary treatment of the wounded: she notes how their images and cultural work displaced the intimate, tactical, and medical attention male orderlies provided for the wounded soldiers. *Military Men of Feeling*, 204–8.

58. Charles Kingsley, "Preface to the Fourth Edition," in *The Works of Charles Kingsley* (Philadelphia: John D. Morris, 1889), xv–xvi. The cited preface is dated February 7, 1856.

59. Kingsley, "Preface to the Fourth Edition," xvi. Catherine Marsh was a well-known philanthropist who devoted herself to the poor both financially and through Biblical education.

60. Charles Kingsley, "The Science of Health," in *Sanitary and Social Lectures and Essays* (London: Macmillan & Co., 1880), 18. Hereafter cited in the text as *SOH*.

61. Charles Kingsley, "The Massacre of the Innocents," in *Sanitary and Social Lectures and Essays* (London: Macmillan, 1880), 151–52. Hereafter cited in the text as *MOI*.

62. Florence Nightingale, *Notes on Nursing: What It Is, and What It Is Not* (New York: D. Appleton, 1860), 13–14. In the vein of literary influences on medicine, Louise Penner argues that the genre of sensation fiction shapes passages such as the above. Penner, *Victorian Medicine and Social Reform*, 24–25.

63. Charles Kingsley, "Mad World, My Masters," *Frasier's Magazine* 57, no. 337 (January 1858), 133. Choi links Kingsley's claim that sanitary reform did not appeal to many individuals to difficulty in seeing the links between action and effect with the narrative logic of contagionism in *Two Years Ago*. Choi, *Anonymous Connections*, 65.

64. Catherine Gallagher, *The Industrial Reformation of English Fiction* (Chicago: University of Chicago Press, 1995), 118. See also Mooney, *Intrusive Inerventions*, 123–25, 180–81.

65. Foucault, *The Birth of the Clinic*, 33.

66. Florence Nightingale, *Florence Nightingale to Her Nurses* (London: Macmillan, 1914), 113–14.

67. Florence Nightingale, *Postscript to George H. De'Ath's Cholera: What Can We Do About It?* (Buckingham: Walford, 1892), 18–19.

68. Gilbert, *Cholera and Nation*, 157. See also Laura Fasik, "Charles Kingsley's Scientific Treatment of Gender" in *Muscular Christianity: Embodying the Victorian Age*, ed. Donald Hall (Cambridge, UK: Cambridge University Press, 1994), 94.

69. Gilbert, 176.

70. "Two Years Ago by Charles Kingsley," *The British Foreign and Evangelical Review* 7, no. 13 (1858): 140.

71. Philip Williamson, "State Prayers, Fasts and Thanksgivings: Public Worship in Britain 1830–1897," *Past & Present* 200, no. 1 (2008): 137, 166.

72. Charles Kingsley, "Morning Sermon on the Day of Humiliation for Cholera [delivered at] Eversley Church," 5 October 1849, Charles Kingsley Papers (1819–1875), Wellcome Archives & Manuscripts, MS.3108, Wellcome Trust Library, UK: 11–12.

73. Gilbert, *Cholera and Nation*, 183.

74. "Two Years Ago," *Putnam's Monthly Magazine of American Literature, Science, and Art* 9, no. 53 (1857): 506.

75. Kingsley, *True Words*, 138.

76. Lyons, *A Treatise on Fever*, 8.

77. See Poovey, *Uneven Developments*, 127.

78. Charles Kingsley, "The Fall," in *Sermons on National Subjects* (London: Macmillan, 1885), 412–422.

79. Hamlin has also identified the relationship between disease, nature, and sin in Kingsley's writings. Hamlin, *Cholera*, 87–89, 94.

80. Gilbert, *Cholera and Nation*, 159, 5.

81. Kingsley, *True Words*, 132.

82. Goodlad, *Victorian Literature and the Victorian State*, 19–21. Foucault also suggests that when we talk about the pastoral, we are talking about the history of the subject. Foucault, *Security, Territory, Population*, 184, 200, 234.

83. Cf. *Alton Locke*: "The only way to write songs—to let some air get possession of one's whole soul, and gradually inspire the words for itself." Charles Kingsley, *Alton Locke* (London: Macmillan, 1862), 189.

84. Charles Kingsley, "The Two Breaths," in *Health and Education* (London: W. Ibster, 1874). Kingsley connects this process to infectious disease: "Sir James Simpson tells in his lectures to the working-classes of Edinburgh, when at a Christmas meeting thirty-six persons danced all night in a small room with a low ceiling, keeping the doors and windows shut. The atmosphere of the room was noxious beyond description; and the effect was, that seven of the party were soon after seized with typhus fever, of which two died" (28).

85. Kingsley, "The Two Breaths," 30. *Carbonic acid* was the nineteenth-century term for carbon dioxide.

86. Charles Kingsley, "Life and Death," in *Twenty-Five Village Sermons* (London: John Parker, 1849), 32. In "The Resurrection," Kingsley contends that it is God's spirit that keeps decay away from Christ's body; that is why his body remains alive and does not submit to physical corruption. Charles Kingsley, "The Resurrection," in *Twenty-Five Village Sermons* (London: John Parker, 1849), 182.

87. Kingsley, "Cholera, 1866," 198.

88. Foucault, *Society Must Be Defended*, 244. See also Cooter's discussion of endemic and epidemic disease, "War and Epidemics," 287–88.

89. Carpenter, *Health, Medicine, and Society*, 34.

90. Frances Kingsley, ed., *Charles Kingsley: His Letters and Memories of His Life*, vol. 2 (London: Macmillan, 1894), 339.

91. The Public Health Act of 1848 gave local health boards the power to regulate environmental health risks such as public works. These laws were productive rather than punitive, as the public had the power to enact local boards if 10 percent of the population petitioned for it. The Sanitary Act of 1866 compelled local boards to act and if they failed to do so, gave towns the power to appoint sanitary inspectors to force the home secretary (the local police authority) to remove "nuisance."

92. Kingsley, "Morning sermon on the Day of Humiliation for Cholera," 11–12.

93. Kingsley would write about this phenomenon in "Cheap Clothes and Nasty," indicating that upper-class consumers were still prey to disease because of the conditions in which goods were produced. Charles Kingsley [Parson Lot, pseud.] *Cheap Clothes and Nasty* (London: Macmillan, 1850).

94. The Great Stink of 1858 was characterized by an unusually hot August with temperatures that made the human waste in the Thames significantly more odorous than normal. Despite Snow's work, people thought the stink to be a cause of disease. Ultimately, the noxious event proved to be a significant factor in the development of a new sewer system.

Chapter 3

1. Here, it is worth parsing the difference between *isolation* and *quarantine* in the most technical sense, as I use quarantine as a broader rubric that encompasses both. Although the terms were and continue to be used interchangeably, in the strictest sense, the former denotes isolation of persons infected, while the latter is defined by the separation and restriction of movement to infected persons and those exposed or possibly exposed to an infectious disease. Isolation tends to occur in hospitals, while quarantine can occur in public or private spaces like a home. On the changing emphasis from quarantine to isolation, see Mooney, *Intrusive Interventions*, 7; Kerr, *Contagion, Isolation, and Biopolitics*, 31–33.

2. For a representative sampling of these overlapping tacks see Arata, "The Occidental Tourist. 'Dracula' and the Anxiety of Reverse Colonization"; Jordan Kistler, "Rethinking the New Woman in *Dracula*," *Gothic Studies* 20, no. 1–2 (2018): 244–56; Carol A. Senf, "'Dracula': Stoker's Response to the New Woman," *Victorian Studies* 26, no. 1 (1982): 33–49; Jack Halberstam, "Technologies of Monstrosity: Bram Stoker's "Dracula," *Victorian Studies* 36, no. 3 (1993): 333–35; Christine Ferguson, *Language, Science and Popular Fiction in the Victorian Fin-de-Siècle: The Brutal Tongue* (Aldershot, UK: Ashgate, 2006); Kathleen L. Spencer, "Purity and Danger: Dracula, the Urban Gothic, and the Late Victorian Degeneracy Crisis," *ELH* 59, no. 1 (1992); Kelly Hurley, *The Gothic Body: Sexuality, Materialism, and Degeneration at the Fin de Siècle* (Cambridge, UK:

Cambridge University Press, 1996); Diana Louis Shahinyan, "That Which Mere Modernity Cannot Kill': The Evolution of Legal Professionalism in Bram Stoker's Dracula," *Journal of Victorian Culture* 23, no 1 (2018): 119–36; Nicholas Daly, "Incorporated Bodies: Dracula and the Rise of Professionalism," *Texas Studies in Literature and Language* 39, no. 2 (1997): 181–203.

3. Daly, "Incorporated Bodies," 185–86.

4. Carol A. Senf, *Science and Social Science in Bram Stoker's Fiction* (London: Greenwood Press, 2002), 22.

5. John William Springthorpe, "The Battle of Life," *Australasian Medical Gazette* 15 (1896); Charles-Edward Amory Winslow, "The War against Disease," *Atlantic Monthly* 91, no. 543 (January 1903); "Unseen Enemies," *London Times*, May 22, 1880, 6e; C. H. Leibbrand, "How London Fights the Microbe," *Windsor Magazine*, May 1899, 657–62.

6. See, for instance, Springthorpe, "The Battle of Life." Choi provides a more in-depth reading of a number of these prose texts in conversation with fiction. Choi, *Anonymous Connections*, 132–37.

7. Bruno Latour documents and outlines the relationship between the French military, government, and Pasteur's laboratory. While relevant and helpful, I take another tack in this project, not only in scope, but in eschewing the confounding metaphorical usages related to war and force in my argument. *The Pasteurization of France* (Cambridge, MA: Harvard University Press), 13–59, 114–16.

8. Winslow, "The War against Disease," 43.

9. Ernest Wende, "The Microscope in the Diagnosis of Diseases of the Skin," *Cincinnati-Lancet*, June 4, 1887, 707. On the shift from the histological focus of "Hospital Medicine" to the cellular and biochemical in "Laboratory Medicine," see Jewson, "The Disappearance of the Sick-Man."

10. In addition to Choi, some of the more sustained readings related to disease and etiology include Jens Lohfert Jørgensen, "Bacillophobia: Man and Microbes in *Dracula*, the *War of the Worlds*, and *The Nigger of the 'Narcissus*,'" *Critical Survey* 27, no. 2 (2015); Ross G. Forman, "A Parasite for Sore Eyes: Rereading Infection Metaphors in Bram Stoker's Dracula," *Victorian Literature and Culture* 44, no. 4 (2016); Emilie Taylor-Brown, "'She Has a Parasite Soul!' The Pathologization of the Gothic Monster as Parasitic Hybrid in Bram Stoker's *Dracula*, Richard Marsh's *The Beetle*, and Arthur Conan Doyle's 'The Parasite,'" in *Monsters and Monstrosity from the Fin de Siècle to the Millennium: New Essays*, eds. Sharla Hutchison and Rebecca A. Brown (Jefferson, NC: McFarland, 2015); Jessica Howell, *Malaria and Victorian Fictions of Empire* (Cambridge, UK: Cambridge University Press, 2018); Martin Willis, "'The Invisible Giant,' 'Dracula,' and Disease," *Studies in the Novel* 39, no. 3 (2007); Tabitha Sparks, "Medical Gothic and the Return of the Contagious Diseases Acts in Stoker and Machen," *Nineteenth-Century Feminisms* 6 (2002); Laura Sagolla Croley, "The Rhetoric of Reform in Stoker's "Dracula": Depravity, Decline, and the Fin-De-Siècle 'Residuum,'" *Criticism* 37, no. 1 (1995).

11. Choi, *Anonymous Connections*, 147.

12. Thomas M. Stuart, "Out of Time: Queer Temporality and Eugenic Monstrosity," *Victorian Studies* 60, no. 2 (2018): 219.

13. Bram Stoker, *Dracula: Authoritative Text, Contexts, Reviews and Reactions, Dramatic and Film Variations, Criticism*, eds. Nina Auerbach and David J. Skal (New York: W. W. Norton, 1997), 106. Hereafter cited parenthetically in the text as *D*.

14. William Shakespeare, *Othello: The Moor of Venice*, ed. Michael Neill (Oxford, UK: Oxford University Press, 2006), 390.

15. John Twyning, *Forms of English History in Literature, Landscape, and Architecture* (Houndmills, UK: Palgrave Macmillan, 2014), 214–15. The Red Cross became an icon of the Crusades after the thirteenth century. While acknowledging that it served as a standard for other nations such as France, Victorian historians addressed the fact that it was an early emblem of English culture. In 1854, George Proctor writes, "The red cross of St. George was our early national emblem, and still proudly floats on the banner which 'a thousand years has braved the battle and the breeze.'" *History of the Crusades: Their Rise, Progress, and Results* (Glasgow, UK: Richard Griffin 1854), 14.

16. "Recent Novels," *Spectator*, July 31, 1897, 151.

17. Twyning, *Forms of English History*, 214.

18. Patrick Brantlinger, *Taming Cannibals: Race and the Victorians* (Ithaca, NY: Cornell University Press, 2011), 67. See also Daniel Pick, *Faces of Degeneration: A European Disorder, c. 1848–c. 1918* (Cambridge, UK: Cambridge University Press, 1999).

19. Stephen Daniels, "Mapping National Identities: The Culture of Cartography with Particular Reference to the Ordnance Survey," in *Imagining Nations*, ed. Geoffrey Cubitt (Manchester: Manchester University Press, 1998), 118–21.

20. Gilbert, *Mapping the Social Body*, 10.

21. Paul Dobraszczyk, "Mapping Sewer Spaces in mid-Victorian London," in *Dirt: New Geographies of Cleanliness and Contamination*, eds. Ben Campkin and Rosie Cox (New York: I. B. Tauris, 2007), 124.

22. Daniels, "Mapping National Identities," 120–21. Todd notes that Jonathan's reference to the ordnance maps are "descendant from military action" and representative "of the evolution from the direct control of colonial intervention in the eighteenth century to the manipulation of signifiers in the nineteenth." Macy Todd, "What Bram Stoker's Dracula Reveals about Violence," *English Literature in Transition, 1880–1920* 58, no. 3 (2015): 383.

23. Daniels, "Mapping National Identities," 120.

24. See Bram Stoker, *Bram Stoker's Notes for Dracula: A Facsimile Edition*, eds. Robert Eighteen-Bisang and Elizabeth Russell Miller (Jefferson, NC: McFarland, 2008), 227, 241, 313.

25. Arata, "The Occidental Tourist," 630.

26. Choi, *Anonymous Connections*, 147.

27. Fred Botting, *Gothic*, 2nd ed. (Florence: Taylor and Francis, 1999), 142; Jack Halberstam, "Technologies of Monstrosity: Bram Stoker's 'Dracula,'" 334–35.

28. The count compromises "their precious asset, the racial purity of their line of descent." Susan Zieger, *Inventing the Addict: Drugs, Race, and Sexuality in Nineteenth-Century British and American Literature* (Amherst: University of Massachusetts Press, 2008), 215.

29. Halberstam, "Technologies of Monstrosity," 337–39.

30. Sander L. Gilman, "Sexology, Psychoanalysis, and Degeneration: From a Theory of Race to a Race to Theory," in *Degeneration: The Dark Side of Progress*, eds. J. Edward Chamberlin and Sander L. Gilman (New York: Columbia University Press, 1985), 87.

31. Brantlinger, *Taming Cannibals*, 79.

32. Arata, "The Occidental Tourist," 627–29.

33. Howell, *Malaria and Victorian Fictions of Empire*, 175.

34. *Oxford English Dictionary Online*, s.v. "Lancet," accessed December 10, 2013, http://www.oed.com/view/Entry/105422?redirectedFrom=lancet&.

35. Choi, *Anonymous Connections*, 146.

36. Foucault, *The History of Sexuality*, 147.

37. Though blood transfusion had been attempted numerous times, effective anticoagulants were not identified until 1894, and it was another twenty-one years before that discovery transferred to mainstream practice. Transfusion was not safe until the discovery of blood types in the early twentieth century. P. Learoyd, "The History of Blood Transfusion Prior to the 20th Century, Part 2," *Transfusion Medicine* 22, no. 6 (2012): 375–76.

38. Howell, *Malaria and Victorian Fictions of Empire*, 175.

39. Willis, "The Invisible Giant," 316.

40. Sparks, "Medical Gothic and the Return of the Contagious Diseases Acts," 94.

41. Sparks, *The Doctor in the Victorian Novel*, 22.

42. Judith R. Walkowitz, *Prostitution and Victorian Society: Women, Class, and the State* (Cambridge, UK: Cambridge University Press, 1980); Judith R. Walkowitz, *City of Dreadful Delight: Narratives of Sexual Danger in Late-Victorian London* (Chicago: University of Chicago Press, 1992); Pamela K. Gilbert, *Disease, Desire, and the Body in Victorian Women's Popular Novels* (Cambridge, UK: Cambridge University Press, 1997).

43. Walkowitz, *Prostitution and Victorian Society*, 48, 76.

44. Walkowitz, 88.

45. Walkowitz, 78; Philippa Levine, "Venereal Disease, Prostitution, and the Politics of Empire: The Case of British India," *Journal of the History of Sexuality* 4, no. 4 (1994): 580.

46. Levine, "Venereal Disease," 583.

47. Léopold Lambert, *Weaponized Architecture: The Impossibility of Innocence* (New York: DPR-Barcelona, 2012), 21–22.

48. Maria Isabel Romero Ruiz, "Fallen Women and the London Lock Hospitals and By-Laws of 1840 (Revised 1848)," *Journal of English Studies* 8, no. 141 (2010): 147.

49. Ruiz, "Fallen Women and the London Lock Hospitals," 147.

50. Walkowitz, *Prostitution and Victorian Society*, 59.

51. Sparks, *The Doctor in the Victorian Novel*, 90.

52. Frank Mort, *Dangerous Sexualities: Medico-Moral Politics in England since 1830* (New York: Routledge & Kegan Paul, 1987), 10–11.

53. Kimeya Baker, "The Contagious Diseases Acts and the Prostitute: How Disease and the Law Controlled the Female Body," *UCL Journal of Law and Jurisprudence* 1, no. 1 (2012): 93.

54. Butler, *The Constitution Violated*, 91.

55. Sparks, "Medical Gothic and the Return of the Contagious Diseases," 87.

56. Sparks, *The Doctor in the Victorian Novel*, 117–19, 112.

57. Christopher Craft, "'Kiss Me with Those Red Lips': Gender and Inversion in Bram Stoker's Dracula," *Representations*, no. 8 (1984): 121–22.

58. *The Era* 7 (August 1987), quoted in Taylor-Brown, "'She Has a Parasite Soul!,'" 27n8.

59. See Nina Auerbach's note in Stoker, *Dracula: Authoritative Text*, 248n6.

60. Todd, "What Bram Stoker's Dracula Reveals about Violence," 363.

61. Matthew L. Newsom Kerr, *Contagion, Isolation, and Biopolitics in Victorian London* (Gewerbestrasse, Switzerland: Palgrave Macmillan, 2018), 60–61. For a more expansive look at the inimicalization of animals specifically as disease vectors (spreaders) and reservoirs, see Christos Lynteris (ed.), *Framing Animals as Epidemic Villains: Histories of Non-Human Disease* (Gewerbestrasse, Switzerland: Palgrave, 2019), 5.

62. Anne Stiles, *Popular Fiction and Brain Science in the Late Nineteenth Century* (Cambridge, UK: Cambridge University Press, 2012), 50–84.

63. James Y. Simpson, in *The Works of Sir James Y. Simpson*, vol. II, ed. W. G. Simpson (Edinburgh: Adam & Charles Black, 1871): 544–45. Emphasis in the original.

64. Kerr, *Contagion, Isolation, and Biopolitics*, 60.

65. William Budd, "Can the Government, Further, Beneficially Intervene in the Prevention of Infectious Diseases?" in *Transactions of the National Association for the Promotion of Social Science: Bristol Meeting 1869*, ed. Edwin Pears (London: Longmans, Green, Reader, & Dyer, 1870), 392.

66. Budd, "Can the Government, Further, Beneficially Intervene," 400. My discussion here follows Kerr's reading of this passage, when he suggests that Budd uses the analogy of war to justify authority and the necessity of controlling contagion. Kerr, *Contagion, Isolation, and Biopolitics*, 61.

67. "Social Science Association," *Lancet* 94, no. 2406 (1869): 522–23. Emphasis added.

68. Budd, "Can the Government, Further, Beneficially Intervene," 396, 399.

69. Editorial, *Times*, October 5, 1869, 7. Emphasis added.

70. Quoted in Aidan Forth, *Barbed-Wire Imperialism: Britain's Empire of Camps, 1876–1903* (Oakland: University of California Press, 2017), 78.

71. Forth, 78–79.

72. "The Black Death," *All The Year Round* no. 569, October 25, 1879, 436–41.

73. "The Black Death," 437, 440–41.

74. Carol Margaret Davison, *Anti-Semitism and British Gothic Literature* (London: Palgrave Macmillan, 2004), 44–45.

75. Maud Ellmann, *The Nets of Modernism: Henry James, Virginia Woolf, James Joyce, and Sigmund Freud* (Cambridge: Cambridge University Press, 2010), 19.

76. Ellmann, *The Nets of Modernism*, 20.

77. Iqbal Akhtar Khan, "Plague: The Dreadful Visitation Occupying the Human Mind for Centuries," *Transactions of the Royal Society of Tropical Medicine and Hygiene* 98, no. 5 (2004): 273. The bacillus was discovered in 1894, but the role of rats was not recognized until 1898, one year after the novel was published.

78. Christopher Herbert, "Rat Worship and Taboo in Mayhew's London," *Representations*, no. 23 (1988): 15. Herbert's reading also indicates that rats were associated with the taboo, primitive, and sexual, and the belief that they consume and produce filth. Consistent with the blurry boundaries between disease theories, it is also important to note both the contagious and the miasmic qualities of the rat. Mayhew, for instance, writes that "Rats have the ability to communicate un-cleanness to whatever they [touch]." Mayhew, *London Labour and the London Poor*, vol. 3, 6. See Herbert, "Rat Worship," 14. As Lynteris notes, even with the bacteriological identification of rats as carriers of plague at the end of the nineteenth century, the idea of rats as carriers or spreaders (along with mosquitoes for yellow fever and malaria) was "itself already complicated by an already-established stratum of signification, by which by the mid-seventeenth century, had led to the introduction of new symbolic and ontological and legal frameworks for thinking about vermin," *Framing Animals as Epidemic Villains*, 3.

79. Charlotte Stoker, typeset transcription, "Account of the Cholera Outbreak in Ireland in 1832," 11076/2/3: 6, Papers of the Stoker Family, Trinity College Archives and Manuscripts.

80. Raymond T. McNally and Radu Florescu, *In Search of Dracula: The History of Dracula and Vampires* (Boston: Houghton Mifflin, 1994), 137.

81. Charlotte Stoker, "Account of the Cholera Outbreak," 1.

82. Willis, "The Invisible Giant," 311.

83. Croley, "The Rhetoric of Reform," 89.

84. Croley, 88.

85. Willis, *Vision, Science, and Literature*, 18.

86. Otis and Choi have made similar arguments about the reproductive and penetrative qualities attached to germ theory. Choi, *Anonymous Connections*, 133–35; Otis, *Membranes*, 5.

87. Jørgensen, "Bacillophobia," 40. See also Willis, "The Invisible Giant."

88. Zieger, *Inventing the Addict*, 229.

89. Budd, "Can the Government, Further, Beneficially Intervene," 390.

90. Taylor-Brown, "She Has a Parasite Soul!" 27n6. See also Douglas Melvin Haynes, *Imperial Medicine: Patrick Manson and the Conquest of Tropical Disease* (Philadelphia: University of Pennsylvania Press, 2001).

91. Emilie Taylor-Brown, "(Re)Constructing the Knights of Science: Parasitologists and Their Literary Imaginations." *Journal of Literature and Science* 7, no. 2 (2014): 62–64. See also Christopher Lawrence and Michael Brown's related history, "Quintessentially Modern Heroes: Surgeons, Explorers, and Empire, c. 1840–1914," *Journal of Social History* 50, no. 1 (2016).

92. Emilie Taylor-Brown, "'Petty Larceny" and 'Manufactured Science': Nineteenth-Century Parasitology and the Politics of Replication" *Replication in the Long Nineteenth Century* eds. Julie Codell and Linda K. Hughes (Edinburgh: Edinburgh University Press, 2018), 73.

93. I am indebted to Taylor-Brown for identifying this periodical source. Taylor-Brown, "(Re)Constructing the Knights of Science," 74. Please find the more extensive development of this argument in Emilie Taylor-Pirie (née Taylor-Brown), *Empire Under the Microscope: Parasitology and the British Literary Imagination, 1885–1935* (London: Palgrave, 2021).

94. Albert F. King, "Insects and Disease: Mosquitoes and Malaria," *Popular Science Monthly* 23 (1883): 644. See Forman, "A Parasite for Sore Eyes," 935.

95. Taylor-Brown, "She Has a Parasite Soul!," 13. See also Forman's reading of tropical medicine vis-à-vis the novel's "textual parasitism." Forman, "A Parasite for Sore Eyes," 927.

96. Willis, *Vision, Science, and Literature*, 23.

Chapter 4

1. Arthur Conan Doyle, "A Study in Scarlet," in *Sherlock Holmes: The Complete Novels and Stories*, vol. I (New York: Bantam Dell, 2003), 4. Hereafter cited parenthetically in the text as SS.

2. Otis, *Membranes*, 6.

3. O'Conner has made a similar argument about the way in which postcolonial criticism has used metaphors of hygiene to articulate the work of empire in relation to colonized peoples. *Raw Material*, 54–57.

4. Brown, "Cold Steel," 158.

5. Joseph W. Childers, "Foreign Matter: Imperial Filth," in *Filth: Dirt, Disgust, and Modern Life*, eds. William A. Cohen and Ryan Johnson (Minneapolis: University of Minnesota, 2006), 205.

6. Brown notes how for eugenicist Karl Pearson wars of conquest served as a "form of preparatory group cathesthics" that kept the nation, in Pearson's words, "up to a high pitch of external efficiency . . . by way of war with inferior races." Quoted in Brown, "Cold Steel," 157.

7. Lawrence Rothfield, *Vital Signs: Medical Realism in Nineteenth-Century Fiction* (Princeton: Princeton University Press, 1992), 141.

8. Jennifer Tucker, "Photography as Witness, Detective, and Impostor: Visual Representation in Victorian Science," in *Victorian Science in Context*, ed. Bernard Lightman (Chicago: University of Chicago Press, 1997), 394.

9. Joseph Bell, "Mr. Sherlock Holmes," in *A Study in Scarlet*, ed. Arthur Conan Doyle (London: Ward, Lock, & Bowden, 1893), 9.

10. Bell, 10.

11. Michael Worboys, *Spreading Germs: Disease Theories and Medical Practice in Britain, 1865–1900* (Cambridge, UK: Cambridge University Press, 2000), 31.

12. Warwick Anderson and Ian R. Mackay, *Intolerant Bodies: A Short History of Autoimmunity* (Baltimore: Johns Hopkins University Press, 2014), 28.

13. See for instance, Rudolph Virchow, "The Huxley Lecture on Recent Advances in Science and Their Bearing on Medicine and Surgery," *Lancet* 152, no. 3919 (1898); G. Murray Humphry et al., "A Discussion on Phagocytosis and Immunity," *British Medical Journal* 1, no. 1625 (1892); Joseph Lister, "An Address on the Present Position of Antiseptic Surgery," *British Medical Journal* 2, no. 1546 (1890); T. Spencer Wells, "The Bradshaw Lecture on Modern Abdominal Surgery," *British Medical Journal* 2, no. 1564 (1890): 1415. Spencer Wells, for instance, writes, "The phagocyte theory of Metchnikoff, or rather his observations upon the wandering cells or leukocytes by which the animal body protects itself against the attacks of bacteria—taking in the bacilli, digesting them, and so preventing their multiplication and diffusion—explains much that was almost incomprehensible in the relations of bacteria to wounds and to infective diseases," "Modern Abdominal Surgery," 1415.

14. John Burdon-Sanderson, "The Croonian Lectures on The Progress of Discovery Relating to the Origin and Nature of Infectious Diseases: Lecture III," *British Medical Journal* 2, no. 1612 (1891): 1084.

15. Burdon-Sanderson, 1086.

16. Cohen, *A Body Worth Defending*, 5. See also Esposito, *Immunitas*, 43. For a more complex understanding of immunity in more recent history that draws on affect, queer theory, animal studies, and new materialism, see Ahuja, *Bioinsecurities*.

17. Although I hesitate to make such an affirmative claim, Alvin Rodin and Jack Key suggest that his description of the leukocytes confirms knowledge

of Metchnikoff, whose first presentation on phagocytosis was published the same year as "Life and Death in Blood," and the engulfing capacity of leukocytes had been observed and published on as early as 1876. Jack D. Key and Alvin E. Rodin, *Medical Casebook of Doctor Arthur Conan Doyle: From Practitioner to Sherlock Holmes and Beyond* (Malabar: R. E. Krieger, 1984), 99.

18. "The Day of a Healthy Man," in *Harmsworth Popular Science*, vol. 1, ed. Arthur Mee (London: Educational Book Co., 1913), 73. The illustrator, G. F. Morrell, was a British artist and scientist who not only drew scientific illustrations but also political and military ones for the periodical press.

19. "The Day of a Healthy Man," 69.

20. Martin Booth, *The Doctor and the Detective: A Biography of Sir Arthur Conan Doyle* (New York: St. Martin's Minotaur, 2000), 101.

21. Arthur Conan Doyle, "Life and Death in the Blood," *Good Words* 24 (March 1883): 178. Hereafter cited parenthetically in the text as *LD*.

22. Quoted in Cohen, *A Body Worth Defending*, 260. Metchninkoff speaks of the leukocytes as phagocytes as they engage in phagocytosis—literally "cell eating."

23. Taylor-Brown cites helminthologist T. Spencer Cobbod: "[Entozoa are] a peculiar fauna, destined to occupy an equally peculiar territory. That territory is the widespread domain of the interior bodies of man and animals. Each animal or 'host' may be regarded as a continent, and each part or viscus of his body may be noted as a district," *Under the Microscope*.

24. Childers, "Foriegn Matter"; Otis, *Membranes*; Christopher Pittard, *Purity and Contamination in Late Victorian Detective Fiction* (Burlington, VT: Ashgate, 2011).

25. Deborah Brunton, *Medicine Transformed: Health, Disease and Society in Europe, 1800–1930* (Manchester: Manchester University Press in association with the Open University, 2004), 243.

26. Willis, *Vision, Science, and Literature*, 36–38.

27. Rothfield, *Vital Signs*, 142.

28. Doyle, "The Adventure of the Copper Beeches," 500.

29. Meegan Kennedy, *Revising the Clinic: Vision and Representation in Victorian Medical Narrative and the Novel* (Columbus: Ohio State University Press, 2010), 157–59.

30. Willis, *Vision, Science, and Literature*, 19.

31. Willis, 18.

32. Otis, *Membranes*, 105.

33. Susan Cannon Harris, "Pathological Possibilities: Contagion and Empire in Doyle's Sherlock Holmes Stories," *Victorian Literature and Culture* 31, no. 2 (2003): 449.

34. Harris, 449.

35. Monkshood is a common name for Aconitum, also known as "wolfsbane," a flower. The active toxin, aconitine, has a history in nineteenth-century

military medicine and imperialism. During the Indian Mutiny of 1857, Indian chefs tried to poison a British detachment by adulterating a soup with it. This account is given in Reginald Garton Wilberforce, *An Unrecorded Chapter of the Indian Mutiny: Being the Personal Reminiscences of Reginald G. Wilberforce, Late 52nd Light Infantry, Compiled from a Diary and Letters Written on the Spot* (London: John Murray, 1894), 88–89. The story goes that when the chefs refused to taste their own preparation, the British troops gave it to a monkey, who subsequently died—a trial reminiscent of Holmes' using a terrier to test a mysterious pill, which turns out to be poison, in *A Study in Scarlet*. In the twentieth century, the Soviets investigated its use as a chemical weapon. Salahuddin Malik, "The Panjab and the Indian 'Mutiny': A Reassessment," *Islamic Studies* 15, no. 2 (1976): 95.

36. Arthur Conan Doyle, *The Parasite: A Story* (New York: Harper and Brothers, 1894), 3.

37. Cohen, *A Body Worth Defending*, 202.

38. Quoted in Cohen, 202.

39. Cohen, 193.

40. See Lisa Cartwright, *Screening the Body: Tracing Medicine's Visual Culture* (Minneapolis: University of Minnesota Press, 1995), 26.

41. Cohen, *A Body Worth Defending*, 202. See also Shira Shmuely, "Curare: The Poisoned Arrow that Entered the Laboratory and Sparked a Moral Debate," *Social History of Medicine*, published online prior to print, accessed March 16, 2019, https://doi.org/10.1093/shm/hky124.

42. According to Eliot S. Valenstein, Bernard began experimenting with the toxin in 1840 after a friend gave him the substance, claiming he had acquired it from an African native. Elliot S. Valenstein, *The War of the Soups and the Sparks: The Discovery of Neurotransmitters and the Dispute over How Nerves Communicate* (New York: Columbia University Press, 2007), 4–5.

43. Arthur Conan Doyle, "The Sign of Four," in *Sherlock Holmes: The Complete Novels and Stories: Volume I* (New York: Bantam Dell, 2003), 162. Hereafter cited parenthetically in the text as *SOF*.

44. Arthur Conan Doyle, "The Adventure of the Speckled Band" in *Sherlock Holmes: The Complete Novels and Stories: Volume I* (New York: Bantam Dell, 2003), 422.

45. For a discussion of this as it relates to orthodox medicine and quackery in Doyle, see Sylvia A. Pamboukian, *Doctoring the Novel: Medicine and Quackery from Shelley to Doyle* (Athens: Ohio University Press, 2012), chapter 4.

46. Arthur Conan Doyle to *The Hampshire County Times*, Portsmouth, 27 July 1887, "Compulsory Vaccination," in *Letters to the Press*, eds. J. M. Gibson and R. L. Green (Iowa City: University of Iowa Press, 1986): 31.

47. Childers, "Foreign Matter," 217.

48. Childers, 218.

49. Doyle, "Compulsory Vaccination."

50. Steve M. Blevins and Michael S. Bronze, "Robert Koch and the 'Golden Age' of Bacteriology," *International Journal of Infectious Diseases* 14, no. 9 (2010): e747.

51. Quoted in Bernd Rosslenbroich, *On the Origin of Autonomy: A New Look at the Major Transitions in Evolution* (New York: Springer, 2016), 26.

52. Cohen, *A Body Worth Defending*, 196, 199.

53. Cohen, 258.

54. Cohen, 196.

55. Bruno Latour, *The Pasteurization of France* (Cambridge, MA: Harvard University Press, 1993), 123.

56. Georges Canguilhem, *The Normal and the Pathological* (New York: Zone Books, 1989), chapter 2.

57. Bernard does not give this example of tuberculosis, but it helps exemplify his theories on pathology. In further detail: the body's macrophages identify the bacteria in the lung alveoli, causing these immune system agents to "attack" the alveoli. The macrophages attempt to engulf the bacteria, but they cannot do so completely, and the bacteria infect the macrophages themselves, feeding on them to reproduce. The immune system forms a wall around the area in which this occurs, known as a granuloma. This either creates scar tissue or causes the cordoned tissue to necrotize, producing the blood, sputum, and dead, non-functioning tissue that ultimately suffocates the individual—instead of the alveolar sacs providing gas exchange, the lungs fill with fluid, making breathing impossible. The case demonstrates how the actual processes that cause signs and symptoms are, in fact, normal physiological functions. Leonard V. Crowley, *An Introduction to Human Disease: Pathology and Pathophysiology Correlations* (Burlington, VT: Jones & Bartlett Learning, 2013), 386–89.

58. Quoted in Cohen, *A Body Worth Defending*, 260.

59. Quoted in Cohen, 260.

60. Anderson and Mackay, *Intolerant Bodies*, 28.

61. Burdon-Sanderson, "The Croonian Lectures on The Progress of Discovery Relating to the Origin and Nature of Infectious Diseases: Lecture III." *Lancet* 138, no. 3560 (1891): 1154. Succinct phrasing quoted here from the abbreviated speech as printed the *Lancet*, but for additional detail see also the more expansive explanation in the speech of the same title in the *British Medical Journal* 2, no. 1612 (1891), 1084–1087.

62. Burdon-Sanderson, "The Croonian Lectures on The Progress of Discovery Relating to the Origin and Nature of Infectious Diseases: Lecture IV," *British Medical Journal* 2, no. 1613 (1891): 1139.

63. Arthur Conan Doyle, "Dr. Koch and His Cure," *Review of Reviews* 2, no. 12 (December 1890): 556. Hereafter cited parenthetically in the text as KC.

64. At the beginnings of pharmacology and in its broadest definition, *chemotherapy* denotes the use of specific chemical agents as treatments for specific diseases.

65. Quoted in Otis, *Membranes*, 33.

66. Thomas Goetz, *The Remedy: Robert Koch, Arthur Conan Doyle, and the Quest to Cure Tuberculosis* (New York: Gotham, 2014), 172.

67. Otis, *Membranes*, 109–10.

68. Rosemary Rees, *Poverty and Public Health, 1815–1948* (Oxford: Heinemann, 2001), 82.

69. This poor health of the Boer War recruits was a well-known interpretation of significance to Victorian and Edwardian culture. See John Peck, *War, the Army, and Victorian Literature* (New York: St. Martin's Press, 1998).

70. Peck, 165.

71. Arthur Conan Doyle, *The Great Boer War* (London: Smith, Elder & Co., 1900), 337. Hereafter cited in the text as *BW*.

72. Howell, notes that the struggle against malaria, for instance, "in colonial environments was explicitly struggled as a struggle between races," citing for instance Ronald Ross's characterization of malaria as "the principle and gigantic ally of Barbarism," *Malarial Fictions of Empire*, 7. Read in this way, the Boer's have been hardened by their survival against disease and pathogenic environment.

73. See Brown, "Cold Steel," 158.

74. Otis, *Membranes*, 94; Peck, *War, the Army, and Victorian Literature*, 166.

75. Arthur Conan Doyle, *The War in South Africa: Its Causes and Conduct* (New York: McClure, Phillips, 1902), 10. Hereafter cited parenthetically in the text as *WS*.

76. Otis, *Membranes*, 94.

77. Otis, 94.

78. V. J. Cirillo, "Arthur Conan Doyle (1859–1930): Physician During the Typhoid Epidemic in the Anglo-Boer War (1899–1902)," *Journal of Medical Biography* 22, no. 1 (2014): 5.

79. Reid, *The Biopolitics of the War on Terror*, 13, 18.

80. Arthur Conan Doyle, *Memories and Adventures* (Cambridge, UK: Cambridge University Press, 2012), 159.

81. Brown, "Cold Steel," 158.

82. Arthur Conan Doyle, "The War in South Africa, the Epidemic of Enteric Fever at Bloemfontein," *British Medical Journal* 2, no. 2062 (1900): 49.

83. Doyle, 49. For the affective dimension of male orderlies from the midcentury, see Furneaux, *Military Men of Feeling*,

84. Brown, "Cold Steel," 169–74.

85. Harold Ellis, *A History of Surgery* (London: Greenwich Medical Media, 2001), 137.

86. Ellis, 137.

87. See Anne Hardy, "'Straight Back to Barbarism': Antityphoid Inoculation and the Great War, 1914," *Bulletin of the History of Medicine* 74, no. 2 (2000): 269.

88. Hardy, 269.

89. Hardy, 284.

90. William Osler, "Bacilli and Bullets": https://www.google.com/books/edition/Bacilli_and_Bullets/Zknc3L3JxgEC?hl=en&gbpv=1&dq=Bacilli+and+Bullets&pg=PA3&printsec=frontcover](London: Oxford University Press, 1914), 8. Emphasis in the original.

91. Hardy, "Straight Back to Barbarism," 288.

92. This argument has notably also been made by Hannah Arendt in her linkage of the racial origins of imperialism to the Holocaust. See *The Origins of Totalitarianism* (New York: Harcourt, Brace & World, 1966). For a more recent analysis from Black studies, questioning the centrality of the concentration camp in the history of biopolitics versus the plantation, see Alexander G. Weheliye, *Habeas Viscus* (Durham, NC: Duke University Press, 2014), 34–36.

93. Forth, *Barbed-Wire Imperialism*, 5, 23.

94. See Arnold, *Colonizing the Body*; Paul Rabinow, *French Modern: Norms and Forms of the Social Environment* (Cambridge, MA: MIT Press, 1989); Frederick Cooper and Ann Laura Stoler, "Between Metropole and Colony," in *Tensions of Empire: Colonial Cultures in a Bourgeois World*, eds. Frederick Cooper and Ann Laura Stoler (Berkeley: University of California Press, 2009).

95. Forth, *Barbed-Wire Imperialism*, 23.

96. Key and Rodin, *Medical Casebook of Doctor Arthur Conan Doyle*, 65.

97. Achille Mbembe, "Necropolitics," *Public Culture* 15, no. 1 (2003): 24.

98. Jane Lewis, "Providers, 'Consumers,' the State and the Delivery of Health Care in Twentieth-Century Britain," in *Medicine in Society: Historical Essays*, ed. Andrew Wear (Cambridge, UK: Cambridge University Press, 1992), 322.

99. Quoted in Peter D. McDonald, *British Literary Culture and Publishing Practice, 1880–1914* (Cambridge, UK: Cambridge University Press, 1997), 168.

100. Bell, "Mr. Sherlock Holmes," 10.

101. Other scholars have identified this story's use of bacteria as a "biological weapon." See, for instance, Setu K. Vora, "Sherlock Holmes and a Biological Weapon," *Journal of the Royal Society of Medicine* 95, no. 2 (2002).

102. Arthur Conan Doyle, "The Adventure of the Dying Detective," in *Sherlock Holmes: The Complete Novels and Stories*, vol. II (2003), 434. Hereafter cited as *DD* parenthetically in the text.

103. Otis, *Membranes*, 9.

104. Upamanyu Pablo Mukherjee, "'Out-of-the-Way Asiatic Disease': Contagion, Malingering, and Sherlock's England," in *Literature of an Independent England: Revisions of England, Englishness, and English Literature*, eds. Claire Westall and Michael Gardiner (New York: Palgrave Macmillan, 2013), 85.

105. Mukherjee, 88. Arendt suggests that the biological justification in Nazism finds its origins in the racial thinking of imperial ideology of nations like Britain, citing writers like Spencer and Huxley. Arendt, *The Origins of Totalitarianism*, 179–80.

106. Harris, "Pathological Possibilities," 463.
107. Mukherjee, "Out-of-the-Way Asiatic Disease," 84.
108. John Collie, *Malingering and Feigned Sickness* (London: Edward Arnold, 1913), 10.
109. Mukherjee, "Out-of-the-Way Asiatic Disease," 87.
110. Collie, *Malingering and Feigned Sickness*, 44.
111. See Cooter, "Of War and Epidemics," 300. On medical metaphor vis-à-vis industrialization, see O'Conner, *Raw Material*.
112. Arthur Conan Doyle, "The Adventure of the Blanched Soldier," in *Sherlock Holmes: The Complete Novels and Stories*, vol. II (New York: Bantam Dell, 2003), 539. Hereafter cited parenthetically in the text as BB.
113. Harris, "Pathological Possibilities," 463.
114. Peck, *War, the Army, and Victorian Literature*, 173.
115. Otis, *Membranes*, 102.
116. Otis, 102.
117. Arthur Conan Doyle, quoted in "This Week: Topics of the Day," *Medical Times and Gazette*, June 16, 1883, 671.
118. Yumna Siddiqi, *Anxieties of Empire and the Fiction of Intrigue* (New York: Columbia University Press, 2008), 68.
119. Harris, "Pathological Possibilities," 463.

Chapter 5

1. Ronald Ross, introduction to *Malaria, a Neglected Factor in the History of Greece and Rome* by William Henry Jones (Cambridge, MA: Macmillan & Bowes, 1907), 14.
2. Martin Bock, *Joseph Conrad and Psychological Medicine* (Lubbock: Texas Tech University Press, 2002); Charlotte Rogers, *Jungle Fever: Exploring Madness and Medicine in Twentieth-Century Tropical Narratives* (Nashville: Vanderbilt University Press, 2012). See Patrick Brantlinger, "Victorians and Africans: The Genealogy of the Myth of the Dark Continent," *Critical Inquiry* 12, no. 1 (1985): 29.
3. Cheryl Hindrichs, "'A Vision of Greyness': The Liminal Vantage of Illness in Heart of Darkness," *Modern Fiction Studies* 65, no. 1 (2019): 179.
4. Jean Aubry to Paul Wohlfart, 1936, "Joseph Conrad (1857–1924), novelist: notes on his health," Wellcome Archives & Manuscripts, MS.8512, Wellcome Trust Library, UK. I am indebted to my colleagues and friends Kathy Hardman and Ryan Sullivan for the translation of the French letter in this file.
5. Brantlinger, "Victorians and Africans," 193.
6. Deborah J. Neill, *Networks in Tropical Medicine: Internationalism, Colonialism, and the Rise of a Medical Specialty, 1890–1930* (Stanford, CA: Stanford

University Press, 2012), 21–23. Although, following other scholars, I discuss the "emergence of tropical medicine" as a late nineteenth-century development, it has much earlier roots. Military tracts on the subject appear as early as the late eighteenth century, such as Benjamin Moseley's *A Treatise on Tropical Diseases: On Military Operations; and on the Climate of the West-Indies* (London: T. Cadell, 1792). It was not, however, until the Scramble for Africa that tropical medicine became an institution.

7. Mbembe, "Necropolitics," 27.

8. Mbembe, 21, 40.

9. Mark S. Bailey, "A Brief History of British Military Experiences with Infectious and Tropical Diseases," *Journal of the Royal Army Medical Corps* 159, no. 3 (2013): 155.

10. Quoted in Adam Hochschild, *King Leopold's Ghost: A Story of Greed, Terror, and Heroism in Colonial Africa* (Boston: Houghton Mifflin, 1998), 44.

11. Hochschild, 123–24.

12. Mbemebe cites quinine as one of the technologies of empire. Mbembe, "Necropolitics," 25. See also Daniel R. Headrick, *The Tools of Empire: Technology and European Imperialism in the Nineteenth Century* (Oxford: Oxford University Press, 1981). In relation to these, although he focuses on the American colonization of the Philippines, Warwick Anderson's landmark work *Colonial Pathologies* (Durham, NC: Duke University Press, 2006) speaks to imperial hygiene as a tool of colonization. It is worth noting that quinine had been in use by the Peruvians, in the form of Cinchona bark, for some time before it was introduced to Europeans in the seventeenth century. After 1820, it could be extracted from the bark into its concentrated alkaloid form.

13. William Cohen, for instance, suggests that quinine's causal link to empire has been overestimated, specifically in the example of French imperialism. William B. Cohen, "Malaria and French Imperialism," *Journal of African History* 24, no. 1 (1983): 23–24.

14. Otis, *Membranes*, 33.

15. Haynes, *Imperial Medicine*, 7.

16. Martin Bock, "Joseph Conrad and Germ Theory: Why Captain Allistoun Smiles Thoughtfully," *Conradian* 31, no. 2 (2006): 7.

17. Joseph Conrad, *The Shadow Line: A Confession* (Garden City: Doubleday, 1917), 130.

18. Federation for the Defence of Belgian Interests Abroad, "The Death of Dr. Dutton," *The Truth on the Congo Free State* no. 21, 15 July 1905, 81.

19. Taylor-Brown, "(Re)Constructing the Knights of Science," 63.

20. Ronald Ross, "The Battle for Health in the Tropics," *Journal of Tropical Medicine and Hygiene* 7 (1904): 187.

21. Ross, introduction to *Malaria, a Neglected Factor* by Jones, 1.

22. Ross, 14.

23. It was actually French physiologist Alphonse Laveran who discovered the plasmodium parasite itself in 1880 while working in a military hospital. He would go on to be recognized and receive a Nobel Prize five years after Ross.

24. Ronald Ross, *Philosophies* (London: John Murray, 1923), 53. The book, originally published in 1910, dates the poem, "Reply," as written on August 21, 1897.

25. Otis, *Membranes*, 5.

26. Quoted in Taylor-Brown, "(Re)Constructing the Knights of Science," 48.

27. Ronald Ross, "Researches on Malaria," *Journal of the Royal Army Medical Corps* 4, no. 4 (1905): 451.

28. Patrick Manson, "The Malaria Parasite," *Journal of the Africa Society* 7, no. 13 (1907): 227. See Taylor-Pirie, *Empire under the Microscope*, forthcoming.

29. Howell, *Malarial Fictions of Empire*, 5–7. Howell's nuanced readings of the structure of malarial narratives, not only considers the inimical and racial antagonism presented, but also the affirmative, subversive possibilities afforded by cyclical fevers such as introspection, malleability, and adaptation, in contrast to many of the pejorative accounts in medical prose, 9–11.

30. Joseph Conrad, *Heart of Darkness: Authoritative Text, Backgrounds and Contexts, Criticism*, ed. Paul B. Armstrong (New York: W. W. Norton, 2006), 14. Hereafter cited in the text as HD.

31. See for instance *Encyclopædia Britannica*, 9th ed. (Chicago: Werner, 1895), s.v. "Malaria." In his novella *Victory*, set in what is now Indonesia, Conrad wrote about "the low, pestilential, mangrove-lined coast" of the protagonist's destination. Joseph Conrad, *Victory* (New York: Modern Library, 1915), xiv. Philip Manson-Bahr, Manson's son in law, notes that Manson also makes connections between the so-called "mangrove fly" and filariasis, a parasitic roundworm spread by black flies and mosquitoes in the early editions of *Manson's Tropical Diseases*. Philip H. Manson-Bahr, *Manson's Tropical Diseases* (New York: W. Wood, 1921), 633.

32. Ian Watt, *Conrad in the Nineteenth Century* (Berkeley: University of California Press, 1979), 219.

33. See, for instance, L. Westenra Sambon, "Acclimatization of Europeans in Tropical Lands," *Geographical Journal* 12, no. 6 (1898): 590.

34. Watt, *Conrad in the Nineteenth Century*, 270.

35. See Paul Johnson Byrne, "'Heart of Darkness': The Dream-Sensation and Literary Impressionism Revisited," *Conradian* 35, no. 2 (2010); Watt, *Conrad in the Nineteenth Century*.

36. The Maxim gun is often referred to as a "central tool of empire," along with railroads and steamships. Daniel R. Headrick, "Sleeping Sickness Epidemics and Colonial Responses in East and Central Africa, 1900–1940," *PLoS Neglected Tropical Diseases* 8, no. 4 (2014): e2772. https://doi.org/10.1371/journal.pntd.0002772. See also Headrick, *The Tools of Empire*, chapter 7. For a

reading of its ambiguous reception with respect to the perceived degenerating martial prowess and troubling destructive power, see Brown, "Cold Steel," 165–69.

37. Neill, *Networks in Tropical Medicine*, 21–22.

38. Neill, 23.

39. John Holt to Ronald Ross, 27 August 1906, "Material on Ross receiving the Officier de l'Ordre de Leopold II, Belgium in August 1906," Sir Ronald Ross Collection, GB 0809 Ross/162/12, London School of Tropical Medicine & Hygiene, London.

40. Brantlinger, "Victorians and Africans," 176.

41. Robert Marks, *The Origins of the Modern World: Fate and Fortune in the Rise of the West* (Lanham, MD: Rowman & Littlefield, 2007), 142. The market was previously dominated by the Dutch.

42. Henry Morton Stanley, *The Founding of the Congo Free State: A Story of Work and Exploration*, vol. II (London: Samson Low, Marston, Searle, & Rivington, 1885), 327.

43. This was an expedition to rescue a German doctor who had been appointed governor of Equatoria (now South Sudan and Uganda) and who was in danger from Mahdist forces. Stanley, still under Leopold's employment, made a deal with Leopold that he would take the longer route up the Congo to further develop it for the king. A number of scholars suggest that the Emin Pasha relief expedition was an inspiration for Marlow and his rescue narrative. See Watt, *Conrad in the Nineteenth Century*, 142.

44. See "Parke on Health in Africa," *London Medical Press and Circular* 108, no. 14 (1894). Parke was recognized outside medical circles and was included among the "distinguished Men and Women of the Time." G. Washington Moon, *Men and Women of the Time: A Dictionary of Contemporaries*, 13th ed. (London: George Routledge & Sons, 1891), 619.

45. Thomas Heazle Parke, *My Personal Experiences in Equatorial Africa, as Medical Officer of the Emin Pasha Relief Expedition* (New York: Charles Scribner's Sons, 1891), 480.

46. Parke, 480.

47. Quoted in Margaret M. Lock and Vinh-Kim Nguyen, *An Anthropology of Biomedicine* (Chichester: Wiley-Blackwell, 2010), 153.

48. Taylor-Brown, "(Re)Constructing the Knights of Science," 65. Brown and Lawerence make a related claim when comparing heroic rhetoric of imperial explorers like Stanley to modern surgeons, in terms of their affinities in practice, professional identity, public representation, and ideology. "Quintessentially Modern Heroes," 2.

49. Taylor-Pirie notes how the discourse of parasitology drew from archetypal "fairy-tale lexis of sword-fighting, dragon slaying, and giant killing," shifting the focus from the colonial subject to the colonial disease. *Empire Under the*

Microscope. This is a rhetoric that did not always turn out to be accurate in terms of the harming of colonial bodies, as Conrad's texts shows.

50. Bock, "Joseph Conrad and Germ Theory," 1.

51. It is possible but not likely that Conrad was referring specifically to the malaria plasmodium that Ross discovered. This research was not widely publicized until 1900, in a letter to the editor of the *Lancet*. See Ronald Ross, "The Relationship of Malaria and the Mosquito," *Lancet* 156, no. 4010 (1900). However, even in early germ theory, germs were often characterized as *parasites* in a broader sense of the term than tropical medicine and parasitology would adopt, which included protozoa (e.g., malaria plasmodium and toxoplasmosis), helminths (e.g., hookworms), ectoparasites (e.g., ticks), and the like.

52. Kiel J. Hume, "Time and the Dialectics of Life and Death in 'Heart of Darkness,'" *Conradian* 34, no. 2 (2009): 69.

53. Mbembe, "Necropolitics," 14.

54. Hume, "Time and the Dialectics," 70.

55. Mbembe, "Necropolitics," 40. Emphasis in the original.

56. Maryinez Lyons, *The Colonial Disease: A Social History of Sleeping Sickness in Northern Zaire, 1900–1940* (Cambridge, UK: Cambridge University Press, 1992), 12.

57. David Sherman, *In a Strange Room: Modernism's Corpses and Mortal Obligation* (Oxford: Oxford University Press, 2014), 16–17.

58. Edward W. Said, *Culture and Imperialism* (New York: Knopf, 1993), 30. Emphasis in the original.

59. Mbembe, "Necropolitics," 36–38.

60. Alex Houen, "Sacrificial Militancy and the Wars around Terror," in *Terror and the Postcolonial: A Concise Companion*, eds. Elleke Boehmer and Stephen Morton (Chichester: Wiley Blackwell, 2010), 131.

61. Arthur Conan Doyle, *The Crime of the Congo* (New York: Doubleday, 1909), 108–9.

62. Hume, "Time and the Dialectics," 65.

63. Allen MacDuffie, "Joseph Conrad's Geographies of Energy," *ELH* 76, no. 1 (2009): 90–91.

64. Lyons, *The Colonial Disease*, 13.

65. Lock and Nguyen, *An Anthropology of Biomedicine*, 148–49.

66. Lock and Nguyen characterize two more phases: the nationalist phase 1960–1980s; and the non-govermental phase, 1980 to the present. Lock and Nguyen, 18.

67. Neill, *Networks in Tropical Medicine*, 105.

68. Lyons, *The Colonial Disease*, 47.

69. I do not suggest that Stanley was the sole agent of the epidemic. Nevertheless, he is consistently identified as contributing to it, much as the violent changes to the environment by colonization more generally contributed; these

changes in terrain and population shaped the ecological factors for epidemics. Lyons, *The Colonial Disease*, 190; Roy Porter, *The Greatest Benefit to Mankind: A Medical History of Humanity* (New York: W. W. Norton, 1997), 476. See also Headrick, "Sleeping Sickness Epidemics and Colonial Responses."

70. Lyons, *The Colonial Disease*, 20. Nutritional deficiencies accounted for a significant portion of tropical disease (and still do). While they are pathogenic in and of themselves, they also lead to depressed immune function and a higher probability of microbial infection. Roger Casement suggests this in his "Congo Report" when he contends that many people fell prey to disease due to privation. Roger Casement, "Mr. Casement to the Marquess of Lansdowne," in *Africa. No. 1 (1904): Correspondence and Report from His Majesty's Consul at Boma Respecting the Administration of the Independent State of the Congo* (London: Harrison & Sons, 1904), 28.

71. Parke, *My Personal Experiences in Equatorial Africa*, 480.

72. See Doyle, *The Crime of the Congo*; Casement, "Mr. Casement to the Marquess of Lansdowne."

73. Hochschild, *King Leopold's Ghost*, 158–66.

74. Esposito, *Immunitas*, 147.

75. Otis, *Membranes*, 109.

76. Joseph Conrad to David Meldrum, 7 January 1902, in *The Collected Letters of Joseph Conrad, Volume 2: 1898–1902*, eds. Frederick R. Karl and Laurence Davis (Cambridge, UK: Cambridge University Press, 1986), 368. See also Martin Bock, "Disease and Medicine," in *Joseph Conrad in Context*, ed. Alan Simmons (Cambridge, UK: Cambridge University Press, 2009), 130.

77. Huxley, "The Connection of the Biological Sciences and Medicine," 429.

78. Quoted in Mannfred A. Hollinger, *Introduction to Pharmacology*, 3rd ed. (Abingdon, UK: CRC Press, 2007), 167.

79. John Parascandola, "The Theoretical Basis of Paul Ehrlich's Chemotherapy," *Journal of the History of Medicine and Allied Sciences* 36, no. 1 (1981): 20, 34.

80. Fèlix Bosch and Laia Rosich, "The Contributions of Paul Ehrlich to Pharmacology: A Tribute on the Occasion of the Centenary of His Nobel Prize," *Pharmacology* 82, no. 3 (2008): 172.

81. Quoted in Lyons, *The Colonial Disease*, 109.

82. Lyons, 109.

83. Lyons, 109.

84. Myriam Mertens, "Chemical Compounds in the Congo: Pharmaceuticals and the 'Crossed History' of Public Health in Belgian Africa (Ca. 1905–1939)" (PhD diss., University of Gent, 2014), 38, http://hdl.handle.net/1854/LU-4443278. See also Lawrence and Brown, "Quintessential Heroes."

85. See Neill, *Networks in Tropical Medicine*, 104.

86. Parascandola, "The Theoretical Basis of Paul Ehrlich's Chemotherapy," 31.

87. S. Riethmiller, "From Atoxyl to Salvarsan: Searching for the Magic Bullet," *Chemotherapy* 51, no. 5 (2005): 239.

88. Parascandola, "The Theoretical Basis of Paul Ehrlich's Chemotherapy," 31.

89. Huxley, "The Connection of the Biological Sciences and Medicine," 355.

90. D'Alembert, Jean le Rond. *Esprit, Maximes et Principes de D'Alembert, de l'Académie Française, &c.* (Paris: Chez Briand, 1789), 295.

91. Neill, *Networks in Tropical Medicine*, 16, 58, 63.

92. Mertens, "Chemical Compounds in the Congo," 33–34.

93. Mertens, 81.

94. Parascandola, "The Theoretical Basis of Paul Ehrlich's Chemotherapy," 35.

95. Lorenzo Zaffiri, Jared Gardner, and Luis H. Toledo-Pereyra, "History of Antibiotics: From Salvarsan to Cephalosporins," *Journal of Investigative Surgery* 25, no. 2 (2012): 68.

96. Paul de Kruif, *The Microbe Hunters* (New York: Blue Ribbon Books, 1926), 355.

97. For instance, consider how de Kruif characterizes Ehrlich's Latinate phrases as "battle cries" or how he describes the first animal test of Ehrlich's Compound 606: " 'Make the injection,' said Paul Ehrlich. And into the ear-vein of that rabbit went the clear yellow fluid of the solution of 606, for the first time to do battle with the disease of the loathsome name," *The Microbe Hunters*, 382.

98. John E. Lesch, *The First Miracle Drugs: How the Sulfa Drugs Transformed Medicine* (Oxford, UK: Oxford University Press, 2007), 5–10.

99. Ghislain Thibault, "Needles and Bullets: Media Theory, Medicine, and Propaganda, 1910–1940," in *Endemic: Essays in Contagion Theory*, eds. Kari Nixon and Lorenzo Servitje (London: Palgrave Macmillan, 2016), 67–92.

Collateral Damage

1. David Edgerton, "War and the Development of the British Welfare State," in *Warfare and Welfare: Military Conflict and Welfare State Development in Western Countries*, ed. Herbert Obinger (Oxford, UK: Oxford University Press, 2018), 201–2.

2. Marlieke E. A. de Kraker, Andrew J. Stewardson, and Stephan Harbarth, "Will 10 Million People Die a Year Due to Antimicrobial Resistance by 2050?" *PLoS Medicine* 13, no. 11(2016): e1002184, https://doi.org/10.1371/journal.pmed.1002184.

3. Brigitte Nerlich, " 'The Post-Antibiotic Apocalypse' and the 'War on Superbugs': Catastrophe Discourse in Microbiology, Its Rhetorical Form and Political Function," *Public Understanding of Science* 18, no. 5 (2009): 575; Nina Singh et al., "How Often Are Antibiotic-Resistant Bacteria Said to 'Evolve' in

the News?," *PLoS ONE* 11, no. 3 (2016): e0150396, https://doi.org/10.1371/journal.pone.0150396.

4. Hannah Landecker, "Antibiotic Resistance and the Biology of History," *Body & Society* 22, no. 4 (2015): 18.

5. John F. Cryan and Timothy G. Dinan, "Mind-Altering Microorganisms: The Impact of the Gut Microbiota on Brain and Behaviour," *National Review of Neuroscience* 13, no. 10 (2012): 701–2. For recent work on this topic in feminist science studies, see Elizabeth A. Wilson, *Gut Feminism* (Durham, NC: Duke University Press, 2016).

6. Nik Brown and Sarah Nettleton. "'There Is Worse to Come': The Biopolitics of Traumatism in Antimicrobial Resistance (AMR)." *The Sociological Review* 65, no. 3 (2017): 6.

7. Michael Howard, quoted in George Jones, "Fighting Talk as Leaders Clash in Commons Showdown," *Telegraph*, April 7, 2005, accessed March 12, 2019, https://www.telegraph.co.uk/news/uknews/1487283/Fighting-talk-as-leaders-clash-in-Commons-showdown.html.

8. Brian Greenwood, "Brexit and What It Means for Global Health," *American Journal of Tropical Medicine and Hygiene* 98, no. 3 (2018): 643–44; Zosia Kmietowicz, "Brexit—Not EU Membership—Threatens the NHS, 60 Eminent Doctors Say," *British Medical Journal* 353 (2016): i3373, https://doi.org/10.1136/bmj.i3373.

9. Jack Guy, "'Dickensian Diseases' are Making a Comeback in the UK," *CNN*, February 2, 2019, accessed March 12, 2019, https://www.cnn.com/2019/02/02/health/dickensian-diseases-britain-scli-gbr-intl/index.html.

10. Samuel Earle, "The Toxic Nostalgia of Brexit," *Atlantic*, October 5, 2017, accessed July 29, 2018, https://www.theatlantic.com/international/archive/2017/10/brexit-britain-may-johnson-eu/542079/.

11. "How Antibiotic Resistance Could Take Us Back to the 'Dark Ages'" *BBC News*, November 1, 2018, accessed March 12, 2019, https://www.bbc.com/news/health-45942574.

12. Lorenzo Servitje, "Gaming the Apocalypse in the Time of Antibiotic Resistance," *Osiris Osiris* 34, no. 1 (2019): 316; Lorenzo Servitje, "'The Path of Most Resistance': *Surgeon* X and the Graphic Estrangement of Antibiosis," in *The Palgrave Handbook of Twentieth and Twenty-First Century Literature and Science*, ed. Neel Ahuja et al. (New York: Palgrave Macmillan, 2020).

13. Margaret B. Planta, "The Role of Poverty in Antimicrobial Resistance," *Journal of the American Board of Family Medicine* 20, no. 6 (2007); Paul E. Farmer et al., "Structural Violence and Clinical Medicine," *PLoS Medicine* 3, no. 10 (2006): e449, https://doi.org/10.1371/journal.pmed.0030449.

14. Aiden Hollis and Peter Maybarduk, "Antibiotic Resistance Is a Tragedy of the Commons That Necessitates Global Cooperation," *Journal of Law and Medical Ethics* 43, no. 3 (2015): 33.

15. Here I follow Peterson and Round's definition. Charisse Petersen and June L. Round, "Defining Dysbiosis and Its Influence on Host Immunity and Disease," *Cellular Microbiology* 16, no. 7 (2014): 1024–25. It's important to specify this provenance, as the term has increased in usage and definitional looseness and overextension, to the point where it is unclear if it is a cause or effect, whether it is a taxonomic or functional definition. Katarzyna B. Hooks and Maureen A. O'Malley, "Dysbiosis and Its Discontents." *mBio* 8, no. 5 (2017): e01492-17, https://doi.org/10.1128/mBio.01492-17.

16. Cliodna A. M. McNulty et al., "Don't Wear Me Out—the Public's Knowledge of and Attitudes to Antibiotic Use," *Journal of Antimicrobial Chemotherapy* 59, no. 4 (2007); Wellcome Trust, *Exploring the Consumer Perspective on Antimicrobial Resistance*, June 2015, accessed March 19, 2019, https://wellcome.ac.uk/sites/default/files/exploring-consumer-perspective-on-antimicrobial-resistance-jun15.pdf.

17. Servitje, "The Path of Most Resistance"; Timothy Morton has also briefly addressed antibiotic resistance as a hyperobject. Morton, *Dark Ecology*, 7, 59.

18. See Catherine Belling, "Dark Zones: The Ebola Body as a Configuration of Horror," in *Endemic*, eds. Kari Nixon and Lorenzo Servitje (London: Palgrave Macmillan, 2016); Douglas Melvin Haynes, "Still the Heart of Darkness: The Ebola Virus and the Meta-Narrative of Disease in The Hot Zone," *Journal of Medical Humanities* 12, no. 2 (2002).

19. Selwyn Duke, "Will the Migrant Caravan Kill Your Child—With Disease?," *New American*, October 28, 2018, accessed March 17, 2019, https://www.thenewamerican.com/usnews/immigration/item/30471-will-migrant-caravan-kill-your-child-with-disease; Jenna Amatulll, " 'Fox & Friends' Host Says Migrant Caravan May Be Bringing 'Diseases' To America," *Huffington Post*, October 29, 2018, accessed March 17, 2019, https://www.huffingtonpost.com/entry/brian-kilmeande-fox-friends-caravan-diseases_us_5bd70a85e4b0a8f17ef9e965.

20. Richard Evans provides a thorough survey of the affordances and problematics associated with using military-conflict and criminal justice analogies to understand the securitization of infectious disease, specifically Ebola. He makes a compelling case for using military analogies vis-à-vis infectious disease in specific circumstances, and contends that we should try to take the analogies seriously rather than try to divorce the language completely: "Given that emerging infectious diseases are linked with the language of armed conflict, we ought to apply our best tools to understand what this analogy means for the ethics of infectious disease response, and where the analogy breaks down." "Ebola: From Public Health Crisis to National Security Threat," 287. While I remain slightly less optimistic of the productive possibilities for using war to articulate scaled infectious disease threats, I would suggest *Medicine Is War* is precisely following Evan's call to understand the martial metaphor, its ethical challenges, and "where it breaks down."

21. Corey Charlton, "Run, They May Have Ebola! Nudist Beach Panic over Migrant Boat from Africa," *Daily Mail*, November 6, 2014, accessed March 14, 2019, https://www.dailymail.co.uk/news/article-2823883/Ebola-scare-Canary-Island-nudist-beach-migrants-Sierra-Leone-arrive-boat-fever-taken-away-dumped-truck-terrified-tourists.html.

22. Sara C. Nelson, "Ebola Zombie 'Risen from the Dead' Is a Horrible Viral Hoax," *Huffington Post UK*, October 6, 2014, accessed March 12, 2019, http://www.huffingtonpost.co.uk/2014/10/06/ebola-zombie-risen-dead-viral-hoax_n_5937728.html.

23. Ahuja, *Bioinsecurities*, 15.

24. See Umberto Pellecchia et al., "Social Consequences of Ebola Containment Measures in Liberia," *PLoS ONE* 10, no. 12 (2015): e0143036, https://doi.org/10.1371/journal.pone.0143036; Mark A. Rothstein, "The Moral Challenge of Ebola," *American Journal of Public Health* 105, no. 1 (2015). See also Adia Benton's reading of the "immuno-logics," of who lived and died in the 2014 West Africa Ebola epidemic. "Race and the immuno-logics of Ebola response in West Africa," *Somatasphere*, September 14, 2014, accessed August 9, 2014, http://somatosphere.net/2014/race-and-the-immuno-logics-of-ebola-response-in-west-africa.html/.

25. Judith Butler, *Notes Toward A Performative Theory of Assembly* (Cambridge, MA: Harvard University Press, 2015), 12.

26. Butler, 12.

27. Butler, 12.

28. Susan L. Smith, *Toxic Exposures: Mustard Gas and the Health Consequences of World War II in the United States* (New Brunswick, NJ: Rutgers University Press, 2019), 97–101.

29. David J. Rothman, *Strangers at the Bedside: A History of How Law and Bioethics Transformed Medical Decision Making* (New Brunswick, NJ: Aldine Transaction, 2009), 30; Jordan Goodman, Anthony McElligott, and Lara Marks, "Making Human Bodies Useful: Historicizing Medical Experiments of the Twentieth Century," in *Useful Bodies: Humans in the Service of Medical Science in the Twentieth Century*, ed. Jordan Goodman, Anthony McElligott and Lara Marks (Baltimore: Johns Hopkins University Press, 2008).

30. Louis S. Goodman et al, "Nitrogen Mustard Therapy: Use of Methyl-Bis(Beta-Chloroethyl)amine Hydrochloride and Tris(Beta-Chloroethyl)amine Hydrochloride for Hodgkin's Disease, Lymphosarcoma, Leukemia and Certain Allied and Miscellaneous Disorders," *JAMA* 132, no. 3 (1946): 126–32.

31. Devra Davis, *The Secret History of the War on Cancer* (New York: Basic Books, 2007), 208–11.

32. Davis, 208–11.

33. Cristian Tomasetti and Bert Vogelstein, "Variation in Cancer Risk among Tissues Can Be Explained by the Number of Stem Cell Divisions," *Science* 347, no. 6217 (2015): 81.

34. Sadaf Sajjad et al., "Psychotherapy through Video Game to Target Illness Related Problematic Behaviors of Children with Brain Tumor," *Current Medical Imaging Reviews* 10, no. 1 (2014): 63. I have made similar claims about the disciplinary function of video games, in our own contemporary moment, with respect to adopting official governmental narratives in response to epidemic threats. See Lorenzo Servitje, "H5n1 for Angry Birds: *Plague Inc.*, Mobile Games, and the Biopolitics of Outbreak Narratives," *Science Fiction Studies* 43, no. 1 (2016): 85–103.

35. Peggy Orenstein, "Surviving Cancer without the Positive Thinking," *Atlantic*, May 7, 2016, accessed March 12, 2019, https://www.theatlantic.com/health/archive/2016/05/surviving-cancer-without-the-positive-thinking/481764/?utm_source=atlfb.

36. Rita Charon, *Narrative Medicine: Honoring the Stories of Illness* (Oxford, UK: Oxford University Press, 2006). For a recent narratological reading of nineteenth-century literature and medicine that also makes a compelling case for the relevance of Victorian literature to narrative medicine, see Wright, *Reading for Health*.

37. Olivia Banner, "Structural Racism and Practices of Reading in the Medical Humanities," *Literature and Medicine* 34, no. 1 (2016): 26–27.

Addendum

1. Matt Watson, Twitter post, August 2020, 1:03 p.m., https://mobile.twitter.com/BioAndBaseball/status/1289970107561783300.

2. World Health Organization, "Pneumonia of Unknown Cause—China," Emergencies Preparedness, Response, January 5, 2020, accessed August 7, 2020, https://www.who.int/csr/don/05-january-2020-pneumonia-of-unkown-cause-china/en/.

3. Gianfranco Spiteri et al., "First Cases of Coronavirus Disease 2019 (COVID-19) in the WHO European Region, 24 January to 21 February 2020," *Eurosurveillance* 25, no. 9 (2020): 1.

4. Derrick Bryson Tyler, "A Timeline of the Coronavirus Pandemic," *New York Times*, August 6, 2020, https://www.nytimes.com/article/coronavirus-timeline.html.

5. Travis Chi Wing Lau, "On Virality, Corona or Otherwise," *Synapsis*, May 15, 2020, https://medicalhealthhumanities.com/2020/05/15/on-virality-corona-or-otherwise/.

6. Angela Rasmussen, Twitter post, February 2020, 12:36 p.m., https://twitter.com/angie_rasmussen/status/1229459742378090496?s=20.

7. Monica Green, Twitter Post, February 2020, 2:16 p.m., https://twitter.com/monicaMedHist/status/1233108570687717376?s=20.

8. Lehigh University, "3.11.20: Lehigh Moves to Remote Learning Temporarily," Lehigh News, March 11, 2020, https://www2.lehigh.edu/news/31120-lehigh-moves-to-remote-learning-temporarily.

9. Suhas Gondia et al., "A Timeline of the Coronavirus Pandemic"; Gondi, Suhas, et al. "Personal Protective Equipment Needs in the USA during the COVID-19 Pandemic," *Lancet*, May 23, 2020, https://doi.org/10.1016/S0140-6736(20)31038-2.

10. Derived from Worldometer, "COVID-19 Coronavirus Pandemic," August 8, 2020, https://www.worldometers.info/coronavirus/.

11. Christos Lynertis, *Framing Animals as Epidemic Villains*, 2.

12. Tonia Poteat et al., "Understanding COVID-19 Risks and Vulnerabilities among Black Communities in America: The Lethal Force of Syndemics," *Annals of Epidemiology* 47 (2020): 1–3.

13. Sirry Alang et al., "Police Brutality and Black Health: Setting the Agenda for Public Health Scholars," *American Journal of Public Health* 107 (2017): 662; Christina Sharpe, *In the Wake: On Blackness and Being* (Durham, NC: Duke University Press, 2006), 13–19.

14. Jerome Viala-Gaudefroy and Dana Linderman, "Donald Trump's 'Chinese Virus': The Politics of Naming," *Conversation*, April 21, 2020, https://theconversation.com/donald-trumps-chinese-virus-the-politics-of-naming-136796.

15. Maria Panaritis, "I Went to the Supermarket and Came Home Shaken," *Philadelphia Inquirer*, March 31, 2020, https://www.inquirer.com/health/coronavirus/coronavirus-covid-19-supermarkets-grocery-stores-shopping-low-inventory-wynnewood-giant-maria-panaritis-20200331.html.

16. Lorenzo Servitje, "Acting Fatally on the Strength of the Martial Metaphor," *Somatosphere*, May 10, 2020, http://somatosphere.net/forumpost/covid19-martial-metaphor/.

17. Jessie Yeung, Adam Renton, and Angela Dewan, "May 6 Coronavirus News," *CNN*, May 6, 2020, https://www.cnn.com/world/live-news/coronavirus-pandemic-05-06-20-intl/index.html, emphasis added.

18. T. J. Tallie, "Asymptomatic Lethality: Cooper, COVID-19, and the Potential for Black Death," *Nursing Clio*, June 8, 2020, https://nursingclio.org/2020/06/08/asymptomatic-lethality-cooper-covid-19-and-the-potential-for-black-death/.

19. Jessie Yeung, Steve George, Zamira Rahim, and Fernando Alfonso, "May 27 Coronavirus News," *CNN*, March 2020, https://www.cnn.com/world/live-news/coronavirus-pandemic-05-27-20-intl/index.html.

20. Charles Kingsley, "The Two Breaths," *Health and Education* (London: W. Ibster, 1874), 30.

21. Michael Daly, "Palm Beach 'Patriots' Are Ready to Die for Their Freedom to Breathe Mask-Free," *Daily Beast*, June 25, 2020, https://www.thedailybeast.com/palm-beach-county-patriots-tell-hearing-they-are-ready-to-die-for-their-freedom-to-breathe-mask-free.

22. Jonathan Levinson et al. "Federal Officers Use Unmarked Vehicles to Grab People in Portland, DHS Confirms," *NPR*, June 17, 2020, https://www.npr.org/2020/07/17/892277592/federal-officers-use-unmarked-vehicles-to-grab-protesters-in-portland; Firmin DeBrabander, "The Great Irony of America's Armed

Anti-Lockdown Protesters," *Atlantic*, May 13, 2020, https://www.theatlantic.com/ideas/archive/2020/05/guns-protesters/611560/.

23. Tsing, Anna Lowenhaupt. *The Mushroom at the End of the World: On the Possibility of Life in Capitalist Ruins* (Princeton, NJ: Princeton University Press, 2015), 2.

24. George Eliot, *Middlemarch* (New York: W. W. Norton, 2000), 514–15.

25. Alissa Wilkinson, "Pandemics Are Not Wars," *Vox*, April 15, 2020, https://www.vox.com/culture/2020/4/15/21193679/coronavirus-pandemic-war-metaphor-ecology-microbiome; Yasmeen Serhan, "The Case against Waging 'War' on the Coronavirus," *Atlantic*, March 31, 2020, https://www.theatlantic.com/international/archive/2020/03/war-metaphor-coronavirus/609049/; Jacob Hagstom, "Stop Calling Covid-19 a War," *Washington Post*, April 20, 2020, https://www.washingtonpost.com/outlook/2020/04/20/stop-calling-covid-19-war/.

26. Benjamin R. Bates, "The (In)Appropriateness of the WAR Metaphor in Response to SARS-CoV-2: A Rapid Analysis of Donald J. Trump's Rhetoric," *Frontiers in Communication* 5 (June 2020), https://doi.org/10.3389/fcomm.2020.00050.

27. Charlotte Brives, "The Politics of Amphibiosis: The War against Viruses Will Not Take Place," *Somatosphere*, April 19, 2020, http://somatosphere.net/2020/the-politics-of-amphibiosis.html.

28. See, for instance, Angela Brown et al, "Membrane Localization of the Repeats-in-Toxin (RTX) Leukotoxin (LtxA) Produced by Aggregatibacter Actinomycetemcomitans." *PLoS ONE* 13, no. 10 (2018): 1–17; Lynette Cegelski et al, The Biology and Future Prospects of Antivirulence Therapies." *Nature Reviews Microbiology* 6, no. 1 (2008): 17–27.

29. Iona Walker, "Beyond the military metaphor: Comparing antimicrobial resistance and the COVID-19 pandemic in the United Kingdom," *Medicine Anthropology Theory* 7, no. 2 (2020): 261–272.

30. Brian Resnick and Umair Irfan, "What Immunity to Covid-19 Might Actually Mean," *Vox*, April 23, 2020, https://www.vox.com/science-and-health/2020/4/23/21219028/covid-19-immunity-testing-reinfection-antibodies-explained.

31. Eliot, *Middlemarch*, 515.

Bibliography

Ackerknecht, Erwin H. "Anticontagionism between 1821 and 1867." *International Journal of Epidemiology* 38, no. 1 (2009): 7–21.
Adair, James M. *Commentaries on the Principles and Practices of Physic.* London: T. Becket, 1772.
Ahuja, Neel. *Bioinsecurities.* Durham, NC: Duke University Press, 2016.
Alang, Sirry, Donna McAlpine, Ellen McCreedy, and Rachel Hardeman. "Police Brutality and Black Health: Setting the Agenda for Public Health Scholars." *American Journal of Public Health* 107, no. 5 (2017): 662–65.
Al-Zahrani, Abdulsalam. "Darwin's Metaphors Revisited: Conceptual Metaphors, Conceptual Blends, and Idealized Cognitive Models in the Theory of Evolution." *Metaphor & Symbol* 23, no. 1 (2008): 50–82.
Amatulli, Jenna. "'Fox & Friends' Host Says Migrant Caravan May Be Bringing 'Diseases' to America." *Huffington Post.* October 29, 2018. Accessed March 17, 2019. https://www.huffingtonpost.com/entry/brian-kilmeande-fox-friends-caravan-diseases_us_5bd70a85e4b0a8f17ef9e965.
Anderson, Warwick. *Colonial Pathologies.* Durham, NC: Duke University Press, 2006.
Anderson, Warwick, and Ian R. Mackay. *Intolerant Bodies: A Short History of Autoimmunity.* Baltimore, MD: Johns Hopkins University Press, 2014.
Arata, Stephen. "The Occidental Tourist: 'Dracula' and the Anxiety of Reverse Colonization." *Victorian Studies* 33, no. 4 (1990): 621–45.
Arendt, Hannah. *The Origins of Totalitarianism.* New York: Harcourt, Brace & World, 1966.
Arikha, Noga. *Passions and Tempers: A History of the Humours.* New York: Ecco, 2007.
Armstrong, Nancy. *Desire and Domestic Fiction: A Political History of the Novel.* Oxford, UK: Oxford University Press, 1989.
Arnold, David. *Colonizing the Body: State Medicine and Epidemic Disease in Nineteenth-Century India.* Berkeley: University of California Press, 1993.

Aubry, Jean. Letter to Paul Wohlfart. 1936. "Joseph Conrad (1857–1924), Novelist: Notes on His Health." Wellcome Archives & Manuscripts. MS.8512. Wellcome Trust Library, UK.

Bailey, Mark S. "A Brief History of British Military Experiences with Infectious and Tropical Diseases." *Journal of the Royal Army Medical Corps* 159, no. 3 (September 2013): 150–57.

Baker, Kimeya. "The Contagious Diseases Acts and the Prostitute: How Disease and the Law Controlled the Female Body." *UCL Journal of Law and Jurisprudence* 1, no. 1 (2012): 88–119.

Banner, Olivia. "Structural Racism and Practices of Reading in the Medical Humanities." *Literature and Medicine* 34, no. 1 (2016): 25–52.

Bates, Benjamin R. "The (In)Appropriateness of the WAR Metaphor in Response to SARS-CoV-2: A Rapid Analysis of Donald J. Trump's Rhetoric." *Frontiers in Communication* 5, no. June (2020): 1–12.

Beer, Gillian. *Darwin's Plots: Evolutionary Narrative in Darwin, George Eliot and Nineteenth-Century Fiction*. 3rd ed. Cambridge, UK: Cambridge University Press, 2009.

Benton, Adia, "Race and the Immuno-logics of Ebola Response in West Africa," *Somatasphere*, September 14, 2014, accessed August 9, 2014, http://somatosphere.net/2014/race-and-the-immuno-logics-of-ebola-response-in-west-africa.html/.

———. "Race and the Immuno-logics of Ebola Response in West Africa," *Somatasphere*, September 14, 2014, accessed August 9, 2014, http://somatosphere.net/2014/race-and-the-immuno-logics-of-ebola-response-in-west-africa.html/.

Bell, Joseph. "Mr. Sherlock Holmes." In *A Study in Scarlet*. Edited by Arthur Conan Doyle, 8–11. London: Ward, Lock, & Bowden, 1893.

Belling, Catherine. "Dark Zones: The Ebola Body as a Configuration of Horror." In *Endemic: Essays in Contagion Theory*. Edited by Kari Nixon and Lorenzo Servitje, 43–66. London: Palgrave Macmillan, 2016.

Bewell, Alan. *Romanticism and Colonial Disease*. Baltimore, MD: Johns Hopkins University Press, 2003.

Bichat, Xavier. *Physiological Researches Upon Life and Death*. Translated by Tobias Watkins. Philadelphia: Smith & Maxwell, 1809.

"The Black Death," *All The Year Round* no. 569, October 25, 1879, 436–41.

Bleakley, Alan. *Thinking with Metaphors in Medicine: The State of Art*. New York: Routledge, 2017.

Blevins, Steve M., and Michael S. Bronze. "Robert Koch and the 'Golden Age' of Bacteriology." *International Journal of Infectious Diseases* 14, no. 9 (2010): e744–e51.

Bock, Martin. "Disease and Medicine." In *Joseph Conrad in Context*. Edited by Alan Simmons, 124–31. Cambridge, UK: Cambridge University Press, 2009.

———. "Joseph Conrad and Germ Theory: Why Captain Allistoun Smiles Thoughtfully." *Conradian* 31, no. 2 (2006): 1–14.

———. *Joseph Conrad and Psychological Medicine*. Lubbock: Texas Tech University Press, 2002.

Booth, Martin. *The Doctor and the Detective: A Biography of Sir Arthur Conan Doyle*. New York: St. Martin's Minotaur, 2000.

Bosch, Fèlix, and Laia Rosich. "The Contributions of Paul Ehrlich to Pharmacology: A Tribute on the Occasion of the Centenary of His Nobel Prize." *Pharmacology* 82, no. 3 (2008): 171–79.

Botting, Fred. *Gothic*. 2nd ed. Florence: Taylor and Francis, 1999.

Brantlinger, Patrick. *Taming Cannibals: Race and the Victorians*. Ithaca, NY: Cornell University Press, 2011.

———. "Victorians and Africans: The Genealogy of the Myth of the Dark Continent." *Critical Inquiry* 12, no. 1 (1985): 166–203.

Brives, Charlotte. "The Politics of Amphibiosis: The War against Viruses Will Not Take Place." *Somatosphere*. April 19, 2020. Accessed August 2, 2020, http://somatosphere.net/2020/the-politics-of-amphibiosis.html.

Brown, Angela, Kathleen Boesze-Battaglia, Nataliya V. Balashova, Nestor Mas Gómez, Kaye Speicher, Hsin Yao Tang, Margaret E. Duszyk, and Edward T. Lally. "Membrane Localization of the Repeats-in-Toxin (RTX) Leukotoxin (LtxA) Produced by Aggregatibacter Actinomycetemcomitans." *PLoS ONE* 13, no. 10 (2018): 1–17. https://doi.org/10.1371/journal.pone.0205871

Brown, Michael. "Cold Steel, Weak Flesh: Mechanism, Masculinity and the Anxieties of Late Victorian Empire." *Cultural and Social History* 14, no. 2 (2017): 155–81.

———. "From Foetid Air to Filth: The Cultural Transformation of British Epidemiological Thought, ca. 1780–1848." *Bulletin of the History of Medicine* 82, no. 3 (2018): 515–44.

———. "'Like a Devoted Army': Medicine, Heroic Masculinity, and the Military Paradigm in Victorian Britain." *Journal of British Studies* 49, no. 3 (2010): 592–622.

———. "Medicine, Reform and the 'End' of Charity in Early Nineteenth-Century England." *English Historical Review* 124, no. 511 (2009): 1353–88.

———. *Performing Medicine: Medical Culture and Identity in Provincial England, c. 1760–1850*. Manchester, UK: Manchester University Press, 2011.

Brown, Nik and Sarah Nettleton. "'There Is Worse to Come': The Biopolitics of Traumatism in Antimicrobial Resistance (AMR)." *The Sociological Review* 65, no. 3 (2017): 493–508.

Brunton, Deborah. *Medicine Transformed: Health, Disease and Society in Europe, 1800–1930*. Manchester: Manchester University Press in association with the Open University, 2004.

Budd, William. "Can the Government, Further, Beneficially Intervene in the Prevention of Infectious Diseases?" In *Transactions of the National Association for the Promotion of Social Science: Bristol Meeting 1869*. Edited by Edwin Pears, 386–402. London: Longmans, Green, Reader, & Dyer, 1870.

Burdon Sanderson, John. "The Croonian Lectures on the Progress of Discovery Relating to the Origin and Nature of Infectious Diseases: Lecture III." *British Medical Journal* 2, no. 1612 (1891): 1083–807.

———. "The Croonian Lectures on the Progress of Discovery Relating to the Origin and Nature of Infectious Diseases: Lecture III." *Lancet* 138, no. 3560 (1891): 1149–54.

———. "The Croonian Lectures on the Progress of Discovery Relating to the Origin and Nature of Infectious Diseases: Lecture IV." *British Medical Journal* 2, no. 1613 (1891): 1135–39.

Burke, Edmund. *A Philosophical Inquiry into the Origin of Our Ideas of the Sublime and Beautiful*. London: N. Hailes, 1824.

Burney, Ian. "Medicine in the Age of Reform." In *Rethinking the Age of Reform Britain 1780–1850*. Edited by Arthur Burns and Joanna Innes, 163–81. Cambridge, UK: Cambridge University Press, 2009.

Butler, Josephine. *The Constitution Violated: An Essay*. Edinburgh: Edmonston & Douglas, 1871.

Butler, Judith. *Notes toward A Performative Theory of Assembly*. Cambridge, MA: Harvard University Press, 2015.

Bynum, W. F. "Nosology" in *The Companion Encyclopedia of the History of Medicine*. Edited by W. F. Bynum and Roy Porter. London: Routledge, 1993.

Bynum, W. F., and Roy Porter, eds. *Companion Encyclopedia of the History of Medicine*. London: Routledge, 1993.

Bynum, William F., Stephen Lock, and Roy Porter, eds. *Medical Journals and Medical Knowledge*. London: Routledge, 1992.

Byrne, Paul Johnson. "'Heart of Darkness': The Dream-Sensation and Literary Impressionism Revisited." *Conradian* 35, no. 2 (2010): 13–29.

Cameron, Lauren. "Mary Shelley's Malthusian Objections in *The Last Man*." *Nineteenth-Century Literature* 67, no. 2 (2012): 177–203.

Campbell, Maurice. *Sherlock Holmes and Dr. Watson: A Medical Digression*. London: Guy's Hospital Gazette Committee, 1951.

Canguilhem, Georges. *The Normal and the Pathological*. New York: Zone Books, 1989.

Carpenter, Mary Wilson. *Health, Medicine, and Society in Victorian England*. Santa Barbara: Praeger, 2010.

———. "Medical Cosmopolitanism: Middlemarch, Cholera, and the Pathologies of English Masculinity." *Victorian Literature and Culture* 38, no. 2 (2010): 511–28.

Cartwright, Lisa. *Screening the Body: Tracing Medicine's Visual Culture*. Minneapolis: University of Minnesota Press, 1995.

Casement, Roger. "Mr. Casement to the Marquess of Lansdowne." In *Africa. No. 1 (1904): Correspondence and Report from His Majesty's Consul at Boma Respecting the Administration of the Independent State of the* Congo, 21–81. London: Harrison & Sons, 1904.
Cegelski, Lynette, Garland R. Marshall, Gary R. Eldridge, and Scott J. Hultgren. "The Biology and Future Prospects of Antivirulence Therapies." *Nature Reviews Microbiology* 6, no. 1 (2008): 17–27. https://doi.org/10.1038/nrmicro 1818
Charlton, Corey. "Run, They May Have Ebola! Nudist Beach Panic over Migrant Boat from Africa." *Daily Mail*. November 6, 2014. Accessed March 14, 2019. https://www.dailymail.co.uk/news/article-2823883/Ebola-scare-Canary-Island-nudist-beach-migrants-Sierra-Leone-arrive-boat-fever-taken-away-dumped-truck-terrified-tourists.html.
Charon, Rita. *Narrative Medicine: Honoring the Stories of Illness*. Oxford, UK: Oxford University Press, 2006.
Chatterjee, Ranita. "Our Bodies, Our Catastrophes: Biopolitics in Mary Shelley's *The Last Man*." *European Romantic Review* 25, no. 1 (2014): 35–49.
Childers, Joseph W. "Foreign Matter: Imperial Filth." In *Filth: Dirt, Disgust, and Modern Life*. Edited by William A. Cohen and Ryan Johnson, 201–24. Minneapolis: University of Minnesota, 2006.
———. *Novel Possibilities: Fiction and the Formation of Early Victorian Culture*. Philadelphia: University of Pennsylvania Press, 1995.
Choi, Tina Young. *Anonymous Connections: The Body and Narratives of the Social in Victorian Britain*. Ann Arbor: University of Michigan Press, 2015.
Chi Wing Lau, Travis. "Inventing Edward Jenner: Historicizing Anti-vaccination." In *The Routledge Companion to Health Humanities*, eds. Paul Crawford, Brian Brown, and Andrea Charise, 120–133. London: Routledge, 2020.
———. "On Virality, Corona or Otherwise," *Synapsis*, May 15, 2020. Accessed August 7, 2020. https://medicalhealthhumanities.com/2020/05/15/on-virality-corona-or-otherwise/.
Cirillo, V. J. "Arthur Conan Doyle (1859–1930): Physician during the Typhoid Epidemic in the Anglo-Boer War (1899–1902)." *Journal of Medical Biography* 22, no. 1 (2014): 2–8.
Cohen, Ed. *A Body Worth Defending: Immunity, Biopolitics, and the Apotheosis of the Modern Body*. Durham, NC: Duke University Press, 2009.
Cohen, William B. "Malaria and French Imperialism," *Journal of African History* 24, no. 1 (1983): 23–36.
Cohen-Vrignaud, Gerard. *Radical Orientalism: Rights, Reform, and Romanticism*. Cambridge, UK: Cambridge University Press, 2015.
Colin, Jonathan. "An Illiberal Descent: Natural and National History in the Work of Charles Kingsley." *History* 96, no. 322 (2011): 167–87.
Colley, Linda. *Britons: Forging the Nation 1707–1837*. New Haven: Yale University Press, 1992.
Collie, John. *Malingering and Feigned Sickness*. London: Edward Arnold, 1913.

Collini, Stefan. "The Idea of 'Character' in Victorian Political Thought." *Transactions of the Royal Historical Society* 35 (1985): 29–50.
Conan Doyle, Arthur. "The Adventure of the Blanched Soldier." In *Sherlock Holmes: The Complete Novels and Stories*, vol. II, 538–58. New York: Bantam Dell, 2003.
———. "The Adventure of the Copper Beeches." In *Sherlock Holmes: The Complete Novels and Stories*, vol. I, 492–518. New York: Bantam Dell, 2003.
———. "The Adventure of the Dying Detective." In *Sherlock Holmes: The Complete Novels and Stories*, vol. II, 428–44. New York: Bantam Dell, 2003.
———. "The Adventure of the Speckled Band." In *Sherlock Holmes: The Complete Novels and Stories*, vol. I, 396–422. New York: Bantam Dell, 2003.
———. Arthur Conan Doyle to the *Hampshire County Times*, Portsmouth, 27 July 1887, "Compulsory Vaccination." In *Letters to the Press*. Edited by J. M. Gibson and R. L. Green, 29–32. Iowa City: University of Iowa Press, 1986.
———. *The Crime of the Congo*. New York: Doubleday, 1909.
———. "Dr. Koch and His Cure." *Review of Reviews* 2, no. 12 (December 1890): 552–60.
———. *The Great Boer War*. London: Smith, Elder, 1900.
———. "Life and Death in the Blood." *Good Words* 24 (March 1883): 178–81.
———. *Memories and Adventures*. Cambridge, UK: Cambridge University Press, 2012.
———. *The Parasite: A Story*. New York: Harper and Brothers, 1894.
———. "The Sign of Four." In *Sherlock Holmes: The Complete Novels and Stories*, vol. I, 121–236. New York: Bantam Dell, 2003.
———. "A Study in Scarlet." In *Sherlock Holmes: The Complete Novels and Stories*, vol. I, 1–120. New York: Bantam Dell, 2003.
———. *The War in South Africa: Its Causes and Conduct*. New York: McClure, Phillips, 1902.
———. "The War in South Africa, the Epidemic of Enteric Fever at Bloemfontein." *British Medical Journal* 2, no. 2062 (1900): 49–53.
Conrad, Joseph. *The Collected Letters of Joseph Conrad, Volume 2: 1898–1902*. Edited by Frederick R. Karl and Laurence Davis. Cambridge, UK: Cambridge University Press, 1986.
———. *Heart of Darkness: Authoritative Text, Backgrounds and Contexts, Criticism*. Edited by Paul B. Armstrong. New York: W. W. Norton, 2006.
———. *The Shadow Line: A Confession*. Garden City: Doubleday, 1917.
———. *Victory*. New York: Modern Library, 1915.
Cooper, Frederick, and Ann Laura Stoler. "Between Metropole and Colony." In *Tensions of Empire: Colonial Cultures in a Bourgeois World*. Edited by Frederick Cooper and Ann Laura Stoler. Berkeley: University of California Press, 2009.

Cooter, Roger. "Of War and Epidemics: Unnatural Couplings, Problematic Conceptions." *Journal for the Society of the Social History of Medicine* 16, no. 2 (2003): 283–302.
Coyer, Megan. *Literature and Medicine in the Nineteenth Century Periodical Press: Blackwood's Edinburgh Magazine, 1817–1858*. Edinburgh: Edinburgh University Press, 2017.
Craft, Christopher. "'Kiss Me with Those Red Lips': Gender and Inversion in Bram Stoker's Dracula." *Representations*, no. 8 (1984): 107–33.
Croley, Laura Sagolla. "The Rhetoric of Reform in Stoker's 'Dracula': Depravity, Decline, and the Fin-De-Siècle 'Residuum.'" *Criticism* 37, no. 1 (1995): 85–108.
Crowley, Leonard V. *An Introduction to Human Disease: Pathology and Pathophysiology Correlations*. Burlington: Jones & Bartlett Learning, 2013.
Cryan, John F., and Timothy G. Dinan. "Mind-Altering Microorganisms: The Impact of the Gut Microbiota on Brain and Behaviour." *National Review of Neuroscience* 13, no. 10 (2012): 701–12.
D'Alembert, Jean le Rond. *Esprit, Maximes et Principes de D'Alembert, de l'Académie Française, &c*. Paris: Chez Briand, 1789.
Daly, Michael. "Palm Beach 'Patriots' Are Ready to Die for Their Freedom to Breathe Mask-Free," *Daily Beast*, June 25, 2020. Accessed August 8, 2020, https://www.thedailybeast.com/palm-beach-county-patriots-tell-hearing-they-are-ready-to-die-for-their-freedom-to-breathe-mask-free.
Daly, Nicholas. "Incorporated Bodies: Dracula and the Rise of Professionalism." *Texas Studies in Literature and Language* 39, no. 2 (1997): 181–203.
Daniels, Stephen. "Mapping National Identities: The Culture of Cartography with Particular Reference to the Ordnance Survey." In *Imagining Nations*. Edited by Geoffrey Cubitt, 112–31. Manchester: Manchester University Press, 1998.
Darwin, Charles. *The Origin of Species by Means of Natural Selection, or the Preservation of Favoured Races in the Struggle for Life*. New York: Signet, 1859 (2003).
Davis, Devra. *The Secret History of the War on Cancer*. New York: Basic Books, 2007.
Davison, Carol Margaret. *Anti-Semitism and British Gothic Literature*. London: Palgrave Macmillan, 2004.
"The Day of a Healthy Man." In *Harmsworth Popular Science*, vol. 1. Edited by Arthur Mee, 67–73. London: Educational Book, 1913.
De Grandis, Giovanni. "On the Analogy between Infectious Diseases and War: How to Use It and Not to Use It." *Public Health Ethics* 4, no. 1 (2011): 70–83.
De Kraker, Marlieke E. A., Andrew J. Stewardson, and Stephan Harbarth, "Will 10 Million People Die a Year Due to Antimicrobial Resistance by 2050?"

PLoS Medicine 13, no. 11 (2016): e1002184. https://doi.org/10.1371/journal. pmed.1002184.

DeBrabander, Firmin. "The Great Irony of America's Armed Anti-Lockdown Protesters."*The Atlantic*. May 13, 2020. Accessed August 8, 2020, https:// www.theatlantic.com/ideas/archive/2020/05/guns-protesters/611560/.

Debrix, François. "The Sublime Spectatorship of War: The Erasure of the Event in America's Politics of Terror and Aesthetics of Violence." *Millennium: Journal of International Studies* 34, no. 3 (2006): 767–91.

DeLacy, Margaret. *The Germ of an Idea: Contagionism, Religion, and Society in Britain, 1660–1730*. Basingstoke, UK: Palgrave Macmillan, 2016.

Dillon, Michael, and Julian Reid. *The Liberal Way of War Killing to Make Life Live*. New York: Routledge, 2009.

Dobraszczyk, Paul. "Mapping Sewer Spaces in mid-Victorian London." In *Dirt: New Geographies of Cleanliness and Contamination*. Edited by Ben Campkin and Rosie Cox, 123–37. New York: I. B. Tauris, 2007.

Donne, John. *Devotions upon Emergent Expressions and Death's Duel*. New York, Cosimo: 2010.

Douglas, Mary. *Purity and Danger: An Analysis of Concepts of Pollution and Taboo*. London: Routledge, 1966.

Duke, Selwyn. "Will the Migrant Caravan Kill Your Child—With Disease?" *New American*. October 28, 2018. Accessed March 17, 2019. https://www.thenew american.com/usnews/immigration/item/30471-will-migrant-caravan-kill-your-child-with-disease.

Earle, Samuel. "The Toxic Nostalgia of Brexit." *Atlantic*. October 5, 2017. Accessed July 29, 2018. https://www.theatlantic.com/international/archive/2017/10/brexit-britain-may-johnson-eu/542079/.

Edgerton, David. "War and the Development of the British Welfare State." In *Warfare and Welfare: Military Conflict and Welfare State Development in Western Countries*. Edited by Herbert Obinger, 202–28. Oxford, UK: Oxford University Press, 2018.

Editorial, *Times*, October 5, 1869, 7.

Eliot, George. *The Mill on the Floss*. New York: W. W. Norton, 1994.

———. *Middlemarch*, New York: W. W. Norton, 2000.

Ellis, Harold. *A History of Surgery*. London: Greenwich Medical Media, 2001.

Ellmann, Maud. *The Nets of Modernism: Henry James, Virginia Woolf, James Joyce, and Sigmund Freud*. Cambridge, UK: Cambridge University Press, 2010.

Encyclopædia Britannica, 9th ed. 24 vols. Chicago: Werner, 1895.

Esposito, Roberto. *Immunitas: The Protection and Negation of Life*. Cambridge, UK: Polity, 2011.

Evans, Nicholas G. "Ebola: From Public Health Crisis to National Security Threat." In *Biological Threats in The 21st Century: The Politics, People, Science and Historical Roots*, edited by Filippa Lentzos, 277–92. London: Imperial College Press, 2016.

Farmer, Paul E. et al. "Structural Violence and Clinical Medicine." *PLoS Medicine* 3, no. 10 (2006): e449. https://doi.org/10.1371/journal.pmed.0030449.
Fasik, Laura. "Charles Kingsley's Scientific Treatment of Gender." In *Muscular Christianity: Embodying the Victorian Age*. Edited by Donald Hall, 91–113. Cambridge, UK: Cambridge University Press, 1994.
Federation for the Defence of Belgian Interests Abroad. "The Death of Dr. Dutton." *The Truth on the Congo Free State* no. 21, 15 July 1905.
Fee, E., and M. E. Garofalo. "Florence Nightingale and the Crimean War." *American Journal of Public Health* 100, no. 9 (2010): 1591.
Ferguson, Christine. *Language, Science and Popular Fiction in the Victorian Fin-de-Siècle: The Brutal Tongue*. Aldershot, UK: Ashgate, 2006.
Fleck, Ludwik, Fred Bradley, Robert K. Merton, and Thaddeus J. Trenn. *Genesis and Development of a Scientific Fact*. Chicago: University of Chicago Press, 2008.
Floyd-Wilson, Mary. *English Ethnicity and Race in Early Modern Drama*. Cambridge, UK: Cambridge University Press, 2006.
Forman, Ross G. "A Parasite for Sore Eyes: Rereading Infection Metaphors in Bram Stoker's Dracula." *Victorian Literature and Culture* 44, no. 4 (2016): 925–47.
Forth, Aidan. *Barbed-Wire Imperialism: Britain's Empire of Camps, 1876–1903*. Oakland: University of California Press, 2017.
Foucault, Michel. *The Birth of Biopolitics: Lectures at the Collège De France, 1978–79*. New York: Palgrave Macmillan, 2008.
———. *The Birth of the Clinic: An Archaeology of Medical Perception*. Translated by A. M. Sheridan Smith. New York: Vintage, 1994.
———. *The History of Sexuality, Volume 1: An Introduction*. Translated by Robert Hurley. New York: Vintage, 1990.
———. *Security, Territory, Population: Lectures at the Collège De France, 1977–78*. New York: Palgrave Macmillan, 2007.
———. *Society Must Be Defended: Lectures at the Collège de France, 1975–76*. Translated by David Macey. New York: Picador, 2003.
Francino, M. P. "Antibiotics and the Human Gut Microbiome: Dysbioses and Accumulation of Resistances." *Frontiers in Microbiology* 6 (2015): 1543.
Francis, Keith A. "Sermons: Themes and Developments." In *The Oxford Handbook of the British Sermon, 1689–1901*. Edited by Keith A. Francis and William Gibson, 31–46. Oxford, UK: Oxford University Press, 2012.
Frank, Arthur. *At the Will of the Body: Reflections on Illness*. New York: Houghton Mifflin, 2002.
Freeman, Barbara Claire. *The Feminine Sublime: Gender and Excess in Women's Fiction*. Berkeley: University of California Press, 1997.
Fuks, Abraham. "The Military Metaphors of Modern Medicine." In *The Meaning Management Challenge: Making Sense of Health, Illness and Disease*. Edited

by Zhenyi Li and Thomas Lawrence Long, 57–69. Oxford, UK: Inter-Disciplinary Press, 2010.

Fulford, Tim, and Debbie Lee. "The Jenneration of Disease: Vaccination, Romanticism, and Revolution." *Studies in Romanticism* 39, no. 1 (2000): 139–63.

Furneaux, Holly. *Military Men of Feeling: Emotion, Touch, and Masculinity in the Crimean War*. Oxford, UK: Oxford University Press: 2016.

Gallagher, Catherine. *The Industrial Reformation of English Fiction*. Chicago: University of Chicago Press, 1995.

Gelven, Michael. *War and Existence: A Philosophical Inquiry*. University Park: Pennsylvania State University Press, 1994.

Gilbert, Pamela K. *Cholera and Nation: Doctoring the Social Body in Victorian England*. Albany: State University of New York Press, 2008.

———. *The Citizen's Body: Desire, Health, and the Social in Victorian England*. Columbus: Ohio State University Press, 2007.

———. *Disease, Desire, and the Body in Victorian Women's Popular Novels*. Cambridge, UK: Cambridge University Press, 1997.

———. *Mapping the Victorian Social Body*. Albany: State University of New York Press, 2004.

Gilman, Sander L. "Sexology, Psychoanalysis, and Degeneration: From a Theory of Race to a Race to Theory." In *Degeneration: The Dark Side of Progress*. Edited by J. Edward Chamberlin and Sander L. Gilman, 72–96. New York: Columbia University Press, 1985.

Godwin, William. *An Enquiry Concerning Political Justice: And Its Influence on Virtue and Happiness*, vol. 2. London: G. G. J. & J. Robinson, 1793.

Goetz, Thomas. *The Remedy: Robert Koch, Arthur Conan Doyle, and the Quest to Cure Tuberculosis*. New York: Gotham, 2014.

Gondi, Suhas, Adam L. Beckman, Nicholas Deveau, Ali S. Raja, Megan L. Ranney, Rachel Popkin, and Shuhan He. "Personal Protective Equipment Needs in the USA during the COVID-19 Pandemic." *Lancet* 395, no. 10237 (2020): e90–91.

Goldfrank, David M. *The Origins of the Crimean War*. London: Longman, 1994.

Goodlad, Lauren M. E. *Victorian Literature and the Victorian State: Character and Governance in a Liberal Society*. Baltimore, MD: Johns Hopkins University Press, 2003.

Goodman, Jordan, Anthony McElligott, and Lara Marks. "Making Human Bodies Useful: Historicizing Medical Experiments of the Twentieth Century." In *Useful Bodies: Humans in the Service of Medical Science in the Twentieth Century*. Edited by Jordan Goodman, Anthony McElligott and Lara Marks, 1–23. Baltimore, MD: Johns Hopkins University Press, 2008.

Goodman, Louis S. et al. "Nitrogen Mustard Therapy: Use of Methyl-Bis(Beta-Chloroethyl)amine Hydrochloride and Tris(Beta-Chloroethyl)amine Hydrochloride for Hodgkin's Disease, Lymphosarcoma, Leukemia and Certain Allied and Miscellaneous Disorders." *JAMA* 132, no. 3 (1946): 126–32.

Greaves, David. *The Healing Tradition: Reviving the Soul of Western Medicine.* San Francisco: Radcliffe, 2004.
Green, Monica. Twitter Post. February 27, 2020. 2:16 p.m. https://twitter.com/monica MedHist.
Greenwood, Brian. "Brexit and What It Means for Global Health." *American Journal of Tropical Medicine and Hygiene* 98, no. 3 (2018): 643–44.
Griffiths, Devin. *The Age of Analogy: Science and Literature between the Darwins.* Baltimore, MD: Johns Hopkins University Press, 2016.
Guy, Jack. "'Dickensian Diseases' Are Making a Comeback in the UK." *CNN.* February 2, 2019. Accessed March 12, 2019. https://www.cnn.com/2019/02/02/health/dickensian-diseases-britain-scli-gbr-intl/index.html.
Hacking, Ian. *The Taming of Chance.* New York: Cambridge University Press, 1990.
Hadley, Elaine. "Nobody, Somebody, and Everybody." *Victorian Studies* 59, no. 1 (2016): 65–86.
Halberstam, Jack. "Technologies of Monstrosity: Bram Stoker's 'Dracula.'" *Victorian Studies* 36, no. 3 (1993): 333–52.
Hall, Catherine. "Men and Their Histories: Civilizing Subjects." *History Workshop Journal*, no. 52 (2001): 49–66.
Hamlin, Christopher. *Cholera: The Biography.* Oxford: Oxford University Press, 2009.
———. *Public Health and Social Justice in the Age of Chadwick.* Cambridge, UK: Cambridge University Press, 1998.
Haraway, Donna. "The Biopolitics of Postmodern Bodies: Determinations of Self in Immune System Discourse." In *Biopolitics: A Reader.* Edited by Timothy Campbell, 274–309. Durham, NC: Duke University Press, 2013.
Hardy, Anne. "'Straight Back to Barbarism': Antityphoid Inoculation and the Great War, 1914." *Bulletin of the History of Medicine* 74, no. 2 (2000): 265–90.
Harris, Susan Cannon. "Pathological Possibilities: Contagion and Empire in Doyle's Sherlock Holmes Stories." *Victorian Literature and Culture* 31, no. 2 (2003): 447–66.
Harrison, Mark. "Differences of Degree: Representations of India in British Medical Topography, 1820–c. 1870." *Medical History Supplement* 20 (2000): 51–69.
———. *Public Health and British India: Anglo-Indian Preventive Medicine, 1859–1914.* Cambridge, UK: Cambridge University Press, 1994.
Haynes, Douglas Melvin. *Imperial Medicine: Patrick Manson and the Conquest of Tropical Disease.* Philadelphia: University of Pennsylvania Press, 2001.
———. "Still the Heart of Darkness: The Ebola Virus and the Meta-Narrative of Disease in The Hot Zone." *Journal of Medical Humanities* 12, no. 2 (2002): 133–45.
Howell, Jessica. *Malaria and Victorian Fictions of Empire.* Cambridge, UK: Cambridge University Press, 2018.

Headrick, Daniel R. "Sleeping Sickness Epidemics and Colonial Responses in East and Central Africa, 1900–1940." *PLoS Neglected Tropical Diseases* 8, no. 4 (2014): e2772. https://doi.org/10.1371/journal.pntd.0002772.
———. *The Tools of Empire: Technology and European Imperialism in the Nineteenth Century*. Oxford, UK: Oxford University Press. 1981.
Helmstadter, Carol, and Judith Godden. *Nursing before Nightingale, 1815–1899*. Farnham, UK: Ashgate, 2011.
Hensley, Nathan K. *Forms of Empire: The Poetics of Victorian Sovereignty*. Oxford, UK: Oxford University Press, 2016.
Herbert, Christopher. "Rat Worship and Taboo in Mayhew's London." *Representations*, no. 23 (1988): 1–24.
Hibbott, Yvonne. "'Bonaparte Visiting the Plague-Stricken at Jaffa' by Antoine Jean Gros (1771–1835)." *British Medical Journal* 1, no. 5642 (1969): 501–2.
Hindrichs, Cheryl. "'A Vision of Greyness': The Liminal Vantage of Illness in Heart of Darkness." *Modern Fiction Studies* 65, no. 1 (2019): 177–206.
"History of the Rise, Progress, Ravages, &c. of the Blue Cholera of India." *Lancet* 17, no. 429 (1831): 241–84.
Hochschild, Adam. *King Leopold's Ghost: A Story of Greed, Terror, and Heroism in Colonial Africa*. Boston: Houghton Mifflin, 1998.
Hodgkin, Paul. "Medicine Is War: And Other Medical Metaphors." *British Medical Journal* 291, no. 6511 (1985): 1820–21.
Hollinger, Mannfred A. *Introduction to Pharmacology*. 3rd ed. Abingdon: CRC Press, 2007.
Hollis, Aiden, and Peter Maybarduk. "Antibiotic Resistance Is a Tragedy of the Commons That Necessitates Global Cooperation." *Journal of Law and Medical Ethics* 43, no. 3 (2015): 33–37.
Holt, John. Letter to Ronald Ross. 27 August 1906. "Material on Ross receiving the Officier de l'Ordre de Leopold II, Belgium in August 1906." Sir Ronald Ross Collection. GB 0809 Ross/162/12. London School of Tropical Medicine & Hygiene, London.
Hooks, Katarzyna B., and Maureen A. O'Malley. "Dysbiosis and Its Discontents." *mBio* 8, no. 5 (2017): e01492-17. https://doi.org/10.1128/mBio.01492-17.
Horner, Avril, and Sue Zlosnik. "The Apocalyptic Sublime: Then and Now." In *Apocalyptic Discourse in Contemporary Culture: Post-Millennial Perspectives*. Edited by Monica German and Aris Mousoutzanis, 57–70. New York: Routledge, 2014.
Houen, Alex. "Sacrificial Militancy and the Wars around Terror." In *Terror and the Postcolonial: A Concise Companion*. Edited by Elleke Boehmer and Stephen Morton, 113–40. Chichester: Wiley Blackwell, 2010.
"How Antibiotic Resistance Could Take Us Back to the 'Dark Ages'" *BBC News*. November 1, 2018. Accessed March 12, 2019. https://www.bbc.com/news/health-45942574.
Hume, Kiel J. "Time and the Dialectics of Life and Death in 'Heart of Darkness.'" *Conradian* 34, no. 2 (2009): 64–74.

Humphry, G. Murray, J. Burdon-Sanderson, E. Klein, and A. A. Kanthack. "A Discussion on Phagocytosis and Immunity." *British Medical Journal* 1, no. 1625 (1892): 373–80.
Hurley, Kelly. *The Gothic Body: Sexuality, Materialism, and Degeneration at the Fin de Siècle*. Cambridge, UK: Cambridge University Press, 1996.
Huxley, T. H. "The Connection of the Biological Sciences with Medicine." *Science* 2, no. 63 (1881): 426–29.
Institute of Medicine Forum on Microbial Threats, *Ending the War Metaphor: The Changing Agenda for Unraveling the Host-Microbe Relationship: Workshop Summary*. Washington, DC: The National Academies Press, 2006.
Irving, James. *A Concise View of the Progress of Military Medical Literature in This Country*. Edinburgh: Stark, 1846.
Ishizuka, Hisao. *Fiber, Medicine, and Culture in the British Enlightenment*. New York: Palgrave, 2016.
Jacob, Hildebrand. "From *The Works* (1735)." In *The Sublime: A Reader in British Eighteenth-Century Aesthetic Theory*. Edited by Andrew Ashfield and Peter de Bolla, 53–54. Cambridge, UK: Cambridge University Press, 1996.
Jameson, James. *Report on the Epidemick Cholera Morbus: As It Visited the Territories Subject to the Presidency of Bengal, in the Years 1817, 1818 and 1819*. Calcutta: Government Gazette Press, 1820.
Jenner, Edward. *A Continuation of Facts and Observations Relative to the Variolae Vaccinae, or Cow Pox*. London: Sampson Low, 1800.
Jewson, N.D. "The Disappearance of the Sick-Man from Medical Cosmology, 1770–1870." *Sociology* 10, no. 2 (1976): 225–44.
Jones, George. "Fighting Talk as Leaders Clash in Commons Showdown." *Telegraph*. April 7, 2005. Accessed March 12, 2019. https://www.telegraph.co.uk/news/uknews/1487283/Fighting-talk-as-leaders-clash-in-Commons-showdown.html.
Jones, J. Jennifer. "The Art of Redundancy: Sublime Fiction and Mary Shelley's *The Last Man*." *Keats-Shelley Review* 29, no. 1 (2015): 25–41.
Jørgensen, Jens Lohfert. "Bacillophobia: Man and Microbes in Dracula, the War of the Worlds, and the Nigger of the 'Narcissus.'" *Critical Survey* 27, no. 2 (2015): 36–49.
Joshi, Priti. "Edwin Chadwick's Self-Fashioning: Professionalism, Masculinity, and the Victorian Poor." *Victorian Literature and Culture* 32, no. 2 (2004): 353–70.
Kassell, Laura. "Magic, Alchemy and the Medical Economy in Early Modern England: The Case of Robert Fludd's Magnetical Medicine." In *Medicine and the Market in England and Its Colonies, c. 1450–c. 1850*. Edited by Mark Jackson, 88–107. London: Palgrave, 2007.
Kelly, Catherine. *War and the Militarization of British Army Medicine, 1793–1830*. London: Pickering & Chatto, 2011.
Kennedy, Meegan. *Revising the Clinic: Vision and Representation in Victorian Medical Narrative and the Novel*. Columbus: Ohio State University Press, 2010.

Kermode, Frank. *The Sense of an Ending: Studies in the Theory of Fiction*. Oxford: Oxford University Press, 2000.
Kerr, Matthew L. Newsom. *Contagion, Isolation, and Biopolitics in Victorian London*. Gewerbestrasse: Palgrave Macmillan, 2018.
Key, Jack D., and Alvin E. Rodin. *Medical Casebook of Doctor Arthur Conan Doyle: From Practitioner to Sherlock Holmes and Beyond*. Malabar, FL: R. E. Krieger, 1984.
Khan, Iqbal Akhtar. "Plague: The Dreadful Visitation Occupying the Human Mind for Centuries." *Transactions of the Royal Society of Tropical Medicine and Hygiene* 98, no. 5 (May 1, 2004): 270–77.
King, Albert F. "Insects and Disease: Mosquitoes and Malaria." *Popular Science Monthly* 23 (1883): 644–63.
Kingsley, Charles. *Alton Locke*. London: Macmillan, 1862.
———. [Parson Lot, pseud.] *Cheap Clothes and Nasty*. Cambridge, MA: Macmillan, 1850.
———. "Cholera, 1866." In *The Water of Life and Other Sermons*, 149–202. London: Macmillan, 1879.
———. "The Fall." In *Sermons on National Subjects*, 412–22. London: Macmillan, 1885.
———. "Lecture III: The Explosive Forces," in *Three Lectures: Delivered at the Royal Institution, on the Ancien Regime as It Existed on the Continent before the French Revolution*, 86–136. London: Macmillan: 1867.
———. "Life and Death." In *Twenty-Five Village Sermons*, 25–34. London: John Parker, 1849.
———. "Mad World, My Masters." *Frasier's Magazine* 57, no. 337 (January 1858): 133–42.
———. "The Massacre of the Innocents." In *Sanitary and Social Lectures and Essays*, 146–52. London: Macmillan & Co., 1880.
———. "Morning sermon on the Day of Humiliation for Cholera [delivered at] Eversley Church." 5 October 1849. Charles Kingsley Papers (1819–1875). Wellcome Archives & Manuscripts. Wellcome Trust Library, UK.
———. "Physician's Calling." In *The Water of Life and Other Sermons*, 14–16. London: Macmillan, 1879.
———. "Preface to the Fourth Edition," in *The Works of Charles Kingsley*, vii–xvii. Philadelphia: John D. Morris & Co., 1889.
———. "The Resurrection." In *Twenty-Five Village Sermons*, 180–90. London: John Parker, 1849.
———. Review of *A History England from the Fall of Wolsey to the Death of Elizabeth* by J. A. Froude. *North British Review* vol. 25 (November 1856): 38–57.
———. "The Science of Health." In *Sanitary and Social Lectures and Essays*, 13–27. London: Macmillan, 1880.
———. "The Study of Natural History for Soldiers." In *Scientific Lectures and Essays*, 180–98. London: Macmillan, 1899.

———. *True Words for Brave Men*. London: Keagan Paul, Trench, 1888.
———. "The Two Breaths." In *Health and Education*, 26–51. London: W. Ibster, 1874.
———. *Two Years Ago*. London: Collins Clear Type Press, 1903.
Kingsley, Frances, ed. *Charles Kingsley: His Letters and Memories of His Life*. 2 Vols. London: Macmillan, 1894.
Kistler, Jordan. "Rethinking the New Woman in *Dracula*." *Gothic Studies* 20, no. 1–2 (2018): 244–56.
Kmietowicz, Zosia. "Brexit—Not EU Membership—Threatens the NHS, 60 Eminent Doctors Say." *British Medical Journal* 353 (2016): i3373. https://doi.org/10.1136/bmj.i3373.
Koch, Robert. "The Crusade against Typhoid Fever." *British Medical Journal* 1, no. 2200 (1903): 503–5.
Kotar, S. L., and J. E. Gessler. *Cholera: A Worldwide History*. Jefferson, NC: McFarland, 2014.
Kousoulis, Antonis A. "Etymology of cholera." *Emerging Infectious Diseases* 18, no. 3 (2012): 540.
Kruif, Paul de. *The Microbe Hunters*. New York: Blue Ribbon Books, 1926.
Lakoff, George, and Mark Johnson. *Metaphors We Live By*. Chicago: University of Chicago Press, 2003.
Lambert, Léopold. *Weaponized Architecture: The Impossibility of Innocence*. New York: DPR-Barcelona, 2012.
Landecker, Hannah. "Antibiotic Resistance and the Biology of History." *Body & Society* 22, no. 4 (2015): 19–52.
Latour, Bruno. *The Pasteurization of France*. Cambridge, MA: Harvard University Press, 1993.
Lawrence, Christopher. *Medicine in the Making of Modern Britain 1700–1920*. New York: Routledge, 1994.
Lawrence, Christopher, and Michael Brown. "Quintessentially Modern Heroes: Surgeons, Explorers, and Empire, c. 1840–1914." *Journal of Social History* 50, no. 1 (2016): 148–78.
Learoyd, P. "The History of Blood Transfusion Prior to the 20th Century, Part 2." *Transfusion Medicine* 22, no. 6 (2012): 372–76.
Lehigh University. "3.11.20: Lehigh Moves to Remote Learning Temporarily." *Lehigh News*, March 11, 2020. Accessed August 1, 2020, https://www2.lehigh.edu/news/31120-lehigh-moves-to-remote-learning-temporarily.
Leibbrand, C. H. "How London Fights the Microbe." *Windsor Magazine*, May 1899, 657–62.
Lesch, John E. *The First Miracle Drugs: How the Sulfa Drugs Transformed Medicine*. Oxford, UK: Oxford University Press, 2007.
Levine, Philippa. "Venereal Disease, Prostitution, and the Politics of Empire: The Case of British India." *Journal of the History of Sexuality* 4, no. 4 (1994): 579–602.

Levinson, Jonathan, Conard Wilson, James Doubek, and Suzanne Nuyen. "Federal Officers Use Unmarked Vehicles to Grab People in Portland, DHS Confirms" *NPR*. June 17, 2020. Accessed August 10, 2020, https://www.npr.org/2020/07/17/892277592/federal-officers-use-unmarked-vehicles-to-grab-protesters-in-portland.

Lewis, Jane. "Providers, 'Consumers,' the State and the Delivery of Health Care in Twentieth Century Britain." In *Medicine in Society: Historical Essays*. Edited by Andrew Wear, 317–45. Cambridge, UK: Cambridge University Press, 1992.

Lindemann, Mary. *Medicine and Society in Early Modern Europe*. Cambridge, UK: Cambridge University Press, 2013.

Lister, Joseph. "An Address on the Present Position of Antiseptic Surgery." *British Medical Journal* 2, no. 1546 (1890): 377–79.

Lo, Vivienne, and Michael Stanly-Baker. "Chinese Medicine." In *The Oxford Handbook of the History of Medicine*. Edited by Mark Jackson, 150–68. Oxford, UK: Oxford University Press, 2011.

Lock, Margaret M., and Vinh-Kim Nguyen. *An Anthropology of Biomedicine*. Chichester, UK: Wiley-Blackwell, 2010.

Lokke, Kari E. "The Last Man." In *The Cambridge Companion to Mary Shelley*. Edited by Esther Schor, 116–34. Cambridge, UK: Cambridge University Press, 2003.

Lynteris, Christos, ed., *Framing Animals as Epidemic Villains: Histories of Non-human Disease*. Gewerbestrasse, Switzerland: Palgrave, 2019.

Lyons, Emily. "O Little Isle!": Landscape, Englishness, and Apocalypse in *The Last Man* and *The War of the Worlds*." *ISLE: Interdisciplinary Studies in Literature and Environment*, isz067 (2019). https://doi.org/10.1093/isle/isz067.

Lyons, Maryinez. *The Colonial Disease: A Social History of Sleeping Sickness in Northern Zaire, 1900–1940*. Cambridge, UK: Cambridge University Press, 1992.

Lyons, Robert Dyer. *A Treatise on Fever or Selections from a Course of Lectures on Fever Being Part of a Course of Theory and Practice of Medicine*. London: Longman, Green, Longman, & Roberts, 1861.

MacDuffie, Allen. "Joseph Conrad's Geographies of Energy." *ELH* 76, no. 1 (2009): 75–98.

Malik, Salahuddin. "The Panjab and the Indian 'Mutiny': A Reassessment." *Islamic Studies* 15, no. 2 (1976): 81–110.

Manson, Patrick. "The Malaria Parasite." *Journal of the Africa Society* 7, no. 13 (1907): 225–33.

Manson-Bahr, Philip H. *Manson's Tropical Diseases*. New York: W. Wood, 1921.

Markovitz, Stefanie. *The Crimean War and the British Imagination*. Cambridge, UK: Cambridge University Press, 2009.

Marks, Robert. *The Origins of the Modern World: Fate and Fortune in the Rise of the West*. Lanham, MD: Rowman & Littlefield, 2007.
Marshall, April D. "Metaphors We Die By." *Semiotica: Journal of the International Association for Semiotic Studies* 161 (2006): 345–61.
Martin, Emily. *Flexible Bodies: Tracking Immunity in American Culture from the Days of Polio to the Age of AIDS*. Boston: Beacon Press, 1994.
Martin, John. *Contributions to Military and State Medicine: First Volume*. London: J & A Churchill, 1881.
Mayhew, Henry. *London Labour and the London Poor*. 4 vols. New York: Dove, 1861–1862. 1968.
Mbembe, Achille. "Necropolitics." *Public Culture* 15, no. 1 (2003): 11–40.
McClintock, Anne. *Imperial Leather: Race, Gender, and Sexuality in the Colonial Conquest*. New York: Routledge, 1995.
McDonald, Lynn. "Florence Nightingale, Statistics and the Crimean War." *Journal of the Royal Statistical Society: Series A (Statistics in Society)* 177, no. 3 (2014): 569–86.
McDonald, Peter D. *British Literary Culture and Publishing Practice, 1880–1914*. Cambridge, UK: Cambridge University Press, 1997.
McNally, Raymond T., and Radu Florescu. *In Search of Dracula: The History of Dracula and Vampires*. Boston: Houghton Mifflin, 1994.
McNulty, Cliodna A. M. et al., "Don't Wear Me Out—The Public's Knowledge of and Attitudes to Antibiotic Use," *Journal of Antimicrobial Chemotherapy* 59, no. 4 (2007): 727–38.
McWhir, Anne. "Mary Shelley's Anti-Contagionism: *The Last Man* as 'Fatal Narrative.'" *Mosaic* 35, no. 2 (2002): 23–38.
Meloni, Maurizio. *Impressionable Biologies: From the Archaeology of Plasticity to the Sociology of Epigenetics*. New York: Routledge, 2019.
Melville, Peter. "The Problem of Immunity in *The Last Man*." *SEL Studies in English Literature 1500–1900* 47, no. 4 (2007): 825–46.
———. *Romantic Hospitality and the Resistance to Accommodation*. Waterloo, ON: Wilfrid Laurier University Press, 2007.
Mertens, Myriam. "Chemical Compounds in the Congo: Pharmaceuticals and the 'Crossed History' of Public Health in Belgian Africa (ca. 1905–1939)." PhD diss., University of Gent, 2014. http://hdl.handle.net/1854/LU-4443278.
Miller, D. A. *The Novel and the Police*. Berkeley: University of California Press, 1988.
Mongoven, Ann. "The War on Disease and the War on Terror: A Dangerous Metaphorical Nexus?" *Cambridge Quarterly of Healthcare Ethics* 15, no. 4 (2006): 403–16.
Moon, G. Washington. *Men and Women of the Time: A Dictionary of Contemporaries*. 13th ed. London: George Routledge & Sons, 1891.

Mooney, Graham. *Intrusive Interventions: Public Health, Domestic Space, and Infectious Disease Surveillance in England, 1840–1914*. Rochester: University of Rochester, 2015.

Morrell, George F. *Health and Disease in Deadly Combat*. CC BY 4.0 license. Wellcome Collection. https://wellcomecollection.org/works/ngc7gs94.

Mort, Frank. *Dangerous Sexualities: Medico-Moral Politics in England since 1830*. New York: Routledge & Kegan Paul, 1987.

Morton, Timothy. *Dark Ecology: For a Logic of Future Coexistence*. New York: Columbia University Press, 2016.

Moseley, Benjamin. *A Treatise on Tropical Diseases: On Military Operations; and on the Climate of the West-Indies*. London: T. Cadell, 1792.

Mukherjee, Upamanyu Pablo. "'Out-of-the-Way Asiatic Disease': Contagion, Malingering, and Sherlock's England." In *Literature of an Independent England: Revisions of England, Englishness, and English Literature*. Edited by Claire Westall and Michael Gardiner, 77–90. New York: Palgrave Macmillan, 2013.

Neill, Deborah J. *Networks in Tropical Medicine: Internationalism, Colonialism, and the Rise of a Medical Specialty, 1890–1930*. Stanford, CA: Stanford University Press, 2012.

Nelson, Richard. *Asiatic Cholera, Its Origin and Spread in Asia, Africa, and Europe, Introduction into America through Canada*. New York: Townsend, 1866.

Nelson, Sara C. "Ebola Zombie 'Risen from the Dead' Is a Horrible Viral Hoax." *Huffington Post UK*. October 6, 2014. Accessed March 12, 2019. http://www.huffingtonpost.co.uk/2014/10/06/ebola-zombie-risen-dead-viral-hoax_n_5937728.html.

Nerlich, Brigitte. "'The Post-Antibiotic Apocalypse' and the 'War on Superbugs': Catastrophe Discourse in Microbiology, Its Rhetorical Form and Political Function," *Public Understanding of Science* 18, no. 5 (2009): 574–88; discussion 88–90.

Nightingale, Florence. *Florence Nightingale on Public Health Care: The Collected Works of Florence Nightingale Volume 6*. Edited by Lynn McDonald. Waterloo, ON: Wilfrid Laurier University Press, 2004.

———. *Florence Nightingale to Her Nurses*. London: Macmillan, 1914.

———. *Notes on Nursing: What It Is, and What It Is Not*. New York: D. Appleton, 1860.

———. *Postscript to George H. De'Ath's Cholera: What Can We Do about It?* Buckingham, UK: Walford, 1892.

O'Conner, Erin. *Raw Material: Producing Pathology in Victorian Culture*. Durham, NC: Duke University Press, 53–59.

Orenstein, Peggy. "Surviving Cancer without the Positive Thinking." *Atlantic*. May 7, 2016. Accessed March 12, 2019. https://www.theatlantic.com/health/archive/2016/05/surviving-cancer-without-the-positive-thinking/481764/?utm_source=atlfb.

Osler, William. "Bacilli and Bullets." London: Oxford University Press, 1914.
Otis, Laura. *Membranes: Metaphors of Invasion in Nineteenth-Century Literature, Science, and Politics.* Baltimore, MD: Johns Hopkins University Press, 1999.
Otter, Chris. *The Victorian Eye: A Political History of Light and Vision in Britain, 1800–1910.* Chicago: University of Chicago Press, 2008.
Oxford English Dictionary Online. s.v. "Lancet." Accessed December 10, 2013. http://www.oed.com/view/Entry/105422?redirectedFrom=lancet&.
"Parke on Health in Africa." *London Medical Press and Circular* 108, no. 14 (April 4, 1894): 377–78.
Paley, Morton D. *The Apocalyptic Sublime.* New Haven, CT: Yale University Press, 1986.
Pamboukian, Sylvia A. *Doctoring the Novel: Medicine and Quackery from Shelley to Doyle.* Athens: Ohio University Press, 2012.
Panaritis, Maria, "I Went to the Supermarket and Came Home Shaken," *Philadelphia Inquirer*, March 31, 2020. Accessed August 8, 2020, https://www.inquirer.com/health/coronavirus/coronavirus-covid-19-supermarkets-grocery-stores-shopping-low-inventory-wynnewood-giant-maria-panaritis-20200331.html.
Parascandola, John. "The Theoretical Basis of Paul Ehrlich's Chemotherapy." *Journal of the History of Medicine and Allied Sciences* 36, no. 1 (1981): 19–43.
Parke, Thomas Heazle. *My Personal Experiences in Equatorial Africa, as Medical Officer of the Emin Pasha Relief Expedition.* New York: Charles Scribner's Sons, 1891.
Parsi, Kayhan. "War Metaphors in Health Care: What Are They Good For?" *American Journal of Bioethics* 16, no. 10 (2016): 1–2.
Pearlman, R. A., and Tyler P. Tate. "Military Metaphors in Healthcare: Who Are We Actually Trying to Help?" *American Journal of Bioethics* 16, no. 10 (2016): 15–17.
Peck, John. *War, the Army, and Victorian Literature.* New York: St. Martin's Press, 1998.
Pellecchia, Umberto et al. "Social Consequences of Ebola Containment Measures in Liberia." *PLoS ONE* 10, no. 12 (2015): e0143036. https://doi.org/10.1371/journal.pone.0143036.
Pelling, Margaret. "The Meaning of Contagion." In *Contagion: Historical and Cultural Studies.* Edited by Alison Bashford and Claire Hooker, 15–39. London: Routledge, 2001.
Penner, Louise. *Victorian Medicine and Social Reform: Florence Nightingale among the Novelists.* New York: Palgrave Macmillan, 2010.
Petersen, Charisse, and June L. Round. "Defining Dysbiosis and Its Influence on Host Immunity and Disease." *Cellular Microbiology* 16, no. 7 (2014): 1024–33.
Pick, Daniel. *Faces of Degeneration: A European Disorder, c. 1848–c. 1918.* Cambridge, UK: Cambridge University Press, 1999.

Pittard, Christopher. *Purity and Contamination in Late Victorian Detective Fiction*. Burlington, UK: Ashgate, 2011.
Planta, Margaret B. "The Role of Poverty in Antimicrobial Resistance." *Journal of the American Board of Family Medicine* 20, no. 6 (2007): 533–39.
Poovey, Mary. *Uneven Developments: The Ideological Work of Gender in Mid-Victorian England*. Chicago: University of Chicago Press, 1988.
Porter, Roy. *The Greatest Benefit to Mankind: A Medical History of Humanity*. New York: W. W. Norton, 1997.
Poteat, Tonia, Gregorio A. Millett, La Ron E. Nelson, and Chris Beyrer. "Understanding COVID-19 Risks and Vulnerabilities among Black Communities in America: The Lethal Force of Syndemics." *Annals of Epidemiology* 47 (2020): 1–3.
Preston, Richard. "The Ebola Wars." *New Yorker*. October 27, 2014. Accessed January 30, 2018. https://www.newyorker.com/magazine/2014/10/27/ebola-wars.
Price, Kim. *Medical Negligence in Victorian Britain: The Crisis of Care under English Poor Law, c. 1834–1900*. London: Bloomsbury, 2016.
Proctor, George. *History of the Crusades: Their Rise, Progress, and Results*. Glasgow: Richard Griffin, 1854.
Puar, Jasbir. "Introduction: Homonationalism and Biopolitics." In *Terrorist Assemblages*. Edited by Jasbir Puar, *Terrorist Assemblages in Queer Time*. Durham, NC: Duke University Press, 2007.
Rabinow, Paul. *French Modern: Norms and Forms of the Social Environment*. Cambridge, MA: MIT Press, 1989.
Rasamussen, Angela. Twitter post. February 17, 2020. https://twitter.com/angie_rasmussen.
"Recent Novels." *Spectator*, 31 July 1897, 150–51.
Rees, Rosemary. *Poverty and Public Health, 1815–1948*. Oxford, UK: Heinemann, 2001.
Reid, Julian. *The Biopolitics of the War on Terror: Life Struggles, Liberal Modernity and the Defence of Logistical Societies*. Manchester, UK: Manchester University Press, 2009.
Resnick, Brian, and Umair Irfan, "What Immunity to Covid-19 Might Actually Mean." *Vox*, April 23, 2020. Accessed August 10, 2020, https://www.vox.com/science-and-health/2020/4/23/21219028/covid-19-immunity-testing-reinfection-antibodies-explained.
Riethmiller, S. "From Atoxyl to Salvarsan: Searching for the Magic Bullet." *Chemotherapy* 51, no. 5 (2005): 234–42.
Roberts, M. J. D. "The Politics of Professionalization: MPs, Medical Men, and the 1858 Medical Act." *Medical History* 53, no. 1 (2009): 37–56.
Rogers, Charlotte. *Jungle Fever: Exploring Madness and Medicine in Twentieth-Century Tropical Narratives*. Nashville, TN: Vanderbilt University Press, 2012.

Rose, Nikolas. "Medicine, History and the Present." In *Reassessing Foucault: Power, Medicine, and the Body*. Edited by Colin Jones and Roy Porter. London: Routledge, 1998.
Rosenberg, Charles E. "Disease in History: Frames and Framers" *Milbank Quarterly* 67, no. 1 (1989): 1–15.
———. *Explaining Epidemics and Other Studies in the History of Medicine*. Cambridge, UK: Cambridge University Press, 1992.
Ross, Ronald. "The Battle for Health in the Tropics." *Journal of Tropical Medicine and Hygiene* 7 (1904): 187–88.
———. Introduction to *Malaria, a Neglected Factor in the History of Greece and Rome* by William Henry Jones, 1–14. Cambridge, MA: Macmillan & Bowes, 1907.
———. *Philosophies*. London: John Murray, 1923.
———. "The Relationship of Malaria and the Mosquito." *Lancet* 156, no. 4010 (1900): 48–50.
———. "Researches on Malaria," *Journal of the Royal Army Medical Corps* 4, no. 4 (1905): 450–74.
Rosslenbroich, Bernd. *On the Origin of Autonomy: A New Look at the Major Transitions in Evolution*. New York: Springer, 2016.
Rothfield, Lawrence. *Vital Signs: Medical Realism in Nineteenth-Century Fiction*. Princeton, NJ: Princeton University Press, 1992.
Rothman, David J. *Strangers at the Bedside: A History of How Law and Bioethics Transformed Medical Decision Making*. New Brunswick, NJ: Aldine Transaction, 2009.
Rothstein, Mark A. "The Moral Challenge of Ebola." *American Journal of Public Health* 105, no. 1 (2015): 6–8.
Ruiz, Maria Isabel Romero. "Fallen Women and the London Lock Hospitals and By-Laws of 1840 (Revised 1848)." *Journal of English Studies* 8, no. 141 (2010): 141–58.
Ryan, Vanessa L. "The Physiological Sublime: Burke's Critique of Reason." *Journal of the History of Ideas* 62, no. 2 (2001): 265–79.
Said, Edward W. *Culture and Imperialism*. New York: Knopf, 1993.
Sajjad, Sadaf et al. "Psychotherapy through Video Game to Target Illness Related Problematic Behaviors of Children with Brain Tumor." *Current Medical Imaging Reviews* 10, no. 1 (2014): 62–72.
Senf, Carol A. " 'Dracula': Stoker's Response to the New Woman." *Victorian Studies* 26, no. 1 (1982): 33–49.
———. *Science and Social Science in Bram Stoker's Fiction*. London: Greenwood Press, 2002.
Servitje, Lorenzo. "Gaming the Apocalypse in the Time of Antibiotic Resistance," *Osiris* 34, no. 1 (2019): 316–37.
———. "H5n1 for Angry Birds: *Plague Inc.*, Mobile Games, and the Biopolitics of Outbreak Narratives." *Science Fiction Studies* 43, no. 1 (2016): 85–103.

———. "'The Path of Most Resistance': Surgeon X and the Graphic Estrangement of Antibiosis." In *The Palgrave Handbook of Twentieth and Twenty-First Century Literature and Science*. Edited by Neel Ahuja et al. (New York: Palgrave, 2020).

———. "Acting Fatally on the Strength of the Martial Metaphor," *Somatosphere*, May 10, 2020. Accessed August 1, 2020, http://somatosphere.net/forumpost/covid19-martial-metaphor/.

Seymore, Robert. *Cholera Tramples the Victor & the Vanquish'd Both*. 1831. Print. 10 cm x 12 cm. Public Domain. http://resource.nlm.nih.gov/101393375.

Shakespeare, William. *Othello: The Moor of Venice*. Edited by Michael Neill. Oxford, UK: Oxford University Press, 2006.

Shahinyan, Diana Louis. "That which Mere Modernity Cannot Kill': The Evolution of Legal Professionalism in Bram Stoker's Dracula." *Journal of Victorian Culture* 23, no 1 (2018): 119–36.

Sharpe, Christina. *In the Wake: On Blackness and Being*. Durham, NC: Duke University Press, 2016.

Shelley, Mary. *History of a Six Weeks' Tour through a Part of France, Switzerland, Germany and Holland: With Letters Descriptive of a Sail Round the Lake of Geneva, and of the Glaciers of Chamouni*. London: T. Hookham, 1817.

———. *The Last Man*. Edited by Pamela Bickley. Hertfordshire, UK: Wordsworth Classics, 2004.

———. "Letters (6) from Mary Shelley to Claire Clairmont." Ashley Manuscripts 19th Century–20th Century. Ashley MS 5023. British Library Archives, London, UK.

Shelley, Percy Bysshe. *Queen Mab: A Philosophical Poem*. New York: Wright & Owen, 1831.

Sherman, David. *In a Strange Room: Modernism's Corpses and Mortal Obligation*. Oxford, UK: Oxford University Press, 2014.

Shmuely, Shira. "Curare: The Poisoned Arrow that Entered the Laboratory and Sparked a Moral Debate." *Social History of Medicine*. Published online prior to print. Accessed March 16, 2019. https://doi.org/10.1093/shm/hky124.

Siddiqi, Yumna. *Anxieties of Empire and the Fiction of Intrigue*. New York: Columbia University Press, 2008.

Simpson, James Y. "A Proposal to Stamp Out Small Pox and other Contagious Diseases." In *The Works of Sir James Y. Simpson*, vol. II. Edited by W. G. Simpson, 543–53. Edinburgh: Adam & Charles Black, 1871.

Singh, Nina, et al. "How Often Are Antibiotic-Resistant Bacteria Said to 'Evolve' in the News?," *PLoS ONE* 11, no. 3 (2016): e0150396. https://doi.org/10.1371/journal.pone.0150396.

Smith, Susan L. *Toxic Exposures: Mustard Gas and the Health Consequences of World War II in the United States*. New Brunswick, NJ: Rutgers University Press, 2019.

Snow, John. "On the Chief Cause of the Recent Sickness and Mortality in the Crimea." *Medical Times and Gazette*, May 12, 1855, 457–58.

———. *On the Mode of Communication of Cholera*. London: John Churchill, 1855.

"Social Science Association." *Lancet* 94, no. 2406 (1869): 522–23.

Sokoloff, Boris. *The Miracle Drugs*. Chicago: Ziff-Davis, 1949.

Sontag, Susan. *Illness as Metaphor*. New York: Vintage Books, 1979.

Sparks, Tabitha. *The Doctor in the Victorian Novel: Family Practices*. Farnham, UK: Ashgate, 2010.

———. "Medical Gothic and the Return of the Contagious Diseases Acts in Stoker and Machen." *Nineteenth-Century Feminisms* 6 (2002): 87–102.

Spencer, Kathleen L. "Purity and Danger: Dracula, the Urban Gothic, and the Late Victorian Degeneracy Crisis." *ELH* 59, no. 1 (1992): 197–225.

Springthorpe, John William. "The Battle of Life." *Australasian Medical Gazette*, vol. 15 (1896): 81–87.

Spiteri, Gianfranco, James Fielding, Michaela Diercke, Christine Campese, Vincent Enouf, Alexandre Gaymard, Antonino Bella, et al. "First Cases of Coronavirus Disease 2019 (COVID-19) in the WHO European Region, 24 January to 21 February 2020." *Eurosurveillance* 25, no. 9 (March 5, 2020): 1.

Stanley, Henry Morton. *The Founding of the Congo Free State: A Story of Work and Exploration: Volume II*. London: Samson Low, Marston, Searle & Rivington, 1885.

Steinlight, Emily. *Populating the Novel: Literary Form and the Politics of Surplus Life*. Ithaca, NY: Cornell University Press, 2018.

Stiles, Anne. *Popular Fiction and Brain Science in the Late Nineteenth Century*. Cambridge: Cambridge University Press, 2012.

Stoker, Bram. *Bram Stoker's Notes for Dracula: A Facsimile Edition*. Edited by Robert Eighteen-Bisang and Elizabeth Russell Miller. Jefferson, NC: McFarland, 2008.

———. *Dracula: Authoritative Text, Contexts, Reviews and Reactions, Dramatic and Film Variations, Criticism*. Edited by Nina Auerbach and David J. Skal. New York: W. W. Norton, 1997.

Stoker, Charlotte. Typeset transcription. "Account of the Cholera Outbreak in Ireland in 1832." Papers of the Stoker Family. Trinity College Archives and Manuscripts.

Strang, Hilary. "Common Life, Animal Life, Equality: The Last Man." *ELH* 78, no. 2 (2011): 409–31.

Stuart, Thomas M. "Out of Time: Queer Temporality and Eugenic Monstrosity." *Victorian Studies* 60, no. 2 (2018): 218–27.

Swenson, Kristine. *Medical Women and Victorian Fiction*. Norman: University of Missouri, 2007.

Sydenham, Thomas. *The Works of Thomas Sydenham, M.D.*, vol. I. Edited by William A. Greenhill. Translated by R. G. Latham. London: Sydenham Society, 1848.

Tallie, T. J. "Asymptomatic Lethality: Cooper, COVID-19, and the Potential for Black Death," *Nursing Clio*, June 8, 2020. Accessed August 8, 2020, https://nursingclio.org/2020/06/08/asymptomatic-lethality-cooper-covid-19-and-the-potential-for-black-death/.

Tauber, Alfred I. *Immunity: The Evolution of an Idea*. Oxford, UK: Oxford University Press, 2017.

Taylor, Jesse Oak. *The Sky of Our Manufacture: The London Fog and British Fiction from Dickens to Woolf*. Charlottesville: University of Virginia Press, 2016.

Taylor-Brown, Emilie. "(Re)Constructing the Knights of Science: Parasitologists and Their Literary Imaginations." *Journal of Literature and Science* 7, no. 2 (2014): 62–79.

———. "'She Has a Parasite Soul!' The Pathologization of the Gothic Monster as Parasitic Hybrid in Bram Stoker's Dracula, Richard Marsh's The Beetle, and Arthur Conan Doyle's 'The Parasite.'" In *Monsters and Monstrosity from the Fin De Siècle to the Millennium: New Essays*. Edited by Sharla Hutchison and Rebecca A. Brown. Jefferson, NC: McFarland, 2015.

Taylor-Pirie, Emilie. *Empire Under the Microscope: Parasitology and the British Literary Imagination, 1885–1935*. London: Palgrave, 2021.

Thibault, Ghislian. "Needles and Bullets: Media Theory, Medicine, and Propaganda, 1910–1940." In *Endemic: Essays in Contagion Theory*. Edited by Kari Nixon and Lorenzo Servitje, 67–92. London: Palgrave Macmillan, 2016.

"This Week: Topics of the Day." *Medical Times and Gazette*, June 16, 1883, 671–72.

Todd, Macy. "What Bram Stoker's Dracula Reveals about Violence," *English Literature in Transition, 1880–1920* 58, no. 3 (2015): 361–84.

Tomasetti, Cristian, and Bert Vogelstein. "Variation in Cancer Risk among Tissues Can Be Explained by the Number of Stem Cell Divisions." *Science* 347, no. 6217 (2015): 78–81.

Tomes, Nancy. *The Gospel of Germs: Men, Women, and the Microbe in American Life* Cambridge, MA: Harvard University Press, 1998.

Tsing, Anna Lowenhaupt. *The Mushroom at the End of the World: On the Possibility of Life in Capitalist Ruins*. Princeton, NJ: Princeton University Press, 2015.

Tucker, Jennifer. "Photography as Witness, Detective, and Impostor: Visual Representation in Victorian Science." In *Victorian Science in Context*. Edited by Bernard Lightman, 378–408. Chicago: University of Chicago Press, 1997.

Twyning, John. *Forms of English History in Literature, Landscape, and Architecture*. Houndmills, UK: Palgrave Macmillan, 2014.

"Two Years Ago." *Putnam's Monthly Magazine of American Literature, Science, and Art* 9, no. 53 (1857): 505–14.

"Two Years Ago by Charles Kingsley." *British Foreign and Evangelical Review* 7, no. 13 (1858): 130–51.

Tyler, Derek Bryson. "A Timeline of the Coronavirus Pandemic," *New York Times*, August 6, 2020, https://www.nytimes.com/article/coronavirus-timeline.html.

"Unseen Enemies." *London Times*. May 22, 1880, 6e.

Valenstein, Elliot S. *The War of the Soups and the Sparks: The Discovery of Neurotransmitters and the Dispute over How Nerves Communicate*. New York: Columbia University Press, 2007.

Viala-Gaudefroy, Jerome, and Dana Linderman, "Donald Trump's 'Chinese Virus': The Politics of Naming," *The Conversation*, April 21, 2020. Accessed August 8, 2020, https://theconversation.com/donald-trumps-chinese-virus-the-politics-of-naming-136796.

Vine, Steven. "Mary Shelley's Sublime Bodies: Frankenstein, Matilda, the Last Man." *English* 55, no. 212 (2006): 141–56.

Virchow, Rudolph. "The Huxley Lecture on Recent Advances in Science and Their Bearing on Medicine and Surgery." *Lancet* 152, no. 3919 (1898): 909–12.

Vora, Setu K. "Sherlock Holmes and a Biological Weapon." *Journal of the Royal Society of Medicine* 95, no. 2 (2002): 101–3.

Wald, Priscilla. *Contagious: Cultures, Carriers, and the Outbreak Narrative*. Durham, NC: Duke University Press, 2008.

Walkowitz, Judith R. *City of Dreadful Delight: Narratives of Sexual Danger in Late-Victorian London*. Chicago: University of Chicago Press, 1992.

———. *Prostitution and Victorian Society: Women, Class, and the State*. Cambridge: Cambridge University Press, 1980.

Walker, Iona. "Beyond the Military Metaphor: Comparing Antimicrobial Resistance and the COVID-19 Pandemic in the United Kingdom," *Medicine Anthropology Theory* 7, no. 2 (2020): 261–272.

Wang, Fuson. "Romantic Disease Discourse: Disability, Immunity, and Literature." *Nineteenth-Century Contexts* 33, no. 5 (2011): 467–82.

———. "We Must Live Elsewhere: The Social Construction of Natural Immunity in Mary Shelley's *The Last Man*." *European Romantic Review* 22, no. 2 (2011): 235–55.

"The War: Naval and Military Intelligence." *Lancet* 63, no. 1599 (1854): 461–62.

Warren, V. L. "The 'Medicine Is War' Metaphor." *HEC Forum* 3, no. 1 (1991): 39–50.

Watt, Ian. *Conrad in the Nineteenth Century*. Berkeley: University of California Press, 1979.

Watson, Matt. Twitter post. August 2, 2020. 1:02 p.m. https://mobile.twitter.com/BioAndBaseball.

Wee, C. J. Wan-ling. *Culture, Empire, and the Question of Being Modern*. Lanham, MD: Lexington Books, 2003.

Wehelye, Alexander R. *Habeas Viscus: Assemblages, Biopolitics, and Black Feminist Theories of the Human.* Durham, NC: Duke University Press, 2014.

Wellcome Trust. *Exploring the Consumer Perspective on Antimicrobial Resistance.* June 2015. Accessed March 12, 2019. https://wellcome.ac.uk/sites/default/files/exploring-consumer-perspective-on-antimicrobial-resistance-jun15.pdf.

Wells, T. Spencer. "The Bradshaw Lecture on Modern Abdominal Surgery." *British Medical Journal* 2, no. 1564 (1890): 1413–16.

Wende, Ernest. "The Microscope in the Diagnosis of Diseases of the Skin." *Cincinnati-Lancet.* June 4, 1887.

West, Benjamin. *Death on the Pale Horse.* 1796. Oil on canvas. 23 3/8 in. x 50 5/8 in. (59.4 x 128.6 cm). Detroit Institute of Arts, Detroit. https://www.dia.org/art/collection/object/death-pale-horse-64796.

Westenra, Sambon, L. "Acclimatization of Europeans in Tropical Lands." *Geographical Journal* 12, no. 6 (1898): 589–99.

Wilberforce, Reginald Garton. An Unrecorded Chapter of the Indian Mutiny: Being the Personal Reminiscences of Reginald G. Wilberforce, Late 52nd Light Infantry, Compiled from a Diary and Letters Written on the Spot. London: John Murray, 1894.

Wilkinson, Alisa. "Pandemics Are Not Wars," *Vox*, April 15, 2020. Accessed August 5, 2020, https://www.vox.com/culture/2020/4/15/21193679/coronavirus-pandemic-war-metaphor-ecology-microbiome.

Williamson, Philip. "State Prayers, Fasts and Thanksgivings: Public Worship in Britain 1830–1897." *Past & Present* 200, no. 1 (2008): 121–74.

Willing, Benjamin P., Shannon L. Russell, and B. Brett Finlay. "Shifting the Balance: Antibiotic Effects on Host–Microbiota Mutualism." *National Review Microbiology* 9, no. 4 (2011): 233–43.

Willis, Martin. "'The Invisible Giant,' 'Dracula,' and Disease." *Studies in the Novel* 39, no. 3 (2007): 301–25.

———. *Vision, Science, and Literature, 1870–1920: Ocular Horizons.* London: Pickering & Chatto, 2011.

Wilson, Elizabeth. *Gut Feminism.* Durham, NC: Duke University Press, 2016.

Winslow, Charles-Edward Amory. "The War against Disease." *Atlantic Monthly* 91, no. 543 (January 1903): 43–52.

Worboys, Michael. *Spreading Germs: Disease Theories and Medical Practice in Britain, 1865–1900.* Cambridge, UK: Cambridge University Press, 2000.

World Health Organization, "Pneumonia of Unknown Cause—China," Emergencies Preparedness, Response, January 5, 2020. Accessed August 7, 2020. https://www.who.int/csr/don/05-january-2020-pneumonia-of-unkown-cause-china/en/.

Worldometer. "COVID-19 CORONAVIRUS PANDEMIC." Worldometer, August 5, 2020. Accessed August 5, https://www.worldometers.info/coronavirus/.

Wright, Erika. *Reading for Health: Medical Narratives and the Nineteenth-Century Novel.* Athens: Ohio University Press, 2016.

Yeung, Jessie, Adam Renton, and Angela Dewan, "May 6 Coronavirus News," *CNN*, May 6, 2020. Accessed August 10, 2020, https://www.cnn.com/world/live-news/coronavirus-pandemic-05-06-20-intl/index.html, emphasis added.

Yeung, Jessie, Steve George, Zamira Rahim, and Fernando Alfonso, "May 27 Coronavirus News," *CNN*, March 2020. Accessed August 8, 2020. https://www.cnn.com/world/live-news/coronavirus-pandemic-05-27-20-intl/index.html.

Zaffiri, Lorenzo, Jared Gardner, and Luis H. Toledo-Pereyra. "History of Antibiotics. From Salvarsan to Cephalosporins." *Journal of Investigative Surgery* 25, no. 2 (2012): 67–77.

Zieger, Susan. *Inventing the Addict: Drugs, Race, and Sexuality in Nineteenth-Century British and American Literature.* Amherst: University of Massachusetts Press, 2008.

Index

Aceh people, 185
Achebe, Chinua, 195
Ackernecht, Edwin, 12
activism, 129
"Adventure of the Blanched Soldier, The" (Doyle), 149, 177, 187
"Adventure of the Dying Detective, The" (Doyle), 149, 184, 187, 191
"Adventure of the Speckled Band, The" (Doyle), 148, 158–61
aesthetics, 32–33, 57, 67, 194
Africa, 20, 113, 141, 188–89, 194–226, 232–33
Afrikaners, 173
Agamben, Giorgio, 127, 180
agriculture, 232
Ahuja, Neel, 233
air quality, 12, 32, 35, 39–41, 44, 98, 100, 138. *See also* miasmas
Alang, Sirry, 291
Alton Locke (Kingsley), 69
American Cancer Society, 236
amphibiosis, 246
AMR (Antimicrobial Resistance), 247
anatomy, 10, 82, 150–51, 160
Enquiry Concerning Political Justice, An (Godwin), 64
Anglo-Afghan Wars, 145

animals, 119, 130–33, 142, 155, 159–64, 220–21, 242, 271n60, 272n77
anthrax, 111, 150, 168
anthropocentrism, 62, 111–12, 119–20, 230–31
anthropomorphism, 14, 143, 253n39
antibiotics, 3, 197, 224–25, 228–31, 235, 242
anticontagionism, 10–13, 25, 33–35, 40–42, 44–46, 51, 70, 83, 202, 233. *See also* contagionism
antimicrobial therapies, 5
antiquity, 109, 113–15, 135
anti-Semitism, 118–19, 136
antivirulence, 236, 246
Antwerp School of Tropical Medicine, 206
apocalypse, 43, 49, 56, 61, 229
architecture, 5, 80
aristocracy, 79–80, 83–85, 88, 122–23
Arnold, David, 126
Asiatic cholera. *See* cholera
atheism, 74
Atlantic, 246

bacteriology, 6, 13, 111–13, 145–58, 170–72, 183, 186, 191
Bainbridge, George, 135–36

Banner, Olivia, 238
Bates, Benjamin, 246
"Battle for the Health of the Tropics, The" (Ross), 199–200
Belgium, 196, 199, 202
Bell, Joseph, 150, 183, 186
Bernard, Claude, 148, 156–60, 163–64, 166–67, 276n42, 277n57
Bewell, Alan, 37, 47
Bichat, Xavier, 10, 14, 82, 94–97, 111, 148, 150–51, 160
bioethics, 4, 6
Bioinsecurities (Ahuja), 233
biological warfare, 176, 181, 183–91
biology, 15, 70–73, 93–95, 100
biomedicine, 15
biopolitics: disease and, 12, 32; Doyle and, 146, 149, 152, 161–65, 171–73; Kingsley and, 72, 83, 93–105; martial metaphor and, 15–19, 56, 66, 234; modernity and, 180–83; Shelley and, 29, 39, 41, 44–45, 49, 54, 59, 61–62; Stoker and, 112, 118, 121–22, 128, 138–39. *See also* Agamben, Giorgio; Foucault, Michel
biosecurity, 240, 242
bioterrorism, 183, 233
bioweapons, 240
Birth of the Clinic, The (Foucault), 91
birth rates, 15
Black Lives Matter, 243
Black people, 6, 33, 41, 65, 242–43, 245
"Blanched Soldier, The" (Doyle), 190–91
Bleak House (Dickens), 11, 90
blood, 113–25, 131, 138, 142, 154–57, 160, 163–67
Bock, Martin, 209
body, the: biopolitics and, 41, 166, 181; colonialism and, 52, 119, 186, 193; disease and, 9–15; Doyle and, 146–47, 151–52, 164, 167, 172, 180; Kingsley and, 82, 86; landscape and, 154–55; martial metaphor and, 5, 16–19, 236; miasmas and, 44–47; necropolitics and, 211; race and, 33, 66; religion and, 98–99; Shelley and, 35, 56; Stoker and, 120–21, 125, 138, 141
Boer people, 174–75, 180–84
Boer Wars, the: Doyle and, 147–48, 162, 172–80, 183–91; martial metaphor and, 20, 113, 123, 219; modernity and, 126, 180–83
Booth, Charles, 116
borders, 11, 117, 183–84
botany, 14
Brantlinger, Patrick, 194–95, 208
Brexit, 229–30
British Medical Journal, 151, 177
British military: Conrad, 194; disease and, 12–14, 35–38; Doyle and, 147–48, 150, 157–58, 173–75, 181, 188–89; Kingsley and, 72, 77–86, 88–89; martial metaphor and, 18–19, 73; medicine and, 2–3, 184; miasmas and, 47, 52; national identity and, 256n75; public health and, 69–70; Shelley and, 31–34, 59, 61; Stoker and, 115, 126
Britishness. *See* Englishness
Brives, Charlotte, 246
Brown, Michael, 6–9, 72
Browning, Robert, 137
Bruce, David, 197–98
brucellosis, 197–98
BSL-4, 244
Budd, William, 133–35, 141, 158, 233
Bullets and Bacilli (pamphlet), 179
Burdon-Sanderson, John, 132, 151, 167
Burke, Edmund, 55–56, 63–64
Burroughs Wellcome and Co., 207–8

Butler, Josephine, 124, 128
Butler, Judith, 234–35
Byron (Lord), 38

cancer, 234–36
Canguilhem, Georges, 166
"Can the Government, Further, Beneficially Interfere in the Prevention . . ." (Budd), 133
capital, 139, 211
capitalism, 213
Cardigan (Lord), 79
Carpenter, Mary Wilson, 77
cartography, 115–17, 154–55
cattle plague, 130–35, 151
CDC, 233, 236
cell theory, 7, 9
Center for Disease Control. *See* CDC
Chadwick, Edwin, 12–13, 16, 51, 69, 80, 86, 116, 138
Charles Kingsley: His Letters and Memories of His Life (Kingsley), 102–3
Chartism, 70
chemical warfare, 235
chemotherapy, 168–69, 196, 206, 220, 223–24, 235–37
Childers, Joe, 147, 162–63, 257
children, 88–89, 95–97, 124, 180–85
China, 136, 239–40, 242–44
Choi, Tina Young, 7, 72, 121
cholera: Doyle and, 146, 171, 176, 180, 186; Kingsley and, 69–73, 147, 152; martial metaphor and, 1–2, 7, 229; as a national enemy, 73–85; religion and, 94, 100; Shelley and, 30–43, 57, 67; Stoker and, 117, 130, 137; women and, 85–93
Cholera Tramples the Victor & the Vanquish'd Both (Seymour), 42–43

Christianity: COVID-19 and, 244–45; Doyle and, 183, 188; Kingsley and, 69–72, 75, 81, 84, 87–88, 93–105; martial metaphor and, 201; Stoker and, 114–15, 136; the sublime and, 59, 61–64
Christianson, Robert, 158
citizenship, 7, 72, 75
civilians, 180–83
civility, 46, 48, 110, 120, 181, 195, 197–203, 232
Clairmont, Clair, 67
class: the CD Acts and, 126–29; disease and, 12, 15; Doyle and, 146–47, 166, 170–73, 176–80, 183–90; Kingsley and, 71, 75–76, 79–84, 88, 93, 103–5; the martial metaphor and, 6, 9, 16; Nightingale and, 86–87; Shelley and, 31–32, 41, 53; Stoker and, 110, 112, 119–20, 123–24, 139–40
climate, 32, 42, 44–55, 59, 201, 203. *See also* seasons; weather
clinic, the, 198
clinical medicine, 5, 25, 228
cocaine, 162
Cohen, Ed, 18, 152, 160, 166
Cold War, 236
Coleridge, Samuel Taylor, 11
Colley, Linda, 256n75
Collie, John, 187
colonialism: biopolitics and, 180–81; the CD Acts and, 126–27; Conrad and, 193–94, 196–97, 202, 209; Doyle and, 155, 159, 165, 169–70, 184–88; Kingsley and, 77, 81; martial metaphor and, 12–15, 20; miasmas and, 46–55; military medicine and, 38–42; necropower and, 210–19; Shelley and, 29–34, 57, 65; Stoker and, 110–25, 135,

colonialism (continued)
  137, 139–44. See also coloniopathy; imperialism
coloniopathy, 194–95, 210–19
Committee on Physical Deterioration, 183
Committee to Inquire into the Prevalence of Venereal Disease in the Army and Navy, 125–26
Conan Doyle, Arthur. See Doyle, Arthur Conan
concentration camps, 149, 173, 181–82, 219–21, 279n92. See also detention
Congo, 194–226
Congo Diary (Conrad), 199
Congo Free State, 198, 206, 215
Congolese. See native people
Conrad, Joseph: civility and, 197–203; imperialism and, 203–10; magic bullets and, 219–25; martial metaphor and, 3, 13–15, 22–23, 113; modernism and, 24, 193–97, 225–26; necropower and, 210–19
"Constitution Violated, The" (Butler), 128
Contagion (film), 242
contagionism: Doyle and, 158–59; Kingsley and, 72, 83; martial metaphor and, 10–11, 18, 25, 233; Shelley and, 33–43, 50, 65; Stoker and, 131–32, 136–37, 139, 141. See also anticontagionism
Contagious Diseases Acts, 109, 113, 125–31, 180, 228
Cooter, Roger, 6
cosmopolitanism, 78
COVID-19, 239–47
cowpox, 11
crime, 89, 119, 157, 163, 168, 183, 185, 187, 190

Crimean War: Doyle and, 146, 178, 188; gender and, 85–86; Kingsley and, 70–79, 83–84, 91–94, 104, 147; martial metaphor and, 2, 20, 45, 109
"Crime of the Congo, The" (Conrad), 196
Croley, Laura, 139
"Crusade against Typhoid Fever, The" (Koch), 1
Crusades, 114–15, 268n14
culture: cholera and, 34, 41, 69–70, 73; Conrad and, 194, 207–8, 211, 216, 221–23, 226; Doyle and, 149–50, 159, 164, 191; Dracula and, 109–10, 114–22, 130, 137, 143–44; Englishness and, 256n75, 257n2; martial metaphor and, 2–8, 13–14, 19, 24–25, 41, 48, 78, 225n53, 227–38; militarism and, 30, 176, 199; Nightingale and, 87–88; the sublime and, 65–67
curare, 160–61

d'Alembert, Jean le Rond, 222
Darwin, Charles, 14, 155, 177, 255n55
death: Conrad and, 193, 196–207, 210–18, 221–24; COVID-19 and, 242–46; Doyle and, 148, 151–52, 155–64, 179–86; individualism and, 164; Kingsley and, 73–75, 78–82, 88–105; martial metaphor and, 10, 14–17, 25; Shelley and, 29, 40, 49–50, 54, 66–67; Stoker and, 114, 131–34, 140; the sublime and, 57–67
Death on the Pale Horse (painting), 57–59
Decameron (Boccaccio), 51
defense. See national defense
Defense Production Act, 242

degeneration, 15, 119–30, 144, 147, 173–78, 184–85, 189, 233
Degeneration (Nordau), 119
de Kruif, Paul, 224
dermatology, 111
Descent of Man, The (Darwin), 14
detection, 145–50, 157–58, 160–64, 168, 171–73, 183, 187, 190–91
detention, 126–27. See also concentration camps
Devotions upon Emergent Expressions (Donne), 8
diagnostics, 150, 172, 190–91
"Diagram of Causes of Mortality of the Army in the East" (Nightingale), 86
Dickens, Charles, 86
diet, 47. See also food
disability, 187
discipline: Bernard and, 164–65; the CD Acts and, 128–30; Doyle and, 158, 166; Kingsley and, 71, 85, 92, 98, 103; martial metaphor and, 12; Stoker and, 112, 121, 138–39
disease: as an enemy, 33–36, 103, 110, 124; the British military and, 37–38; Conrad and, 195, 202–3; Doyle and, 185–87; Kingsley and, 71, 79, 98–99; martial metaphor and, 2–6, 19, 25, 29, 66–67; medicine and, 7–15; religion and, 96–97; Shelley and, 31–33, 39, 48, 52; the sublime and, 55–56, 59; war and, 69, 75. See also infectious disease
doctor-patient relationship, 3, 5–6, 238. See also patient care
domesticity, 16, 71, 85–88, 91–93, 96
Donne, John, 8
Donovan, Charles, 197–98
donovanosis, 198

Doyle, Arthur Conan: bacteriology and, 149–58; biological warfare and, 183–90; biopolitics and, 180–83; the Boer War and, 123, 172–80; imperialism and, 145–49; martial metaphor and, 3, 13, 20, 52, 113, 126, 196, 229; toxicology and, 158–68; tuberculosis and, 168–72
Dracula (Stoker): the CD Acts and, 125–30; etiology and, 130–43; imperialism and, 113–25, 146; martial metaphor and, 22–23, 48, 109–13, 143–44, 157, 173–75, 184, 189, 209, 233
drainage, 12, 42, 45, 116
Dr. Ehrlich's Magic Bullet (de Kruif), 226
drug-receptor theory, 168, 220
drug use, 162–63
Dutch, the, 174–75, 185, 189
"Dying Detective, The." See "Adventure of the Dying Detective, The" (Doyle)
dysbiosis, 231
dysentery, 74

"Earthly and Heavenly Wisdom, Or Stoop to Conquer" (Kingsley), 95
East India Company, 36, 209
Ebola, 1, 232–34, 236
"Ebola Wars, The" (Preston), 1
ecology, 4, 6, 11, 37, 59, 62, 139, 214, 228, 246–47
economics, 51–54, 81, 104, 214, 230, 232
education, 92, 129, 229–30
Egypt, 171
Ehrlich, Paul, 164, 172, 196, 219–26
Eliot, George, 4, 82, 246–47
Ellman, Maud, 136
empire. See colonialism; imperialism

endemics, 15–16, 100, 121, 180
Ending the War Metaphor: The Changing Agenda for Unraveling the Host-Microbe Relationship, 5
end of life care, 4
Englishness: Conrad and, 193; culture and, 256n75, 257n2; disease and, 32, 49; Doyle and, 146–48, 155, 158, 162–63, 166–67, 172–75, 185, 190–91; Kingsley and, 72, 77–78, 102; martial metaphor and, 13, 46; Stoker and, 111–12, 116, 118–20, 135, 143. *See also* national identity
enteric fever, 174, 191
entrepreneurialism, 71
environment: the body and, 164, 167; Conrad and, 195, 209–10, 215–16; disease and, 12–14, 30, 43, 49; martial metaphor and, 231–32; medicine and, 4, 9; miasmas and, 44–48; Shelley and, 37, 57; Stoker and, 137–38, 140, 143
epidemics: Conrad and, 196–97, 201, 206, 214, 220–22; Doyle and, 171, 180; endemics and, 255n60, 257n5; Kingsley and, 69–78, 83–84, 92–94, 97–101; martial metaphor and, 6, 9, 15–16, 20–21, 24, 229, 233, 242, 245; Shelley and, 31–37, 40, 46–48, 50–51, 56, 64; Stoker and, 113, 117, 128, 135–36
epidemiology, 6, 104
epilogics, 239–47
Esposito, Roberto, 217
ethics, 4, 32, 59–63, 67, 227
etiology, 10–13, 32, 34–38, 130–43
etymology, 121
eugenics, 14, 31, 119
Evans, Richard, 233
evolution, 14, 69, 119–20, 124, 143, 174–75, 228, 231, 246–47

experimental medicine, 148, 156–68, 186, 235

"Fall, The" (Kingsley), 97
family, 87, 104, 234
famine, 180
Farr, William, 69, 80, 86, 100
Federation for the Defence of Belgian Interests Abroad, 199
femininity, 92, 100, 121, 188
feminism, 124, 129
fermentation, 111
Fit to Fight (film), 225
Floyd, George, 243–44
Floyd-Wilson, Mary, 47
flu, 40
Fludd, Robert, 8
folklore, 110, 118, 136
food, 42, 61, 181, 214. *See also* diet
Force Publique, 198
foreignness: disease and, 15, 54, 56; Doyle and, 156, 158–59, 162–63, 171, 183, 188; martial metaphor and, 3, 232; Shelley and, 38, 41, 44, 47, 52–53; Stoker and, 111–13, 127, 135–36, 140, 142–43
forensics, 158, 160, 163, 191. *See also* detection
Forth, Aidan, 180
Foucault, Michel, 15–16, 25, 61, 91, 97–100, 122, 180, 183, 196, 222–23
Founding of the Congo Free State, The (Stanley), 207
Fox News, 232
Framing Animals as Epidemic Villains (Lynteris), 242
France, 116, 169, 174, 202–3
Francis, Keith A., 76
Frasier's Magazine, 90
free trade, 11
French Revolution, 59
Froude, James Anthony, 75

futurity, 112, 119–20, 230

Galton, Francis, 15, 119
Gamp, Sarah, 86
gardening, 9
gaze, the. *See* medical gaze, the
gender: the CD Acts and, 128–29; Conrad and, 194; Kingsley and, 71–73, 79, 81, 85, 95–97, 100, 104–5, 147; martial metaphor and, 13; Shelley and, 65; Stoker and, 111–14, 119, 144. *See also* masculinity
genealogy, 117–18, 122, 127, 188
geohumoralism, 47
George (Lieutenant Colonel), 115–16
Germany, 7, 169, 173, 195, 198
germ theory: Conrad and, 201–3; disease and, 7, 10, 13; Doyle and, 155, 164–65; Kingsley and, 103; martial metaphor and, 6, 14, 25; Shelley and, 35, 50; Stoker and, 110–13, 139, 141, 143
Gilbert, Pamela, 7, 72, 94, 97
Gilman, Sander, 119
global health, 229–30, 233, 240
Godwin, William, 32, 62–63, 67
Goethe, 137
Good Words, 152
Gothic literature, 110, 112, 134, 143, 157, 188–89, 216, 225
governance: biopolitics and, 12, 54, 61, 165–66, 181; Conrad and, 196; COVID-19 and, 245; disease and, 11, 15, 32, 169; Doyle and, 149, 171, 180, 185; Kingsley and, 71–72, 81, 91, 97, 100, 103; martial metaphor and, 16, 233–34; medicine and, 3, 25; Shelley and, 39, 44–45; Stoker and, 112, 120, 127–28, 132–34, 141
Great Boer War, The (Doyle), 149, 174, 181

Great Stink of 1858, 104–5
Green, Monica, 241
Greg, W. R., 96
Gros, Antoine-Jean, 38
guerrilla warfare, 95, 175, 181
Guide to Health in Africa (Parke), 207

Haraway, Donna, 247
Hardy, Ann, 179
Harmsworth Popular Science, 153, 163
health. *See* global health; public health
Health and Disease in Deadly Combat (Morrell), 153
health care, 6, 230, 234
Heart of Darkness (Conrad), 24, 193–225, 232
Hensley, Nathan, 17
Herberty, Sidney, 91
heredity, 14–15, 120, 123–24
heroism, 4–6, 72–74, 81–82, 104, 177–78, 197, 237
heteronormativity, 129
Hindrich, Cheryl, 194
Hippocratic medicine, 160
History of England from the Fall of Wolsey to the Death of Elizabeth, A (Froude), 75
History of the Rise, Progress, Ravages, &c. of the Blue Cholera of India, 36
HIV, 228
Holocaust, 180, 279n92
Holt, John, 206
homicide. *See* murder
horror fiction, 216
hospitals, 10, 44–45, 126–27
Hot Zone, The (Preston), 1, 232
Howard, Michael, 229
Howell, Jessica, 123, 201
humanities. *See* medical humanities
Hume, Kiel, 211
humoral medicine, 9–12, 25, 30, 34, 44–55, 151, 228

Huxley, Thomas, 22, 168, 172, 196, 219–20, 222
hydroxychloroquine, 242
hygiene: Doyle and, 168, 176, 181–82; Kingsley and, 70, 73, 87, 95, 98–100, 104, 147; martial metaphor and, 2–3, 5, 16–17; miasmas and, 44–46, 48; Stoker and, 112, 122–23, 129, 139

iatromechanics, 9–10
identity. *See* Englishness; national identity
Illness as Metaphor (Sontag), 3, 6
immigration, 6, 51–53, 119, 227, 229, 232–33
immunity: Doyle and, 145–49, 151–52, 155, 162–68, 170–72, 175, 179, 191; martial metaphor and, 1, 7, 18–19, 90, 217, 228, 236, 247; Shelley and, 40–41, 65
imperialism: bacteriology and, 149–58; Conrad and, 194–95, 198, 203–10; Doyle and, 145–49, 158, 161–62, 165–67, 171–75, 178–81, 185–91; Kingsley and, 77, 81, 104–5; martial metaphor and, 7, 20, 230; necropower and, 210–19; plagues and, 53–54; Shelley and, 31, 36, 38–39, 51, 61; Stoker and, 109–10, 113–25, 139, 141–42. *See also* colonialism
In Darkest Africa (Stanley), 207
India, 20, 31–37, 47, 141, 158–59, 180, 197–99, 209, 230, 275n35
Indian Mutiny of 1857, 275n35
individualism: biopolitics and, 164–66; Doyle and, 179–80; Kingsley and, 82, 90, 99; martial metaphor and, 16, 19, 29, 230–31, 234; Stoker and, 127, 134
industrialization, 15, 31, 57, 81, 104, 136–37, 139, 256n64

infectious disease: Doyle and, 149, 165, 172, 176, 180, 183; Kingsley and, 74, 86, 94; martial metaphor and, 2–6, 13–16, 234; Shelley and, 30, 33; Stoker and, 113, 130–43
Infectious Futures (anthology), 229
infrastructure, 5
"(In)Appropriateness of the WAR Metaphor in Response to SARS-CoV-2, The" (Bates), 246
insects, 202–3, 212–13
Introduction to the Study of Experimental Medicine, An (Bernard), 159
"Invasion of the Fortress of Health, The" (Fludd), 8
Irfan, Umair, 247
ivory, 215

Jacobite Rebellion, 115–16
Jameson, James, 35
Jenner, Edward, 11, 30
Jews, 119, 136–37
Jewson, N. D., 9–10
Johnson, Mark, 4
John Watson, 145–48, 162–68, 171–74, 184–85, 188, 191
Jones, Alfred, 205
Jones, Jennifer, 63
Jones, William H., 200
Joshi, Priti, 80
journalism, 8, 78, 146, 150. *See also* news media; press
Journal of a Plague Year (Defoe), 51
Journal of the Royal Army Medical Corps (Ross), 201

Kant, Immanuel, 55, 64
Kennedy, Meegan, 156
King, Albert, 141–42
Kingsley, Charles: blood and, 163–64; cholera as an enemy and, 73–85; COVID-19 and, 244–45; disease

and, 14–16; martial metaphor and, 1–3, 69–73, 109–11, 157, 177, 182, 184, 201, 229, 237; masculinity and, 147, 152; miasmas and, 45, 145; sanitation and, 139, 155, 170; women and, 85–93
Kingsley, Fanny, 102–3
Koch, Robert, 1, 13, 110–11, 149–52, 155–56, 159–64, 167–72, 197–98, 219, 224
Koch's Cure (Doyle), 169
Krauger, Paul, 173

labor, 30, 81, 91, 96, 104–5, 173, 187, 196, 210–19
Ladies' Sanitary Association, 88, 95
Lakoff, George, 4
Lambert, Léopold, 127
Lancet (periodical), 8–9, 35, 37, 74, 84, 134–35, 151
landscape, 154–55, 202–3
language. *See* rhetoric
Last Man, The (Shelley): cholera and, 69, 78, 137; imperialism and, 120, 146; martial metaphor and, 29–33; miasmas as invasion and, 44–55; military medicine and, 34–43; plagues and, 232; the sublime and, 55–67
Latour, Bruno, 165–66
Lau, Travis Chi Wing, 240
Laveran, Charles, 141
law: the CD Acts and, 125–30; Doyle and, 150, 162; immunity and, 152, 167; Kingsley and, 80, 97–99; martial metaphor and, 17–19; Stoker and, 131–34, 139
Leopold II (King of Belgium), 198–99, 201, 205–8, 211–15, 221
leprosy, 188–90, 232–33
Lewisite, 235
liberalism: biopolitics and, 67, 164–66; contagionism and, 11–12, 35–36;

COVID-19 and, 245; Doyle and, 179; Kingsley and, 70–71, 80–81, 83–88, 93, 96; the martial metaphor and, 16–17, 228–29, 231; Stoker and, 139
Liberia, 233
"Life and Death" (Kingsley), 98–99
"Life and Death in Blood" (Doyle), 148, 152–54, 157–59, 167–70, 174
Liverpool School of Tropical Medicine, 220–21
Livingstone, David, 207
Lock, Margaret, 213, 223
Loeffler, Friedrich August Johannes, 111
Lombroso, Cesare, 119
London, 116, 120, 139, 145, 163
London and Liverpool Schools of Tropical Medicine, 204–5
London School of Tropical Medicine and Hygiene, 110, 206, 208
lumpenproletariats, 170–71, 183–85
lynchings, 245
Lynteris, Christos, 242
Lyon, Emily, 48
Lyons, Robert Spencer Dyer, 77–78, 95, 221

magic bullets, 22, 24, 172, 219–26, 235, 242. *See also* pharmaceutical torpedoes
malaria, 130, 141–42, 193, 198, 200–201, 213, 220
Malaria, a Neglected Factor in the History of Greece and Rome (Jones), 200
Malay, 141
Malingering and Feigned Sickness (Collie), 187
Malthusian economics, 15, 54, 59, 61–62
Manson, Patrick, 141–42, 197, 199, 201, 203, 208–9, 220

"Man with the Twisted Lip, The" (Doyle), 166
mapping. *See* cartography
marriage, 85–93, 97, 147
Marsh, Catherine, 88
martial metaphor: biological warfare and, 183–91; biopolitics and, 15–19, 180–83; the Boer War and, 172–80; the CD Acts and, 125–30; cholera and, 73–85; civility and, 197–203; COVID-19 and, 239–47; disease and, 7–15; gender and, 85–93; imperialism and, 113–25, 203–10; Kingsley and, 69–73, 103–5; magic bullets and, 219–25; medicine and, 1–7; miasmas and, 44–55; military medicine and, 34–43; modern impacts of, 227–38; modernism and, 193–97, 225–26; necropower and, 210–19; religion and, 93–103; Shelley and, 29–33; Stoker and, 109–13, 130–44; the sublime and, 55–67; toxicology and, 158–68; tuberculosis and, 168–72. *See also* medico-military war
Martin, John, 58
Martin Chuzzlewit (Dickens), 86
martyrdom, 212
masculinity: Doyle and, 188; Kingsley and, 69–70, 72, 78–84, 87, 93, 100, 147; martial metaphor and, 6, 9; militarism and, 45–46; Stoker and, 110, 122, 129
masks, 244, 247. *See also* N95 masks
"Massacre of the Innocents, The" (Kingsley), 88, 95
Mbembe, Achille, 180, 182, 196–97, 211–12
McClintock, Anne, 31
McDermid, Val, 229
McLean's Monthly Sheet of Caricatures, 42–43

McWhir, Ann, 36
measles, 182
Medical Act of 1858, 8, 81
medical gaze, 10, 14, 25, 104, 122, 150–51, 156
medical humanities, 3–6, 227, 238, 241
medical practitioners: Doyle and, 148, 156, 171, 185, 191; Kingsley and, 70, 72, 81–83, 86–88, 91–93, 102–3; martial metaphor and, 8–11, 237–38; Stoker and, 109, 114
medical professionals. *See* medical practitioners
medical science, 2–3, 5, 19. *See also* humoral medicine
medical technology, 1–2, 5, 113, 121–22, 149–51, 168
medical writing: Doyle and, 146, 157, 159, 166–67, 191; martial metaphor and, 7, 11, 15, 19, 37, 110, 134–35, 195
Medicina Catholica, 8
medicine. *See* martial metaphor
medico-military war, 93, 101, 141, 158, 168, 171. *See also* martial metaphor
Meldrum, David, 219
Memories and Adventures (Doyle), 177
Men Against Death (De Kruif), 224
Metchnikoff, Elie, 151–54, 165, 167
Methodism, 101
Mexico, 230
miasmas: Conrad and, 201–2; etiology and, 10–14; as invasion, 44–55; Kingsley and, 72–75, 79, 83, 94, 98–101, 104, 147, 155; martial metaphor and, 18, 170, 244; Shelley and, 32–33, 35, 38–43, 65; Stoker and, 130, 137–41; the sublime and, 58–59

Index / 331

Microbe Hunters (De Kruif), 224–25
microbiology, 13, 25
microbiome, 228, 242, 250n8
microscopy, 13, 111, 143–45, 150–57, 164, 168–70, 208
Middlemarch (Eliot), 82, 246–47
militarism: anticontagionism and, 45; Doyle and, 149; medicine and, 8–9, 29; public health and, 73; sanitation and, 69; Shelley and, 30, 38, 45–46; Stoker and, 112, 133; the sublime and, 59, 61
military. *See* the British military
military fitness, 183–91
military industrial complex, 228, 236
military medicine: Conrad and, 196; Doyle and, 152, 173, 176; Kingsley and, 87, 104; martial metaphor and, 2–3, 6–7, 234–35; Shelley and, 32–43; Stoker and, 125, 141, 143
military science, 78, 235
military technology, 116
Mill, John Stuart, 71
Mill on the Floss, The (Eliot), 4
Milton, John, 100–101
Miracle Drug, The (Sokoloff), 224
miscegenation, 139
modernism: civility and, 197–203; Conrad and, 193–97, 225–26; imperialism and, 203–10; magic bullets and, 219–25; necropower and, 210–19. *See also* modernity
modernity: biopolitics and, 126, 180–83; martial metaphor and, 17, 25, 32, 112; Shelley and, 31, 57; Stoker and, 109, 120, 127, 135–39, 144. *See also* imperialism; modernism
Montagu, Mary Wortley, 11
Mooney, Graham, 6, 85, 251

morality, 16, 25, 63, 104, 124, 126, 245
morbidity, 30, 145
mortality, 30, 61, 138, 145. *See also* death
motherhood, 85–93, 96, 124
MRSA, 229
murder, 89–90, 161, 186
mustard gas, 235

N95 masks, 241. *See also* masks
Napoleonic Wars, 20, 30, 38, 53, 59, 116
Napoleon Visiting the Pesthouse at Jaffa (Gros), 38
NASA, 236
National Academies of Science, Engineering, and Medicine, 5, 228
National Cancer Act, 236
national defense: biopolitics and, 166; disease and, 49, 54; Doyle and, 146, 148, 151, 178, 188; medicine and, 2–3; public health and, 130; Stoker and, 116, 121, 131, 142; the sublime and, 60. *See also* self-defense
National Endowment for Science Technology and the Arts, 229
National Health Service, 227–28, 230
national identity, 15, 20, 30, 71, 116, 135, 147, 191. *See also* Englishness
nationalism: martial metaphor and, 151; COVID-19 and, 242, 245; Kingsley and, 77, 84; martial metaphor and, 6, 18, 32, 64, 229–30, 233–34; Stoker and, 112, 114, 120, 144
national security. *See* national defense
native, 211

native people, 140, 193, 195–96, 198, 202, 206, 208–9, 212, 214, 220–21
natural selection, 14
nature, 11, 55–67, 88–89, 93–105, 184
navy, the. *See* Royal Navy
Nazis, 180, 186
nCoV. *See* COVID-19
necropolitics, 17, 196–97, 210–19
Neill, Deborah, 196, 214
Nelson, Richard, 57
news media, 232, 240–43. *See also* journalism
Nguyen, Vinh-Kim, 213, 223
Nightingale, Florence, 12, 16, 69, 72, 83, 86–93, 98, 264n57
Nixon, Richard, 236
Nordau, Max, 15, 119
Northumberland and Durham Medical Society, 199–200
nosology, 82
Notes on Hospitals (Nightingale), 86
Notes on Matters Affecting the Health, Efficiency and Hospital . . . (Nightingale), 86
Notes on Nursing (Nightingale), 86
Notes toward a Performative Theory of Assembly (Butler), 234
nuclear warfare, 235
nursing, 85–93, 147
Nursing Clio, 246

obstetrics, 133
ocean, the, 48, 55, 59–60, 137, 232
O'Conner, Erin, 7, 57, 256n64
"Ode to the West Wind" (Shelley), 47–48
oncology, 235
On the Origin of Species (Darwin), 14
opium, 161
Ordnance Survey, 115–16

Orientalism, 47
Osler, William, 179
Otis, Laura, 7, 145, 147, 198
Otter, Chris, 71

Paley, Morton, 58
pandemics. *See* cholera; epidemics
panopticon, 165
Paradise Lost (Milton), 100–101
"Parasite: A Story, The" (Doyle), 159
parasites, 113, 119, 130, 139, 141–43, 145, 155, 194, 202–3
Park, Edmund, 2
Parke, Thomas Heazle, 197, 207–9, 218
Pasha, Emin, 207, 214
Pasteur, Louis, 13, 111, 197
pathography, 236
pathology, 7, 10, 97, 103, 113
patient care, 86. *See also* doctor-patient relationship
patriarchy, 124–25, 129
patriotism, 30, 174, 177–78
Paul, Ron, 234
Pearson, Karl, 15
Penday, Amar, 186
penicillin, 224, 228
Penner, Louise, 86
people of color, 242
personal protective equipment, 241
pestilence, 10–11, 39, 55–67, 75, 93, 137–38
pharmaceutical torpedoes, 22, 25, 149, 168, 172, 203. *See also* magic bullets
pharmacology, 5, 149, 161–63, 170–72, 196–97, 208, 235
Philippines, 230
phrenology, 119
Physical Committee on Degeneration, 191
physicians. *See* medical practitioners

"Physician's Calling, The" (Kingsley), 81, 102
physiognomy, 119
physiology, 98, 156
"Pied Piper of Hamlin, The" (Browning), 137
plagues: biopolitics and, 61, 180; Shelley and, 31–33, 38–39, 42, 47, 49–50, 55; Stoker and, 130; the sublime and, 56–57; as a weapon, 186–87
poison. *See* toxicology
policing, 32, 80, 86, 125, 127, 166, 191, 243–45
politics, 2–6, 11, 109, 144
pollution, 138–40, 147
Poor Laws, 8, 51, 80, 82–84, 170, 180
Popular Science Monthly, 141
population, 16, 32, 45, 61, 72, 120, 122, 127–28, 180
populism, 6, 18
poverty, 12, 51, 128–29, 230; miasmas and, 44
Practical Hygiene (Park), 2
press, 207, 227–28
Preston, Richard, 1, 232
primitivism, 193, 195, 232–33
Privy Council, 94, 135
Proctor, George, 268n14
propaganda, 179
prostitution. *See* sex work
pseudoscience, 119, 245
psychological warfare, 182
Puar, Jasbir, 18
public health: biopolitics and, 83, 165, 182; the CD Acts and, 127–30; COVID-19 and, 234, 244; Doyle and, 152, 170, 177–80, 182; gender and, 85–86; imperialism and, 39; Kingsley and, 69–70, 73, 83, 87, 93; martial metaphor and, 2–6, 16, 19, 25, 233; quarantine and, 11; Stoker and, 109, 112, 125. *See also* global health
Public Health Act of 1848, 13, 104
punishment, 25, 61, 76, 97–103, 124–25, 127

quarantine: the CD Acts and, 127–29; contagionism and, 35–36, 39–41, 51; COVID-19 and, 241, 247; disease and, 11–12; Doyle and, 188–89; forcible, 220–21; Kingsley and, 83, 109; martial metaphor and, 233; Stoker and, 113, 131–33, 136–37
Queen Mab (Shelley), 64
quinine, 198–99, 206–7, 216, 219–20

race: biopolitics and, 66, 183; the CD Acts and, 127–29; cholera and, 77, 229; Conrad and, 194–95, 198, 205, 211–12, 215; COVID-19 and, 240, 242–43, 245; disease and, 12, 15; Doyle and, 146–47, 149–50, 155, 170, 173–74, 183, 187–88; Kingsley and, 88; martial metaphor and, 3, 6, 13–14, 20, 25, 233; Shelley and, 31–32, 39–41, 44, 47, 65; Stoker and, 110–13, 118–21, 124, 130, 136, 139, 141, 144
radiation, 236–37
rape, 129
Rasmussen, Angela, 240
rats, 136–38
Red Cross, 268n14
ReframeCovid, 246
Reid, Julian, 17
religion: COVID-19 and, 244–45; Doyle and, 174–75; Kingsley and, 69, 71, 73, 93–103, 201; martial metaphor and, 25; Stoker and,

religion *(continued)*
    111, 113–25, 143; the sublime and,
    59, 61–64
Re-Mission 2 (video game), 237
*Report on the Epidemick Cholera
    Morbus . . .* (Jameson), 35
reproduction, 30, 97, 112, 119–20,
    125, 140–41, 143, 190
Republicans, 234
resistance, 212
Resistance (McDermid), 229
Resnick, Brian, 247
Review of Reviews, 168
rhetoric: bacteriology and, 154–58;
    COVID-19 and, 242, 245–46;
    disease and, 37, 46, 50, 89;
    imperialism and, 208, 212;
    militarization of medical, 2–3, 22,
    89, 110, 127–28, 133–35, 146–49,
    170–71, 176–77, 237; military,
    12–13, 72–74, 82, 87, 114; religion
    and, 97, 114; social order and, 6,
    88, 124; of war, 21, 45, 112, 187,
    236
rhinovirus, 236
rights, 212, 245
rinderpest. *See* cattle plague
romance, 73, 154–56
Romanticism, 33, 37, 55–58, 62, 65
Rose, Nikolas, 5
Rosebury, Theodor, 246
Rosenberg, Charles, 5, 73
Ross, Ronald, 141–42, 193–94, 197,
    199–201, 203, 206, 208–9, 218,
    220, 224
Royal Army College at Netley, 176
Royal Army Medical Corps, 178–
    79
Royal College of Surgeons, 82, 110
Royal Commission on the Health of
    the Army, 125
Royal Navy, 60–61

Royal Society of Tropical Medicine
    and Hygiene, 198
Russia, 1, 45, 74, 78, 83–85, 136,
    216
Ryan, Vanessa, 56

Said, Edward, 195, 212
Sanitary Act, 104
Sanitary Report (Chadwick), 13
sanitation: Doyle and, 155, 170,
    176, 181; Kingsley and, 69–76,
    79–80, 83, 88–90, 94–96, 100–101,
    104–5; martial metaphor and,
    11–13, 16; Nightingale and, 86–87;
    Shelley and, 32–33, 41; Stoker
    and, 116, 126, 138–39. *See also*
    anticontagionism
SARS-CoV-2. *See* COVID-19
scarlet fever, 90
Schaff, Pamela, 243
science, 25, 46, 70, 122–23, 137,
    141, 157–58, 172, 199, 230. *See
    also* medical science; military
    science
science fiction, 154, 216, 229
Scramble for Africa. *See* Africa
Seacole, Mary, 86
seasons, 49–50
self-defense, 4, 152, 164–65. *See also*
    national defense
Series of Catastrophes and Miracles, A
    (Williams), 237
sermons, 70–71, 76, 81, 94, 97–99,
    102
sewage, 80, 105, 116
sexuality: disease and, 272n77; Doyle
    and, 183, 189–90; Stoker and,
    110, 112–13, 118–29, 131, 144;
    women's, 23, 90, 225
sexually transmitted diseases. *See*
    venereal disease
sex work, 96, 109, 126–28

Seymour, Robert, 42–43, 58
Shadow Line, The (Conrad), 199
Sharpe, Christina, 291
Shelley, Mary: imperialism and, 120, 146; martial metaphor and, 3, 29–33, 69–70, 165; miasmas and, 44–55; military medicine and, 34–43; the sublime and, 55–67
Shelley, Percy, 32, 45, 47–48, 56, 59, 62–64, 67
Sherlock Holmes, 13, 145–48, 155–72, 175–77, 183–88, 190–91
Sign of the Four, The (Doyle), 148, 159, 162, 170
Simpson, James Young, 133–35, 158, 233
sin, 93–105
Sinton, John, 198
slavery, 39, 211
sleeping sickness, 198, 206, 213, 220
smallpox, 11, 30, 113, 130, 132–34, 141, 233
Smiles, Samuel, 71
Smith, Thomas Southwood, 12–13
Snow, John, 69, 79–80, 86, 117
social Darwinism, 177
social distancing, 247
social media, 240–41
social order, 5, 45–48, 53–55, 70, 79, 96, 111, 123, 146–47, 193
Sokoloff, Boris, 224
soldiers: Doyle and, 173, 175–80, 187, 191; experimental medicine on, 235; Kingsley and, 70–72, 75–78, 85, 90, 94–95; Shelley and, 37, 41–42, 182–83; Stoker and, 109, 114
Somatosphere, 246
somnambulism, 123
Sontag, Susan, 3, 6, 13
South Africa, 23, 146, 149, 173, 180–83, 186, 189

South African War, 187
sovereignty, 59, 62, 111–12, 127–28, 165, 170, 180
Spain, 174
Sparks, Tabitha, 128, 130
species, 65
Spectator, 115
Spencer, Herbert, 14–15, 119
spirituality, 9, 71–73, 98
staining, 164, 219
Stanley, Henry Morton, 197, 206–9, 214, 218
state, the: cholera and, 75, 94; disease and, 55, 80; Doyle and, 146, 157, 166; Kingsley and, 85, 99; martial metaphor and, 15–19, 25; public health and, 71; Shelley and, 30, 45–46; Stoker and, 112, 137
states of exception, 18–19, 127, 129, 180–81, 245
statistics, 15, 86, 95, 104, 116, 140
Steinlight, Emily, 66
Stoker, Bram: the CD Acts and, 125–30; colonialism and, 52, 113–25; etiology and, 130–43; imperialism and, 113–25, 146; martial metaphor and, 3, 13, 96, 109–13, 143–44, 163, 165–66, 173, 184, 229; miasmas and, 48
Stoker, Charlotte, 137–38
"Stolen Bacillus, The" (Wells), 185–86
Stoler, Ann, 126
Storks, Henry (Lord), 126
Study in Scarlet, A (Doyle), 145, 148, 150, 159, 161, 163, 174, 183, 188
"Study of Natural History for Soldiers, The" (Kingsley), 77
subjects, 15–17, 55, 67, 71–73, 81, 96, 103–4, 139, 162–65, 186
sublime, the, 33, 43, 48, 55–67

suicide, 212
Superbugs (video game), 229
Surgeon X (graphic novel), 229
surgery, 2, 34–36, 80–83, 88, 91, 145, 149
surveillance: biopolitics and, 165–66; Doyle and, 190; Kingsley and, 83, 92, 95; martial metaphor and, 17; Nightingale and, 86; Stoker and, 122, 124–25, 133, 139
Sydenham, Thomas, 8
syphilis, 109, 125, 127, 130, 223–24, 228–29

Tallie, T. J., 244
Tauber, Alfred, 13
Taylor-Brown, Emilie, 154–55, 209, 268, 273, 283
Taylor-Pirie, Emilie (née Taylor-Brown), 142, 209
teachers, 92
Tea Party, the, 234
technology. *See* medical technology
terrorism, 234. *See also* bioterrorism
thanopolitics, 17, 61, 66
theocracy, 111
theology, 71–73, 93–105, 152
therapeutics, 2
Thomas, Henry Wolfesteran, 220–21
Times (*New York Times*), 135
Todd, J. L., 208
Todd, Macy, 132
Tomes, Nancy, 255n53
Tonga, 159, 161, 166, 171
torpedoes. *See* pharmaceutical torpedoes
toxicology, 145–48, 158–69, 172, 186, 190
trade, 11, 35–36, 51, 139
transfusion, 142
Transylvania, 115
Treatise on Fever (Lyons), 95
Treatise on Fever, A (Lyons), 77

tropical medicine, 34, 113, 140–42, 190, 193–226. *See also* the tropics
tropics, the, 12, 29, 31, 46–47, 52, 135, 158, 175, 188. *See also* tropical medicine
True Words for Brave Men (Kingsley), 76
Trump, Donald, 232, 240–41, 243–44, 246
Truth on the Congo Free State, The (periodical), 199
trypanosomiasis, 197–98, 222–23
Tsing, Anna Lowenhaupt, 245
tuberculosis, 1, 13, 149, 152, 164–72, 232–33
Tucker, Jennifer, 150
Turner, J. M. W., 58
Twitter, 241
"Two Breaths, The" (Kingsley), 98
Two Years Ago (Kingsley), 11, 69–75, 78–85, 88, 91–94, 97, 100–105, 152
Twyning, John, 114–15
typhoid, 1, 79, 168, 174, 176, 178–79, 188. *See also* typhus
typhus, 32, 38, 45, 74. *See also* typhoid

Uganda, 221
Union Jack, 114
United States, 6, 225, 228, 232–33, 242, 244–45
United States, 53
urbanization, 12, 15, 81, 104–5, 136, 139
urban spaces, 31, 44–45
US Army Chemical Weapons Division, 235
utopianism, 55–56, 62

vaccination, 11, 30–32, 65, 111, 147, 161–72, 176–80, 191, 220
"Vampire of Sussex, The" (Doyle), 161

vampires, 112–15, 118–25, 129–31, 136–45, 232
venereal disease, 11, 109, 119, 124–30
ventilation, 12
Victoria (Queen), 264n57
violence: the CD Acts and, 127–30; martial metaphor and, 6, 11, 14, 17–18, 32, 83, 181; Stoker and, 109–12, 121–25, 131–32
Virchow, Rudolph, 13
vivisection, 132, 159, 179
Vox, 246

Wald, Priscilla, 18
Walker, Iona, 246
Walking Dead, The (television show), 243
Walkowitz, Judith R., 128
Wang, Fuson, 32
war. *See* martial metaphor
War in South Africa: Its Causes and Conduct, The (Doyle), 149, 181
War on Cancer, 236
War on Drugs, 6
Washington Post, 246
water, 12, 79–80, 176, 181, 184, 186, 232. *See also* the ocean
Water Babies, The (Kingsley), 69
Watt, Ian, 195, 204
weapons, 120–21, 125, 155, 161–63, 166–68, 171, 184–86, 196, 203, 235
weather, 41, 46, 48, 61. *See also* climate
Weber, Max, 25
Weheliye, Alexander G., 279

Wellcome Trust, 229
Wells, H. G., 185–86
Wende, Ernest, 111
West, Benjamin, 57–59
"Who Causes Pestilence?" (Kingsley), 76
Wilberforce, Reginald Garton, 275n35
Williams, Mary Elizabeth, 237
Willis, Martin, 143, 157
Wintle, S. B. (Colonel), 161
women: the CD Acts and, 127–30; concentration camps and, 180, 182; Kingsley and, 71–72, 81, 85–93, 96–97, 103; Stoker and, 109–13, 118–25, 144
Wordsworth, William, 11
World Health Organization, 239–40
World War One, 179–80, 228, 235
World War Two, 224, 228, 235
World War Z (film), 233
Wright, Almroth, 176–77
Wright, Erika, 243
writing, 131–32

xenophobia, 31, 40, 64, 110, 118, 127, 136–39, 226, 229, 233

Yeast (Kingsley), 69
yellow fever, 32

Zieger, Susan, 141
zombies, 233
zoology, 14
zoonotic disease, 228, 240
zoöphagy, 132
Zulu people, 175